Understanding Drugs of Abuse

The Processes of Addiction, Treatment, and Recovery

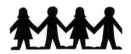

Understanding Drugs of Abuse

The Processes of Addiction, Treatment, and Recovery

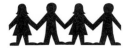

Mim J. Landry
Health and Human Services Division
Macro International
Silver Spring, Maryland

Foreword by **David E. Smith, M.D.**
Founder and Medical Director
Haight Ashbury Free Clinics
San Francisco, California
President-Elect, American Society of Addiction Medicine

Preface by **Martha A. Morrison, M.D.**
Medical Director
Talbott Recovery System
Atlanta, Georgia
Author of *White Rabbit: A Doctor's Story of Her Addiction and Recovery*

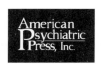

Washington, DC
London, England

Copyright © 1994 Mim J. Landry
ALL RIGHTS RESERVED
Manufactured in the United States of America on acid-free paper
03 02 01 00   5 4 3 2
First Edition

American Psychiatric Press, Inc.
1400 K Street, N.W., Washington, DC   20005

Library of Congress Cataloging-in-Publication Data
Landry, Mim J., 1954–
    Understanding drugs of abuse : the processes of
addiction, treatment, and recovery / Mim J. Landry : preface by
Martha A. Morrison : foreword by David E. Smith.
      p.   cm.
    Includes bibliographical references and index.
    ISBN 0-88048-533-7
    1. Drug abuse. 2. Drug abuse—Treatment. I. Title.
RC564.29.L36   1993
616.86—dc20   93-26208
                                                                              CIP

British Library Cataloguing in Publication Data
A CIP record is available from the British Library.

Contents

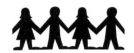

List of Tables

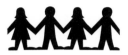

List of Figures

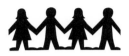

Foreword

A Message to Health Care Professionals

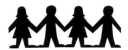

During the early 1960s, while a graduate student in pharmacology and a medical student at the University of California at San Francisco, I developed a fascination with psychopharmacology. While I injected rats with drugs such as LSD and amphetamines, young people a few blocks away were experimenting with these same drugs.

Scientists and physicians such as myself attempted to make sense of what we observed. In many ways, we were like cultural anthropologists observing and documenting a subculture and its drug scenes. We documented the toxic effects of psychoactive drugs. We developed treatment strategies, some of which we learned from the drug users themselves, including talk-down therapy for psychedelic drug bad trips. We learned about addiction.

In 1965, as director of the Alcohol and Drug Abuse Screening Unit at San Francisco General Hospital, it was painfully obvious to me that most people, including physicians, considered alcoholics to be unworthy of medical attention. Medically shunned, they were considered incurable, or nearly so. In fact, we physicians who treated alcoholic people were often as despised as our patients. The barriers to appropriate treatment for alcoholism were numerous.

Sadly, the rejection by society and mainstream medicine of people addicted to illicit drugs was even more severe. The polarization over drug use was fueled primarily by political and personal opinions, as well as clashing values of morality, rather than scientific and medical understanding. As a physician, I found it imperative but strange to fight for patients' rights to medical treatment of addiction to illicit drugs, rather than incarceration and punishment.

Such was the political, medical, and general climate when I founded the Haight Ashbury Free Medical Clinic during the Summer of Love in 1967. At the time, it was not considered a good career move for a young physician.

Today, treatment programs across the country fiercely compete with each other to treat the same addicted people who were shunned and considered incurable during the 1960s. People such as Betty Ford have forever made addiction treatment more acceptable and accessible. Her efforts complement the motto of the Haight Ashbury Free Clinics, recently echoed by President Clinton: "Health care is a right, not a privilege." Currently, there is a wide variety of treatment options. In most areas, low-cost, nonprofit, or free government treatment is available.

During those early days of addiction medicine, the primary focus of treatment was on the medical management of problems that resulted from chronic use of alcohol and other drugs. Further, many of us incorrectly believed that addiction was the result of underlying psychiatric problems. The theory stated that if somehow these psychiatric problems could be effectively cured, the addiction would resolve. In our experience, this did not prove to be true. Also, during those early days, the "nature versus nurture" argument was a quarrel that attempted to force the question: Is addiction caused by genetic or environmental factors?

During the past 25 years, there has been a virtual explosion of research regarding the genetic, psychological, emotional, environmental, pharmacologic, and neurochemical aspects of addiction. Indeed, during that time, we have learned more about brain chemistry as it relates to addiction than during the entire history of science prior to that.

Researchers such as Kenneth Blum, Ph.D., at the University of Texas in San Antonio are currently investigating the role of specific genes in the development of addiction to alcohol and other drugs.

He and others are also investigating the neurochemical basis for addiction, both in terms of preaddiction neurotransmitter deficits as well as postaddiction neurochemical dysfunction. Considerable research has been under way in regard to the relationship between psychiatric disorders and addiction, as well as environmental factors that increase the likelihood of exposure to drugs and subsequent addiction.

Thus, perhaps the most important development in the field of addiction medicine has been the realization that addiction is a biopsychosocial disease. The nature versus nurture argument has been replaced by the awareness that addiction is the result of "nature plus nurture." Indeed, addiction is the result of a complex interplay between numerous biological factors and several environmental factors. In turn, addiction has a powerful effect on many biopsychosocial factors.

The awareness that addiction is a biopsychosocial disease has had a powerfully positive effect on treatment. Today, addiction treatment places an emphasis on the process of addiction, rather than an emphasis on the specific drug of choice. Also, addiction treatment mirrors the biopsychosocial nature of addictive disease. Thus, in addition to the medical management of problems related to chronic drug use, comprehensive addiction treatment also addresses psychological, emotional, social, cognitive, and even spiritual well-being.

Also, the awareness that addiction is a biopsychosocial disease goes a long way to reduce the stigma of addiction. Today, addiction treatment is humanistic and humane. Far from being ostracized, the medical specialty of addiction medicine is now part of mainstream medicine.

Addiction medicine specialist groups such as the American Society of Addiction Medicine have important roles in educating the general public and health care professionals about the nature and treatment of addiction. Perhaps most important, this group, along with organizations such as the National Council on Alcoholism and Drug Dependence, carries the message of hope that treatment and recovery from the disease of addiction are possible.

As a parent, I share the fear that many families have these days: the specter that our children will develop problems with mood-altering drugs. Fortunately, my children are all doing well. They have stayed away from drugs. But the fear remains. As a parent, I have become increasingly aware of the critical need for family education and support.

As a member of a Twelve-Step recovery group, I have grown to understand the spiritual dimension of the recovery process. Recovery from my own adolescent and young adult alcohol problems and dealing with the premature death of my parents during my teenage years have led me to the realization that complete recovery must have a spiritual dimension.

These personal experiences have supported my professional knowledge that recovery from addiction includes spiritual, psychological, and emotional growth as well as medical management of the physical aspects of addiction. Although there are many paths to recovery for both the individual and the family, I have found the Twelve-Step approach, with its attention to spirituality, to be the best and most effective strategy.

Health care professionals, even those who work in the addiction field, often have specific areas of expertise and general knowledge in other areas. Some health care professionals in recovery may rely too much on their own experiences. As a physician specialist in addiction medicine, I recognize the need for a familiarity with basic pharmacologic principles, knowledge about the specific drugs of abuse, and thorough understanding of the processes of addiction, treatment, relapse, and recovery.

This book is a comprehensive guide for all who want to learn more about the drugs of abuse, the addiction process, treatment, and recovery. It can be a useful guide and reference text.

David E. Smith, M.D.
Founder and Medical Director, Haight Ashbury Free Clinics
Associate Clinical Professor, Occupational Health and Clinical
*   Toxicology, University of California, San Francisco*
Alternate Delegate to the American Medical Association representing
*   the American Society on Addiction Medicine*
President-Elect, American Society on Addiction Medicine

Preface

A Message to Family Members

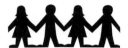

Drug abuse and addiction are powerful forces. With the wrath and fury of hurricanes, the impact they have on families is no less destructive than the impact they have on the drug user. Entire families can be destroyed in the aftermath of addiction.

The good news is that recovery and healing from this destruction are indeed possible. Families can defend themselves from the deafening winds of silence and fear. They can repair the aftermath of pain and shame. With help, families can learn to rebuild themselves.

Indeed, families can learn, grow, and teach others. And they can support one another. Recovery from addiction is possible for the drug user and for the family.

I should know. No stranger to the disease of addiction, I am a recovering addict and alcoholic as well as a psychiatrist and a specialist in addiction medicine. I work with addicted adolescents as well as adolescents with psychiatric and substance use disorders. I work with their families.

I understand that families in a crisis find it difficult to believe that recovery is within reach. But treatment and recovery from addiction are possible. The family can be put back together.

The first step is education. Use this book to educate yourself and your family. Learn about the drugs of abuse and the processes of addiction, treatment, and recovery. Learn to get help for the addicted person in your family. Learn to get help for yourself. There is much wisdom in these chapters.

Recovery is possible. One day at a time.

Martha A. Morrison, M.D.
Medical Director, Talbott Recovery System, Atlanta, Georgia
Author of White Rabbit: A Doctor's Story of Her Addiction and
    Recovery

Acknowledgments

On June 7th, 1967, in a working-class neighborhood of San Francisco, as a block-long line of young people passed a cheerful, handwritten sign proclaiming the opening of the Haight Ashbury Free Medical Clinic, a very special chapter in the history of drug abuse treatment and research began. More than 25 years later, with robust corporate and civic leadership, a new generation of staff and volunteers continue a tradition of humanistic concern, innovative treatment, and vital research. It is appropriate to acknowledge David E. Smith, M.D., for his vision, his pioneering role as founder, and his continued role as medical director of the greatly expanded Haight Ashbury Free Clinics system.

I am deeply indebted to him for providing me with a sound philosophical basis for understanding the drugs of abuse and the processes of addiction and recovery. Many of his ideas can be found here. I appreciate our continued medical writing collaboration, his guidance, our friendship, and our shared and relentless loyalty to the San Francisco Forty-Niners.

I grow increasingly aware of the profound effect that the Haight Ashbury Free Clinics have had on me and am thankful for having been on the receiving end of the brilliant educational efforts of Darryl Inaba, Pharm.D., director of the clinics' Drug Detoxification and Aftercare Project. Similarly, I am gratified to have been exposed to the splendid scholarship and shrewd wit of John Newmeyer, Ph.D. Thanks to George Dykstra for hiring and humoring me.

A warm thanks to Martha A. Morrison, M.D., for her contributions to this book and to the field of adolescent addiction. I am indebted to Ernest C. Reed, Jr., M.D., for sharing his insights with me regarding addiction, treatment, and recovery. He has had a strong impact on my understanding of addiction—and on this book.

I am appreciative to the following people for their chapter introductions: Ken Blum, Ph.D.; Max A. Schneider, M.D., C.A.D.C.; Joseph C. McCarthy, M.D.; Jerry Beck, Dr.P.H.; Lori Karan, M.D.; Donna Jackson, M.F.C.C.; Eileen Kulp, A.C.S.W., L.C.S.W.; Rose Ann Soloway, R.N., M.S., Ed., C.S.P.I.; Nancy Miller, R.N.; Paul Ehrlich, M.A.; John Steinberg, M.D.; Ernest C. Reed, Jr., M.D., M.P.H.; and Clarence T.

I am particularly indebted to Claire Reinburg, Editorial Director, and Carol C. Nadelson, M.D., Editor-in-Chief, of American Psychiatric Press, Inc., for their advocacy and energetic support of this project. Claire was a marvelous navigator through the oft-murky publication bayou and brought joy and humor to the endeavor.

I was honored to have the manuscript reviewed by Norman S. Miller, M.D., Associate Professor and Chief of Addiction Programs, Department of Psychiatry, College of Medicine, Neuropsychiatric Institute at the University of Illinois at Chicago. His comments and recommendations were exceptionally helpful and generous.

My gratitude to Carolyn Davis, Beth Lindeman, Bill Atkins, and Marty Kotler at Macro International for their support of this project and for their good cheer. Thanks also to Julie Withers, Will Hoffmann, and Maryanna Johnson for reviewing parts of the manuscript.

An extraordinary and warm thanks to Marlene Jack for her unending encouragement and friendship during and since the writing of this book. Finally, my parents and family in the Deep South are proof that Cajuns are indeed gracious, generous, and loving. Thanks for everything.

About the Author

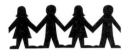

Mim J. Landry is a medical education specialist in addiction and psychiatry and works for the Health and Human Services Division at Macro International, Inc., a professional services and management company in Silver Spring, Maryland. Mr. Landry is part of the Macro International team that helps to develop protocols for the treatment of substance use and psychiatric disorders on behalf of the federal government's Center for Substance Abuse Treatment.

Mr. Landry graduated cum laude from the University of San Francisco, where he was a Louise M. Davies Scholar and a member of the Alpha Sigma Nu National Honor Society. He attended graduate school at John F. Kennedy University in Orinda, California, with course work in clinical psychology and addiction studies. He worked at the Haight Ashbury Free Clinics in San Francisco for 8 years, and was the director of the Free Clinic's Training and Education Project.

Mr. Landry's articles have appeared in the *Journal of Psychoactive Drugs*, the *Journal of the American Board of Family Practice, Family Practice Recertification, California Nursing Review*, and the *Journal of Psychiatric Research*. He is a coauthor of *The New Drugs: Lookalikes, Designer Drugs, and Drugs of Deception*. He contributed to the books *Treating Cocaine Dependence* and *The Addictions: Multidisciplinary Perspectives and Treatments* and collaborated on a chapter on substance use disorders in *Review of General Psychiatry*. Mr. Landry was a member of the American Psychiatric Association Task Force on the Treatment of Psychiatric Disorders, which produced *Treatments of Psychiatric Disorders*. He is an Associate Member of the Association for Medical Education and Research in Substance Abuse (AMERSA) and a member of the Alcohol and Drug Problems Association of North America (ADPA) and the American Medical Writers Association (AMWA).

Introduction to Part One

Pharmacologic Aspects of Addiction

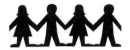

Five thousand years B.C., perhaps copying the behaviors of their pack animals, Andean men discovered the stimulating and nutritious properties of the coca plant. Today, some Peruvian Indians continue to chew coca leaves for gentle stimulation and suppression of appetite, while their city-dwelling relatives seize the fierce fury of cocaine with chemical extraction methods and smoke it.

One group relies on the delicate stimulation to combat fatigue while engaged in grueling, exhausting labor. Many of the other group have long stopped working. Rather, they exist in a murky world of agitated, restless paranoia. Natural chemicals in their brain, normally in a fragile balance, are horribly imbalanced. The imbalances cause an unbelievable and entirely unquenchable thirst for more cocaine. The desire for cocaine satiation seems stronger than the need for food and water. Indeed, it is.

Somewhere in an Oakland, California, hospital, a premature infant finds no solace in clinging to life. The body of her 19-year-old mother is marked with tiny holes from the unclean needles used to inject cocaine. Fortunately, the infant cannot see the handiwork of her father's cocaine-induced rage, and cannot understand a dark irony.

An area of her mother's brain that once processed neurochemical stimulation of pleasure and euphoria—and then became the incessant siren for intense drug hunger—has become the final resting place for a bullet fired during a moment of lost impulse control. If the bullet had not been fired in anger during her father's cocaine rage reaction, perhaps it would have been fired in a final act of depression and hopeless agony caused by her mother's cocaine withdrawal.

If the infant can survive the agonizing cocaine withdrawal and a complete hatred of physical contact, a human immunodeficiency virus (HIV) antibody test will likely predict an early death. She is the hospital's first baby of the new year.

A businessman stands frozen with irrational fears near the entrance of a subway, unable to board the train he has taken home uncounted times before. His heart beats out of control, his hands are sweaty, his legs tremble from the weight of his apprehensions, and he fears that he will lose control.

His distress increases over the next few weeks, and he has a sense of dread when merely thinking about crowded situations. He fears leaving the safety of his home. Scared that he is losing his mind, he has a physical examination and is diagnosed as having a panic disorder. His physician prescribes a sedative-hypnotic drug called alprazolam, a benzodiazepine commonly called Xanax. As the drug is consumed, alprazolam molecules are able to increase the activity of nerves that inhibit or suppress symptoms of anxiety. Increasing the activity of these inhibitory nerves results in a depression of the arousal and emotional centers of the brain, which is overactive during the businessman's panic attacks.

After he takes the medication for 3 weeks as prescribed, the cycle of anxiety and panic is broken. More aware of his high anxiety levels, he exercises and participates in a stress program to keep the panic and phobias at bay. He considers his experience with the medication a blessing.

Later, during a family crisis, his wife self-medicates her anxieties and emotional turmoil with her husband's leftover prescription. In contrast to her husband, she experiences a loss of control over the drug and a powerful compulsion for more. She continues to use the drug despite obvious adverse consequences. In contrast to her husband, she has a family history of addiction.

Near Big Sur, California, a young couple sit facing each other, seemingly unaware of the powerful waves of water beating on the well-worn cliffs. The psychedelic drug they have consumed causes their speech to be more rapid than normal. They experience an empathic, insightful bond with each other. Their unconscious defense mechanisms seem to have temporarily vanished. They seem eager to look more closely at their own behavior and attitudes. They will later describe their experience as one of enhanced empathy and insight, the effects of which appear to last beyond the psychedelic drug experience.

A friend of the young couple seems to be wrestling with demons seen only by her. Frightened by the distortions in sensory perception, scared by the intensity of emotions, and terrorized by unwanted insights about herself, she flees from her demons. Like the young couple, she will continue to experience the effects of her psychedelic drug experience past this day.

At first glance, differences in drug experiences defy explanation. How can the same coca plant produce a mild stimulation when its leaves are chewed but generate a relentless thirst for more when smoked? How can the same sedative-hypnotic molecule help one man to live life more fully by temporarily eliminating his panic attacks, while unleashing compulsion and loss of control in his wife? By what mechanism does the same psychedelic drug prompt experiences of heightened empathy and self-awareness in one group, but provoke distressing episodes of hallucinatory madness in another group?

Although some differences in drug experiences are difficult to understand, the examples above are frankly simple. For instance, routes of drug administration have tremendous effects on drug experiences. Inhaling large clouds of potent cocaine vapor into the brain through the lungs is incomprehensibly more potent than ingesting cocaine through the stomach by chewing leaves with a low cocaine content.

Differences in the development and progression of addiction are associated with numerous risk factors, including a family history of addiction. Although the husband experiences a beneficial response to a sedative-hypnotic drug, his high-risk wife experiences an explosive, addictive reaction. Similarly, responses to psychedelic drugs, more than to most drugs, are greatly affected by environmental, psychological, and emotional factors.

After working during most of the 1980s at the historic Haight Ashbury Free Clinics in San Francisco, I concluded that one lesson stands out above all: Our understanding of contemporary drug problems and drug treatment trends, changes, and fads must take into account the history of drug abuse. Drugs such as crack cocaine and ice amphetamine arrived on the scene with more press coverage than a public relations business could ever provide. They were portrayed as completely new drugs, rather than existing drugs consumed differently. Despite such media attention, alcoholism continues to kill far more people than cocaine or amphetamines ever did or ever will.

Nearly every drug of abuse that will be introduced in the near future will be closely related to a drug that exists today. There may be differences: Perhaps the so-called new drug may be ingested differently, or there may be subtle molecular changes. But likely, the drug will share many more similarities than differences with an existing drug.

The study of drugs of abuse and addiction requires an understanding of a number of principles, many of them relatively simple. Accordingly, Part One of the book is an overview of the pharmacologic aspects of psychoactive drug use and addiction. Chapter 1 begins with definitions of and differences between drug abuse and drug addiction. The effects of addiction on health are described, including impairment of physical, cognitive, psychological, emotional, social, and spiritual health. Risk factors for addiction are outlined, including psychiatric, behavioral, demographic, familial, social, and genetic risk factors.

Similarly, pharmacologic risk factors are summarized, including physical dependence, tolerance, withdrawal, cross-tolerance, and the upper-downer syndrome. Importantly, the different routes of drug administration are described, including inhalation, nasal snorting, injection, and oral ingestion. Chapter 1 also provides a basis for understanding the role of the nervous system in terms of feeling, behavior, and thinking, as those are significant areas of impact by psychoactive drugs.

The remainder of Part One describes the four basic groups of mood-altering drugs: stimulants, depressants, psychedelics, and inhalants. For example, Chapter 2 provides an explanation of the stimulants, including cocaine, the amphetamines, look-alike stimulants, and stimulant drugs of deception. The chapter also explains how stimulant drugs affect people's behavior, mood, and psychiatric states and describes the patterns of stimulant use and the type of drug states that are caused by stimulants.

Chapter 3 is a discussion of the two types of depressant drugs: sedative-hypnotics and opioids. Accordingly, there is a discussion about the effect of sedative-hypnotics on anxiety, the effect of opioids on pain, and the depressant-drug states.

Chapter 4 provides a basis for understanding one of the most unusual group of psychoactive drugs: the psychedelics. In particular, this chapter explains the primary elements of the psychedelic experience. Also described are the patterns of psychedelic drug use, the LSD-related drugs, the psychedelic amphetamines, phencyclidine (PCP), and the psychedelic effects of marijuana.

Part One ends with Chapter 5, which includes a discussion of the inhalant drugs. The inhalants are described in terms of the three major inhalant types: volatile solvents, volatile nitrite inhalants, and inhalation anesthetics.

Overall, Part One of this book provides the reader with an overview of the process of addiction, the drugs of abuse, and their effects on psychological, emotional, and behavioral functioning.

Chapter 1

Basic Principles of Drug Use

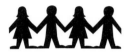

Addiction is not merely the chronic use of a drug. Addiction involves the compulsion to use drugs, a loss of control over the time and amount of drug use, and continued drug use despite negative consequences. These adverse consequences may include impairment in physical, cognitive, psychological, emotional, social, and spiritual health. From a medical perspective, addiction is characterized as a chronic, progressive, relapsing, and potentially fatal disease. The development and progression of addictive disease can be influenced by a number of factors, such as the type and strength of the drug, the route of administration, various individual risk factors, and assorted environmental influences. Understanding the basic principles of drug use is an important step in understanding addiction.

Ernest C. Reed, Jr., M.D., M.P.H.
Medical Director, New Beginnings at Serenity Lodge
Chemical Dependency Treatment Programs
Chesapeake, Virginia

■ Why Do People Use Drugs?

Young children twirl around in circles until they are dizzy and then fall to the ground, laughing and feeling giddy. Moments later they jump up and do it again. A teenage boy becomes nervous and anxious as he builds up the courage to ask a girl out on his first date. After school, he races home to excitedly tell his friends about his experience. On the same day, one person wins the lottery while another loses her job. Every day, people have experiences that alter their mood and feelings. Some experiences cause subtle changes in mood, whereas other experiences cause tremendous mood changes.

Drugs of abuse can have similar effects because they produce changes in mood by stimulating or depressing natural brain chemicals called neurotransmitters. *Neurotransmitters* are naturally occurring chemicals in the brain that are necessary for the transmission of nerve messages in the nervous system. Some neurotransmitters cause nerve messages to travel quickly, whereas others help to slow messages down. Neurotransmitters are responsible for the normal activity of the brain, including emotions, thinking, perception, and behavior.

Consider a person being robbed at gunpoint. Because of the danger involved, it is likely that both the thief and the victim will experience an increased heart rate, shortness of breath, a trembling sensation, muscle tension, and a surge in energy. The victim might describe her feelings as anxiety and fear. In contrast, the thief may describe his feelings as excitement and power. Their interpretation of the experience is different, but both may experience the same symptoms and signs caused by a rapid release of certain neurotransmitters.

The body tries to remain in a state of homeostasis or balance. With a healthy diet and life-style, the body may be able to keep these neurotransmitters in balance. However, severe elevations or depletions of certain neurotransmitters cause anxiety, depression, psychosis, mania, and other psychiatric problems. A drug is capable of having an effect on a person's emotions, thinking, perception, and behavior precisely because of its ability to exert an effect on these neurotransmitters. Thus drugs are able to mimic psychiatric problems such as anxiety, depression, psychosis, and mania. Certain drugs are also able to inhibit psychiatric problems. For example, alcohol decreases anxiety, and stimulants temporarily reduce depression. Drugs also can cause euphoria. Drugs such as crack cocaine or ice amphetamine cause a particularly stimulating euphoria. Drugs such as heroin cause a euphoria that includes an absence of pain and problems. Other drugs such as LSD do not cause euphoria as much as they provoke changes in perception, thinking, and consciousness that many people find pleasurable.

The types of drugs that are most commonly abused are psychoactive drugs. *Psychoactive drugs* are chemicals, substances, and medicine that have a generally rapid effect on people's mood, emotions, behavior, and thinking. For example, changes in mood include stimulation, sedation, and euphoria. Behavioral changes can include an acceleration or retardation of movement or activity. Changes in thinking can include a speeding or slowing of thinking, as well as delusions, hallucinations, and illusions.

Some medications such as antidepressants are able to modify people's mood after several days or weeks, but are not considered psychoactive because they do not cause rapid or euphoric changes in mood. Thus, medications such as antidepressants can be described as *mood regulators*. Similarly, antipsychotic medications cause normalization of the thinking process but do not cause rapid mood alteration or euphoria.

Why do people use drugs? There is no single answer to this question. Many people use drugs to experience the euphoria. Some people experiment with drugs once or a few times and never go any further. Other people use drugs to help deal with social interactions, to decrease anxiety or pain, or to fight insomnia. Athletes may use stimulants or steroids for performance enhancement. Factory workers may use stimulants to stay alert or depressants to drown out the drudgery. Whatever the reason, the user experiences a temporary change in brain chemistry and subsequent changes in mood, emotion, thinking, and behavior.

■ What Is Drug Abuse?

For many people, drug abuse and addiction are emotionally charged issues. People often have deeply held personal theories about the nature and causes of these problems. But in psychiatry and addiction medicine, definitions and diagnoses of medical problems must be objective, not based on personal, social, or political theories, which often change.

For example, during the 1960s, drug abuse was popularly defined as the use of drugs that are illegal and not condoned by the general population. By this definition, the use of illegal drugs (e.g., marijuana) was considered drug abuse, whereas the use of legal drugs (e.g., alcohol) was not.

Since that time, there has been a tremendous amount of medical research regarding our understanding of drug abuse and addiction. Based on this research, current definitions of drug problems are objective and clinical and are designed to help in the identification and treatment process.

Drug abuse is defined as the use of psychoactive drugs in such a way that it seriously interferes with a person's life, including physical, psychological, occupational, legal, educational, spiritual, or social functioning.[1] The key concept regarding drug abuse is evidence of impairment. This impairment can include a family fight, working while hung over, or spending rent money on cocaine. Drug abuse also includes behaviors that are risky or hazardous, such as driving or taking care of children, while intoxicated. In these cases, people are making poor decisions that can easily lead to disaster: they are taking drug-induced risks.

Drug abuse includes a wide range of behaviors. At the low end of the continuum, a person becomes intoxicated, experiences a hangover, dislikes it, and never uses any drug again. At the other end, an individual experiences a pattern of drug-induced impairment over many years. Thus, some people experience drug abuse patterns, whereas others have only rare drug abuse experiences. Fortunately, most people who abuse drugs "grow out of it," often in response to adverse consequences caused by the drugs.

■ What Is Addiction?

People who are addicted often say: "I'm not addicted; I only drink on weekends." Others say: "I can't be an addict; I only smoke marijuana, and you can't get addicted to marijuana." Still others claim: "I'm not an addict; I don't use nearly as much as she does!" Many people mistakenly believe that addiction relates primarily to how frequently the drug is being used, what type of drug is being used, the amount of drug being consumed, or how long a drug has been used. Although these are important factors, they do not define addiction.

Rather, *addiction* can be described as a progressive, chronic, primary disease that is characterized by compulsion, loss of control, continued drug use despite adverse consequences, and distortions in normal thinking, such as denial.[2] To understand addiction, it is important to explore each of these issues.

Addiction is a progressive disorder. If addiction is untreated, it generally gets worse, not better. Spouses who wait for their husbands to "get better" will eventually notice that the severity of the addiction will worsen over time, not go away. In medicine, the word *chronic* is the opposite of *acute,* the latter word meaning having a rapid onset and a short course. Although addiction may have a rapid onset for some people, it is generally of long duration. Thus, addiction is described as chronic.

Addiction is a primary disorder. Addiction is described as primary, meaning it is not merely the symptom of some other medical or psychiatric problem such as anxiety.[3] Other problems (such as anxiety) may be the reason for someone's initial drug use. But once the process of addiction begins, the addiction is viewed as a primary disorder that requires treatment as a separate and independent problem.

Addiction is a disease. A disease is a pathological (or abnormal) condition accompanied by several characteristic symptoms and signs that are exhibited by most people who have that condition. Diseases generally have a predictable prognosis; in other words, the course and end result of the disorder can be predicted. Many diseases (such as cancer) have hereditary, behavioral, and environmental causes and influences. Disease also means an involuntary disability, meaning that state of illness is not deliberately pursued.

Addiction involves craving and compulsion. Compulsion is the overwhelming preoccupation, desire, or drive to use a psycho-active drug. This compulsion may take the form of obsessive thinking about the next drug use experience or planning to obtain additional drugs.[4] Drug compulsion may take the form of simple drug hunger or of drug-seeking or drug-hoarding behavior.

Loss of control. Addiction invariably involves the loss of control over drug consumption or loss of control over drug-induced behavior, or both. Because the loss of control worsens over time, people in early stages of addiction may have some control over their drug use, but the control generally fades with time. There are exceptions, such as maintenance alcoholism. In addition to uncontrolled drug use, loss of control may emerge as the loss of control over drug-influenced behavior such as impulsive actions, verbal or physical violence, and impulsive sexual behavior.

Continued use despite adverse consequences. A hallmark feature of addiction is the tendency for continued drug use despite adverse consequences. Drug-induced problems, such as arrest for driving while intoxicated, would prompt many people to stop or alter their drug use. In contrast, addicted people literally can't "just say no," and continue to use drugs despite job loss, family trauma, or health problems.

Distortions of thinking. The most common distortion in thinking caused by addiction is denial. Denial can take many forms: denial that a drug problem exists, denial that the problem is severe, and denial that help is required. People with addiction generally deny that the adverse consequences they experience are caused by their drug use. Rather, they often believe that they use drugs because of these problems.

Denial is not the same as lying. When applied to addiction, denial is an unconscious defense mechanism that protects people from the harsh reality of their addiction. People who deny what others can plainly see may honestly believe what they say. Addicted people can lie, but the denial process itself is not purposeful lying.[5]

Is It Addiction?

People often want to know if their family member, student, friend, or patient is addicted. Health care professionals use the *Diagnostic and Statistical Manual of Mental Disorders* of the American Psychiatric Association[6] to make the appropriate diagnosis. Table 1–1 contains a questionnaire based on those criteria. The American Psychiatric Association states that answering yes to three or more of these criteria is indicative of addiction. Although this questionnaire is not a substitute for a thorough evaluation, diagnosis, and assessment, it can provide important information concerning a patient's likelihood of addiction.

Table 1–1. Addiction assessment questionnaire

❏ On many occasions, I have used more drugs than I intended, or used drugs for longer periods of time than I intended. (yes/no)

❏ I have tried (or wanted to try) to cut down or control my drug use. (yes/no)

❏ I have spent a great amount of time using drugs, recovering from the effects of drugs, or trying to obtain drugs. (yes/no)

❏ During times when I was or should have been at work, school, or home, I have frequently been intoxicated or experiencing withdrawal symptoms. (yes/no)

❏ Because of my drug use, there have been important social and occupational activities given up or reduced, either to spend time with other drug users or to use drugs in isolation. (yes/no)

❏ Despite realizing that my drug use was causing ongoing physical, psychological, or social problems (or making such problems worse), I continued to use. (yes/no)

❏ Sometimes I have had to use about twice the amount of drugs to get the same effect as before. (yes/no)

❏ There have been times when I experienced withdrawal symptoms after I stopped using drugs. (yes/no)

❏ There have been times when I used drugs in order to avoid withdrawal symptoms. (yes/no)

Source. Adapted with permission from DSM-III-R (American Psychiatric Association 1987).

What Are the Effects of Addiction?

Addiction can affect every aspect of people's lives: their physical, cognitive, psychological, emotional, social, and spiritual health. Because addiction is progressive, these areas of functioning also progressively worsen. Impairment in each of these areas has a particular pattern of symptoms and time course.

Physical health. Drug-induced deterioration of physical health is often a gradual process, measured over years. Thus, physical health is often the last aspect of health to deteriorate, but the first to return to normal. In fact, physical recovery after detoxification often makes people feel that they are "cured," prompting them to leave treatment against medical advice.

Cognitive health. Cognition refers to reasoning, judgment, intuition, memory, and perception. Examples of impaired cognition include intoxication, short-term memory problems, periods of amnesia, deterioration of concentration, and various neurological problems. Impairment of cognitive health can be short-term and long-term.

Psychological health. Addicted people often perceive their environment inaccurately. They may distort what they hear, misperceive what they see, and misinterpret events around them. Mild symptoms include irritability and frustration. Severe symptoms include suspiciousness, paranoia, and delusions.

Emotional health. The emotional health of addicted people is often characterized by extremes; negative emotions are frequent. They are often filled with anger, hate, and resentments. Addicted people may lack love, joy, warmth, and intimacy. They may not have experienced hope in a long time, which is something that should be nurtured during the treatment and recovery process.

Social health. Addicted people's social health often deteriorates rapidly. As drug cravings become stronger, the quest for social interactions weakens. Old friends may be ignored and replaced by drug-using acquaintances. As the addiction progresses, problems at work, with the family, and with friends will progressively worsen. Legal and financial problems may emerge or escalate.

Spiritual health. For people with addiction, life is centered around obtaining, using, and recovering from the effects of drugs. They may feel disconnected from others, no longer a part of their world. They may feel that their lives are without meaning and that there is no higher or spiritual purpose to their lives. They may feel that there is no power greater than themselves to which they can turn for help.

What Are Addiction Risk Factors?

If a husband and wife are both tall, anxious professional chefs, there is an increased likelihood that their children will become tall and anxious and will know how to cook. The influence on the children is both hereditary and environmental. Similarly, there are factors that increase the likelihood or probability of drug use, abuse, and addiction. Addiction risk factors are not guarantees of future addiction; they are rather predictors and indicators of potential addiction.

Psychiatric risk factors. Psychiatric problems may play several roles in the development of addiction.[7] Such problems are often the reason for initial drug use, as well as a reason to maintain drug use. For example, people may drink alcohol to reduce panic and anxiety symptoms. Although there is no evidence of an "addict personality" that leads to addiction, there is a cluster of personality traits that result from addiction, such as low stress tolerance, negative self-image, inadequacy, isolation, and depression.

Behavioral risk factors. Early antisocial, delinquent behavior such as conduct disorder is associated with early drug abuse and addiction.[8] Poor academic performance and a lack of educational commitment are also associated with an increased likelihood of abuse. Abuse often follows a period of negative attitudes toward self and others, social involvement with other troubled peers, and evidence of socially unacceptable behavior to achieve self-worth and gratification.

Demographic risk factors. Demographics relate to the statistical study of populations. Certain demographic factors are associated with abuse and addiction. For instance, men generally have higher rates of abuse and addiction than women.[9] Some ethnic and cultural groups, such as African Americans and Hispanics, have higher rates than other groups.[10] Living in the inner city—where economic, educational, and occupational disadvantages are common—is associated with an increased likelihood of abuse and addiction.

Family risk factors. Parents and other family members can increase the likelihood of children's drug use and abuse through modeling and example. There is an increased chance for abuse and addiction when children can see that other family members abuse alcohol and other drugs and personally accept this behavior.[11] Inconsistent parental discipline, lack of family warmth, and having parents who lack parental skills are all associated with early involvement with alcohol and other drugs.[12] A recent study noted that parental alcoholism influenced adolescent substance use through stress and negative affect, through decreased parental monitoring, and through increased temperamental emotionality (which was associated with heightened negative affect).[13]

Social risk factors. Similarly, children are influenced by their peers' use of alcohol and other drugs, as well as by their peers' attitudes regarding use. Adolescents who have friends with access to alcohol and other drugs have increased exposure and, thus, an increased probability of becoming users themselves. Adults are often influenced by their peers as to which specific drug they choose.

Genetic risk factors. It has long been known that there is a genetic component that influences the likelihood of becoming addicted to alcohol after drinking it. For instance, sons and daughters of alcoholic individuals are three to four times more likely to develop alcoholism than people without a family history of alcoholism.[14] Similarly, addiction to other drugs is also associated with a family history of alcoholism.[15] A family history of addiction is one of the most influential factors, suggesting a high risk for developing addiction.

People with a type of alcoholism that is characterized by an early onset have lower levels of a neurotransmitter called serotonin. Thus, some alcoholic individuals may have a preexisting deficit of this neurotransmitter, and alcohol use may be an attempt to reverse this neurotransmitter imbalance.[16] Indeed, one type of alcoholism may be related to the deficiency of serotonin, whereas another type of alcoholism may result from a different biological deficit.[17]

■ Pharmacologic Risk Factors

Pharmacology is the study of drugs and their effects on the body. Several pharmacologic factors increase the risk for continued use, abuse, and addiction.

Physical Dependence, Tolerance, and Withdrawal

Each drug category (stimulant, depressant, and psychedelic) represents a different type of effect on the central nervous system. For example, stimulants excite central nervous system activity, whereas depressants suppress this activity. Similarly, there are differences within each category. Thus, among depressants, the sedatives decrease anxiety, the hypnotics promote sleep, and the opiates decrease pain. But at higher doses, these three drug types can cause similar intoxication; chronic use will cause variations of a depressant tolerance, physical dependence, and withdrawal.

Drugs differ in regard to the ease with which physical dependence, tolerance, and withdrawal can develop. *Physical (or tissue)* dependence describes the biological adaptation of the body to long-term exposure to a drug. The first time it is exposed to a drug, the body may have a strong reaction, such as intoxication. But after chronic consumption of a drug, the body physically adjusts to it, often stopping the production of natural neurochemicals that are similar to the drug of abuse. In other words, the body begins to expect the presence of a chronically used drug. In addition, the body becomes tolerant to the effects of the drug.

Tolerance describes the physical process during which the same amount of a drug begins to have a decreasing effect. As tolerance develops, increasing amounts of the drug must be consumed to create the same effect.[18] Once physical dependence and tolerance have developed, withdrawal will occur if the drug is abruptly stopped. The stimulants and depressants are well known for the development of physical dependence, tolerance, and withdrawal syndromes. The desire to avoid withdrawal will tend to prolong drug use; the development of tolerance will tend to increase drug use.

Drug withdrawal is the physical process during which the body adapts to the absence of a drug on which it is physically dependent. Because withdrawal is physically and psychologically uncomfortable, the chronic drug user is compelled to use more drugs to avoid the withdrawal effects. Many drugs promote two separate but sometimes overlapping types of withdrawal: acute and prolonged withdrawal.

Acute withdrawal is the cluster of symptoms that occur for the first few days, up to about a week. They begin shortly after stopping or reducing consumption of most drugs to which physical dependence and tolerance have developed. For instance, acute cocaine withdrawal occurs during the first few days after the cessation or reduction of cocaine intake. This is a period of intense depression, fatigue, agitation, irritability, insomnia, or excessive sleeping.

Subacute (or prolonged) withdrawal describes a syndrome that may begin shortly after acute withdrawal, or may occur spontaneously a few weeks or even months after the last use of the drug, but that nonetheless represents additional physical adaptation to the absence of the drug.[19] For example, subacute cocaine withdrawal may suddenly emerge a few weeks or months after the last use of cocaine. The individual may experience intense craving for cocaine, as well as insomnia, agitation, and perhaps depression. Subacute withdrawal, also called prolonged' or protracted withdrawal, has been identified among people addicted to alcohol, heroin, cocaine, and the benzodiazepines and may occur with most drugs of abuse.

Acute withdrawal from any drug is a particularly intense physical and emotional experience. It is often a medical emergency. Thus, withdrawal is often treated under medical care. Acute withdrawal can be anticipated and prepared for. In contrast, subacute withdrawal episodes are often unexpected and unanticipated. People may experience multiple episodes of subacute withdrawal, each lasting a few days. Because drug craving is invariably a component of this syndrome, subacute withdrawal episodes are times of high risk for returning to drug use. Also, because there may be a lapse of time between the acute withdrawal and the subacute withdrawal, the connection between the symptoms and the previous drug use may not seem obvious.

Cross-Tolerance and the Upper-Downer Syndrome

People who use drugs generally use more than one drug. This is called polydrug abuse or polydrug addiction. The most common polydrug pattern involves alcohol, marijuana, and cocaine. One aspect of polydrug use relates to cross-tolerance. *Cross-tolerance* is the pharmacologic ability of one drug to have generally the same effect on the nervous system as another drug.[20] For instance, alcohol and the antianxiety medication diazepam (Valium) are surprisingly similar in effect: they are both sedative-hypnotics. People who have developed a tolerance to alcohol have (often unknowingly) developed a tolerance to diazepam. In other words, people who have developed a tolerance to alcohol can use diazepam to ward off the alcoholic withdrawal, and vice versa.

Although some drugs—such as alcohol and diazepam—are almost fully cross-tolerant, other drugs—such as alcohol and marijuana—are partially cross-tolerant. (As will be described more fully later, marijuana has both depressant and psychedelic effects.) Drugs that are partially and fully cross-tolerant are frequently substituted for one another, depending on the circumstances. People who have a polydrug addiction to marijuana and alcohol will increase use of one of the drugs if access to the other is diminished. For example, when people addicted to both marijuana and alcohol are prevented from drinking alcohol, they will typically increase their marijuana use. The reverse is also true. Thus, cross-tolerance explains in part the frequent substitution of drugs that have similar pharmacologic actions.

Addicted people often develop a preference for drugs that have a specific pharmacologic action, such as a preference for stimulants or opiates. The preference may be quite specific, such as a preference for cocaine rather than amphetamines, and even for cocaine that is smoked rather than snorted. The preferred drug can be called the *primary drug of choice*. For example, people may prefer alcohol as their primary drug of choice, but use diazepam while at work (because it can't be detected on the breath) and smoke marijuana in the morning on weekends (because they don't want to drink early in the day).

People often have a *secondary drug of choice,* or a drug that is frequently used in combination with the primary drug of choice. The secondary drug, which may be pharmacologically similar to the primary drug, may be used to enhance or prolong the effects of the primary drug. On the other hand, the secondary drug of choice may have effects that are pharmacologically opposite to those of the primary drug and may be taken to diminish certain effects of the primary drug. For example, alcohol is a common secondary drug used to decrease the overstimulation, agitation, and insomnia caused by cocaine.

When alcohol is consumed to decrease cocaine overstimulation, the alcohol also reduces the cocaine euphoria. Thus, additional cocaine may be consumed to intensify the euphoria. More cocaine causes more stimulation, creating the need for more alcohol, and so on. This cycle of stimulant-depressant-stimulant-depressant use is called the *upper-downer syndrome* and is summarized in Table 1–2.

The upper-downer syndrome is an attempt to create a balance between stimulation and depression of the nervous system. The balance is temporary because the stimulants and the depressants have different time courses. Thus, people who have simultaneously ingested cocaine and alcohol may not feel intoxicated and may appear relatively normal to nonprofessionals. However, because cocaine's stimulant effects diminish more rapidly than alcohol's depressant effects, users begin having slurred speech and pronounced incoordination and appear to be drunk.

The upper-downer syndrome tends to increase the amounts ingested of both drugs, often to dangerous levels. Without the stimulant, people would probably pass out because of the large amounts of alcohol. Without the alcohol, they might become extremely anxious, agitated, violent, and psychotic.

Also, people who engage in an upper-downer cycle are at higher risk for developing tolerance to and physical dependence on the secondary drug of choice without realizing it. Thus, people addicted to both cocaine and alcohol may develop tolerance to and physical dependence on both drugs and experience a cocaine-alcohol withdrawal syndrome on cessation of drug use.

Routes of Drug Administration

Another important pharmacologic risk factor is the route of drug administration. Psychoactive drugs are mood altering precisely be-

Table 1–2. The upper-downer cycle

Sequence	Action	Result
1	Use a stimulant	Feel euphoric Become overstimulated
2	Use a depressant	Become less stimulated Feel less euphoric
3	Use more stimulant	Feel more euphoric Become overstimulated
4	Use more depressant	Become less stimulated Feel less euphoric
5	Repeat cycle	High doses of stimulant High doses of depressant A "balance" is attempted

Note. The upper-downer cycle often begins with a stimulant as the primary drug of choice. Symptoms of overstimulation may occur, such as anxiety, agitation, nervousness, restlessness, and paranoia. A depressant such as alcohol can be used to diminish the overstimulation; it will also diminish the euphoria. The individual may repeat the upper-downer cycle until large amounts of both drugs have been consumed.

cause of their ability to alter temporarily the normal balance of central nervous system activity: they are mood altering because of their ability to have an effect on the brain. The route of drug administration affects the speed at which drugs get to the brain, as well as how much of the drug actually gets there. Thus, the route of administration has an enormous impact on the drug experience and on the risks of becoming addicted.

The brain is constantly fed oxygen and nutrients through a network of blood vessels that surround the brain. These blood vessels are part of the circulatory system that brings blood to all parts of the body. They can also carry psychoactive drugs. There are several ways for drugs to enter the bloodstream.

Drugs, like other substances, occur in one of three different forms: liquid, solid, or gas. Some drugs such as alcohol are always liquid, whereas other drugs such as diazepam are sold in both solid (pill) and liquid (injectable) forms. Also, drugs such as heroin or cocaine can exist in solid, liquid, and even gas vapor forms.

Inhaling. When water boils, water particles exist in both the steam vapors and in the boiling water. Some drugs such as nitrous oxide (laughing gas) are always in a gas form. Other drugs are in a liquid form, but have vapor-like fumes, such as butyl nitrite, gasoline, and paint thinner. Other drugs such as marijuana and tobacco can be lit on fire, creating a smoke that can be inhaled.

In making freebase cocaine or heating crack cocaine, people are changing the cocaine from a solid substance into a gas vapor. The crack smoke is actually a gas vapor that contains cocaine particles. When this vaporized drug is inhaled, it enters the lungs and is absorbed into the bloodstream through tiny blood vessels in the lungs. There are millions of these tiny blood vessels, and they are able to channel large amounts of the vaporized drug into the bloodstream. Because of the location of the lungs, the drug is pumped into the heart and quickly routed into the brain and rest of the body. An inhaled drug can reach the brain within 7 seconds.

Snorting. Snorting is not the same as inhaling. Snorting involves ingestion of a powdered drug into the tiny blood vessels in the nasal passages. There are far fewer blood vessels in the nasal passages than in the lungs; therefore, snorting drugs channels less of the drug into the bloodstream than inhaling. Thus, snorting is less efficient than inhaling, and a snorted drug takes from 3 to 5 minutes to reach the brain in only modest concentrations.

Injecting. Many drugs such as cocaine, heroin, and some pills can be prepared in a liquid form and injected directly into the body. Drugs can be injected directly into the bloodstream (intravenous), into the muscles (intramuscular), and under the skin (called "skin-popping" or subcutaneous injection).

Injection is the most dangerous way of putting drugs into the body because the body's natural filtering system is bypassed. Because drugs such as cocaine and heroin generally contain impurities, and because needles are often unsterile, impurities can be put directly into the body, raising the risk for infection and other problems. Also, sharing needles creates a risk of transmission of several dangerous viruses such as hepatitis and human immunodeficiency virus (HIV), which causes the acquired immunodeficiency syndrome (AIDS).

Oral ingestion. Liquids (such as alcohol) and solids (such as pills) are swallowed, passed through the esophagus and stomach, and absorbed into the tiny blood vessels in the small intestines. Along the way, drugs must first pass through acids in the stomach and enzymes in the mouth. These enzymes and acids break down food into nutrients and can break down some drugs, making the drugs weaker. Also, because these drugs have to travel slowly through the stomach and intestines, it takes about 20–30 minutes for them to reach the brain.

Other drug routes. Drugs can enter the blood system through specific areas of the body that have great numbers of tiny blood vessels. These areas are called mucous membranes. Examples of areas with mucous membranes that people use to insert or apply drugs include the rectum, the vagina, the eyes, and under the tongue.

Different routes of drug administration affect how quickly drugs reach the brain and how much of a drug actually reaches the brain. Thus, smoking cocaine has an even greater impact on the brain than does snorting cocaine. The faster that a drug gets to the brain and the higher the percentage of a drug that reaches the brain, the greater the euphoria and the higher the risk of addiction. Table 1–3 summarizes the primary routes of drug administration and reaction time.

■ Summary

Neurotransmitters are naturally occurring brain chemicals that are necessary for the transmission of nerve messages in the nervous system. Because these chemicals are essential to the healthy functioning of emotions, thinking, perception, and behavior, any change in their natural balance can affect these areas of life. Psychoactive drugs are mood altering because they are able to create an imbalance in these neurotransmitters, thus creating changes in emotions, thinking, perception, and behavior. Drug abuse is the use of a psychoactive drug

Table 1–3. Route of drug administration

Route	Summary and reaction time
Inhaling	Drug in vapor form is inhaled through mouth and lungs into circulatory system, reaching the brain within 7 seconds.
Snorting	Drug in powdered form is snorted into the nose. Some of the drug lands on the nasal mucous membranes, is absorbed by blood vessels, enters the bloodstream, and reaches the brain in about 4 minutes.
Injection	Drug in liquid form directly enters the body through a needle. Intravenous injection reaches the brain in about 20 seconds. Intramuscular or subcutaneous injection reaches brain in about 4 minutes.
Oral ingestion	Drug in solid or liquid form passes through esophagus and stomach and finally to the small intestines. It is absorbed by blood vessels in the intestines and reaches the brain about 30 minutes after ingestion.
Other routes	Drugs can be absorbed through areas that contain mucous membranes. Drugs can be placed under the tongue, inserted anally and vaginally, and administered as eyedrops.

in such a way that it seriously interferes with a person's life, including physical, psychological, occupational, legal, educational, spiritual, and social functioning. Drug addiction is a progressive, chronic, primary disease that includes the compulsion to use a drug, loss of control over use of the drug, continued use of the drug despite adverse consequences, and distortions in thinking such as denial. Drug addiction risk factors include behavioral, demographic, family, social, and genetic risk factors.

Physical dependence describes the biological adaptation to long-term exposure to a drug, including the reduced production of neurotransmitters that are similar to the drug of addiction. Drug withdrawal is the physical process by which the body tries to adapt to the absence of a drug on which it has become dependent. Acute withdrawal occurs shortly after cessation of chronic use of a drug. Subacute withdrawal may begin shortly after cessation, or it may occur spontaneously weeks or even months after acute withdrawal. Cross-tolerance is the pharmacologic ability of one drug to have the same effect generally on the nervous system as another drug: for example, someone tolerant to alcohol has developed cross-tolerance to Valium. Some drugs such as marijuana and alcohol are partially cross-tolerant.

Addicted people generally have a preferred or primary drug of choice and one or more secondary drugs of choice that may be pharmacologically similar to their primary drug or may have opposite pharmacologic properties. Secondary drugs may be used to enhance, prolong, or diminish the effects of the primary drug. People often engage in an upper-downer cycle in which large amounts of the stimulant and depressant are consumed. Psychoactive drugs must enter the brain to alter mood and behavior. They can enter the brain through inhaling, snorting, injection, and oral ingestion.

■ References

1. Smith DE, Landry MJ: Psychoactive substance use disorders: drugs and alcohol, in Review of General Psychiatry, 2nd Edition. Edited by Goldman HH. Norwalk, CT, Appleton & Lange, 1988

2. Landry M: Addiction diagnostic update: DSM-III-R psychoactive substance use disorders. Journal of Psychoactive Drugs 19:379–381, 1987

3. Morse RM, Flavin DK: The definition of alcoholism. Journal of the American Medical Association 268:1012–1014, 1992

4. Modell JG, Glaser GB, Cyr L, et al: Obsessive and compulsive characteristics of craving for alcohol in alcohol abuse and dependence. Alcoholism: Clinical and Experimental Research 16(2):272–274, 1992

5. Shelp EE, Perl M: Denial in clinical medicine: a reexamination of the concept and its significance. Archives of Internal Medicine 145:697–699, 1985

6. American Psychiatric Association: Diagnostic and Statistical Manual of Mental Disorders, Third Edition, Revised. Washington, DC, American Psychiatric Association, 1987

7. Landry MJ, Smith DE, McDuff D, et al: Anxiety and substance use disorders: a primer for primary care physicians. Journal of the American Board of Family Practice 4:47–53, 1991

8. Hawkins JD, Lischner DM, Jenson JM, et al: Delinquents and drugs: what the evidence suggests about prevention and treatment programming, in Youth at Risk for Substance Abuse. Edited by Brown B, Mills A. Rockville, MD, Alcohol, Drug Abuse, and Mental Health Administration, 1987

9. Regier DA, Boyd JH, Burke JD, et al: One-month prevalence of mental disorders in the United States. Archives of General Psychiatry 45:977–986, 1988

10. Alcohol, Drug Abuse, and Mental Health Administration: Drug Abuse and Drug Abuse Research. Rockville, MD, National Institute on Drug Abuse, 1991

11. Baumrind D: Familial antecedents of adolescent drug use: a developmental perspective, in Etiology of Drug Abuse: Implications for Prevention (National Institute on Drug Abuse Research Monograph No 56). Edited by Jones CL, Battjes RJ. Rockville, MD, National Institute on Drug Abuse, 1985, pp 13–44

12. Kandel DB, Simcha-Fagan O, Davies M: Risk factors for delinquency and illicit drug use from adolescence to young adulthood. Journal of Drug Issues 60:67–90, 1986

13. Chassin L, Pillow DR, Curran PJ, et al: Relation of parental alcoholism to early adolescent substance use: a test of three mediating mechanisms. Journal of Abnormal Psychology 102:3–19, 1993

14. Goodwin DW: Is Alcoholism Hereditary? New York, Ballantine, 1988

15. Cadoret RJ, Troughton E, O'Gorman TW, et al: An adoption study of genetic and environmental factors in drug abuse. Archives of General Psychiatry 43:1131–1136, 1986

16. Buydens-Branchey L, Branchey MH, Noumairi D, et al: Age of alcoholism onset, II: relationship to susceptibility to serotonin precursor availability. Archives of General Psychiatry 46:231–236, 1989

17. Goodwin FG: Alcoholism research: delivering on the promise. Public Health Reports 103(6):569–574, 1988

18. Harris RA, Buck KJ: The process of alcohol tolerance and dependence. Alcohol Health and Research World 14:105–110, 1990

19. Geller A: Protracted abstinence, in The American Society of Addiction Medicine: Syllabus for the Review Course in Addiction Medicine. Washington, DC, American Society of Addiction Medicine, 1990

20. Inaba DS, Cohen WE: Uppers, Downers, All Arounders. Ashland, OR, Cinemed, 1989

Table 2–1. The stimulant drugs

Stimulant drug type	Specific stimulant drugs

Cocaine	Cocaine hydrochloride (intranasally snorted powder)
	Cocaine free base (smokable cocaine)
	  Free base cocaine (inhaled during preparation)
	  Crack cocaine (preprepared, heated, and inhaled)

Amphetamines	Amphetamine sulfate (generic) Dextroamphetamine sulfate (Dexedrine) Methamphetamine hydrochloride (Desoxyn) Ice (recrystallized, smokable methamphetamine) Amphetamine plus dextroamphetamine (Biphetamine) Psychedelic amphetamines (MDA, MDMA, MDE, etc.)
Amphetamine analogues and related CNS stimulants	Benzphetamine (Didrex) Caffeine (coffee, No Doz, Vivarin, some Anacin products) Diethylpropion (Tenuate) Ephedrine (Primatene Mist, Bronkaid Mist) Epinephrine (Primatene Mist Solution) Mazindol (Sanorex) Methylphenidate (Ritalin) Pemoline (Cylert) Phentermine (Fastin) Phendimetrazine (Trimtabs) Phenmetrazine (Preludin) Phenylpropanolamine (Acutrim, Dexatrim, and Dimetapp) Propylhexedrine
Nicotine	Cigarettes, cigars, pipe tobacco Chewing tobacco Nicotine gum (Nicorette) Nicotine patches (Nicoderm) Snuff

Note. MDA = 3,4-methylenedioxyamphetamine;
MDMA = *N*-methyl-3,4-methylenedioxymethamphetamine;
MDE = *N*-ethyl-3,4-methylenedioxyamphetamine;
CNS = central nervous system.

Chapter 2

The Stimulant Drugs

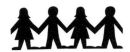

The stimulants are some of the most commonly used drugs throughout the world. They include legal and illegal variants. Since the legal drug caffeine, found in coffee and sodas, is ubiquitous and socially accepted, some people don't realize that it is indeed a drug. Stimulants can be found in cold and flu preparations where they are used as bronchodilators and to counteract the sedation of antihistamines. Stimulants are promoted on television as weight reduction pills, although their effectiveness is extremely short-lived and of little true help. Stimulants such as cocaine and the amphetamines are ever-present street drugs. Modifications in route of administration have given the world crack cocaine and ice amphetamine, perhaps the most noxious of all street drugs. Interestingly, stimulants provoke the activity of normal brain chemicals called neurotransmitters, causing mood changes. Sadly, they can also provoke intense compulsion, profound loss of control, enduring use despite adverse consequences, and a devastating crash and craving.

Max A. Schneider, M.D., C.A.D.C.
Clinical Associate Professor, University of California at Irvine
Past President, American Society of Addiction Medicine
Medical Director, St. Joseph Hospital
Orange, California

■ Introduction

Fluctuations in mood, mental and physical energy, and ability to handle stress are normal aspects of life. People become elated during exciting events and depressed after sad events. They can often identify times of the day when their ability to concentrate is at its best and worst. There are times when people feel confident and have the physical energy to tackle tough problems. On the other hand, there are times when people lack the energy to perform normal tasks and feel overwhelmed by small problems.

These fluctuations in mood, energy, and activity are often reactions to environmental changes such as other people and events. They may be reactions to changes in the diet, becoming ill, experiencing physical trauma, or participating in sports. Whatever internal or external influences may play a role in these normal fluctuations, there is a corresponding fluctuation in the activity of the central nervous system. These fluctuations can be drastically manipulated through the use of drugs.

■ The Stimulants

Drugs that increase the activity of the central nervous system and promote emotional and behavioral stimulation are called the stimulants. The stimulants vary in terms of their ability to create euphoria, the relative strength of the stimulation, the length of time that they produce stimulation, and the way in which they excite the central nervous system. Despite these differences, they are all able to stimulate the central nervous system and to stimulate mental and physical activity.

As drugs of abuse, stimulants are far more similar than they are different. For example, cocaine and amphetamines were indistinguishable in experiments with experienced human users of stimulants as well as with animals trained to distinguish between drugs.[1] Indeed, some of the more significant differences among stimulant experiences are not pharmacologic, but rather are differences in routes of administration.

Cocaine, Freebase, and Crack

Cocaine that has traditionally been sold on the street as a white powder is cocaine hydrochloride. Because cocaine hydrochloride is normally sold in powdered form, is soluble in water, and is absorbed by the nasal mucous membranes, the preferred method of administration has been intranasal snorting, although it can be taken orally or intravenously.

When consumed orally, cocaine must first pass through acids and enzymes of the gastrointestinal system before absorption by the intestines. Accordingly, oral consumption of cocaine results in a less rapid onset of stimulation and a less intense euphoria.

When snorted, cocaine is absorbed by the mucous membranes, enters the bloodstream, and reaches the brain in about 4 minutes. The peak subjective effects occur within 15–20 minutes. Intravenously injected cocaine will reach the brain in about 4 minutes, with substantial effects lasting about a half hour.

Snorted cocaine causes a stronger euphoria than orally consumed cocaine. Because intravenously injected cocaine can release a higher concentration of cocaine directly into the bloodstream, it causes an even stronger euphoria than snorting or oral consumption. Thus, the impact of the drug (specifically, the strength of the euphoria and the overall stimulation) varies greatly depending on whether the cocaine is swallowed, snorted, or injected. An even more powerful euphoria and stimulation effect is created by yet another drug delivery system: cocaine smoking.

Smokable cocaine. Because cocaine hydrochloride vaporizes at such a high temperature (195°C), it cannot be smoked. Rather, it must be converted to cocaine free base, which will vaporize at a much lower temperature (98°C). Thus, cocaine can exist in two chemical states: a water-soluble powder or liquid that can be snorted or injected and a smokable, free base state.

There are two ways to convert cocaine hydrochloride into a free base state. A traditional method called "freebasing" is a chemical process that involves preparing cocaine in an alkaline solution such as ammonia or baking soda and then extracting the free base using volatile solvents such as ether. Cocaine users inhale the cocaine vapor as it is extracted. The extreme flammability of ether makes this a dangerous process. Free base cocaine has been available only to people with freebase kits and fairly large amounts of cocaine.

Crack cocaine, which involves conversion of cocaine hydrochloride into a free base by using baking soda and water, has revolutionized the preparation, marketing, selling, and use of cocaine.[2] Most significant is the preparation of smokable free base cocaine ahead of time and making available small pieces of smokable cocaine. The marketing of crack has been effective and distressing because cocaine in its most addictive, smokable form is now available in small units at prices low enough that it can be bought for little money, even by children.

The euphoria resulting from smoking cocaine in the free base state is extremely intense and very rapid. The critical feature of cocaine smoking is the route of administration: through the lungs to the brain within 7 seconds, often before the pipe leaves the lips of the cocaine smoker.

Whereas much cocaine hydrochloride is wasted during intranasal snorting, when cocaine is smoked, nearly all of the cocaine smoke is able to enter the lungs. In addition, the composition of free base cocaine smoke in pure cocaine is about 93% cocaine particles and about 7% vapor,[3] meaning that a very high percentage of available cocaine can actually reach the lungs and brain (in contrast to the rather small percentage of intranasally snorted cocaine that can reach the brain). Thus, smoking cocaine results in a very rich concentration of cocaine in the blood traveling to the brain. Also, free base cocaine is fat soluble, allowing for very quick passage into the brain. Peak blood levels of cocaine and subjective effects are almost immediate. Consequently, the individual becomes very high, very quickly. Within a few minutes, a small amount of inhaled cocaine free base (50 milligrams) can produce peak blood concentrations that are nearly as great as the maximum achieved 40 minutes after nasal insufflation of twice the amount (100 milligrams) of crystalline cocaine hydrochloride.[4]

Contrary to a popular street drug mythology, free base cocaine is not pure cocaine. When cocaine free base is extracted from cocaine hydrochloride, impurities are not removed. Frequently, impurities are purposefully put into the cocaine hydrochloride as fillers and can survive the extraction process. When the cocaine is smoked, both cocaine and impurities enter the bloodstream.

Cocaine + alcohol = cocaethylene. Only when cocaine is consumed with alcohol, a cocaine metabolite (or breakdown product) called cocaethylene is produced.[5] In contrast to other cocaine metabolites, cocaethylene is psychoactive and causes euphoria, reinforcement, and self-administration. In fact, it is more euphoric, rewarding, and lethal than cocaine. Thus, when people drink alcohol and consume cocaine, they actually experience the effects of three drugs, not two.

Amphetamines, Speed, and Ice

The amphetamines are a group of chemically related stimulant drugs that cause similar psychological, physiological, and behavioral effects. As a group, the amphetamines are related to the naturally occurring neurotransmitters epinephrine and norepinephrine, known also as adrenaline and noradrenaline. Like cocaine, amphetamines cause a dose-related range of effects, from alertness, confidence, and increased well-being to euphoria, impulsiveness, and agitation. Similarly, chronic use of high doses will result in psychomotor agitation and stimulant psychosis. There are three primary amphetamines: amphetamine sulfate (commonly called amphetamine), dextroamphetamine, and methamphetamine. Biphetamine is simply a combination of dextroamphetamine and amphetamine.

The amphetamines were introduced in 1931 as over-the-counter nasal decongestants and later as appetite suppressants. Medical uses have included the treatment of obesity, depression, narcolepsy, and attention-deficit disorder.[6] Today, the only accepted medical indications for amphetamines are the treatment of attention-deficit hyperactivity disorder in children and the treatment of narcolepsy. They are no longer recommended for use as an appetite suppressant or to combat fatigue.

Although amphetamines and cocaine have fundamentally similar psychological and behavioral effects, they differ in terms of the duration of stimulant activity. Although cocaine-induced stimulation may last for 30–40 minutes, amphetamines can cause stimulation for 3–6 hours.[7] As a result, the period of euphoria, distorted thinking, and impaired behavior is lengthy. The lengthy stimulation frequently leads to the use of depressants such as alcohol to decrease overstimulation.

Amphetamines can be obtained in powder, pill, and liquid forms. Some derivatives are made in clandestine labs, whereas others are produced by pharmaceutical companies for prescribing. Except for impurities, there is no chemical difference between legal and illegal amphetamines. Street names for amphetamines include "speed" and "crank."

Smokable amphetamine. Most amphetamine users choose oral or intravenous routes of administration. However, just as cocaine hydrochloride can be prepared for smoking, methamphetamine can be synthesized into a crystalline smokable form. The smokable version of amphetamine is called ice amphetamine.

The 10- to 15-minute-long crack cocaine euphoria and stimulation often prompt a binge episode that involves smoking more cocaine every 10–15 minutes. In comparison, ice amphetamine stimulant intoxication can last between 12 and 24 hours. One smoke of the pipe causes a profound, massive stimulation. People with tolerance to the stimulant effects may be able to work inexhaustibly for 10–20 hours. Other individuals may experience severe agitation, anxiety, hallucinations, and delusions of persecution. As the stimulation wears off, the user experiences extraordinary depression, craving for more drug, and lethargy.

Methamphetamine was developed by the Japanese in 1893 and was provided during World War II (1939–1945) by Japan's military leaders for weary soldiers and munitions-plant workers. This led to an explosive stimulant epidemic resulting in over 500,000 Japanese methamphetamine addicts by 1954.[8] Banned by Japan in the 1950s, many methamphetamine labs moved to South Korea, which is currently a major international supplier of methamphetamine, including the latest variant, ice amphetamine.

Appetite Suppressants, Look-Alikes, and Drugs of Deception

Some stimulants have a less powerful effect than cocaine and amphetamines. However, less powerful does not mean safe. When the dosage is increased, these agents produce powerful central nervous system stimulation. Some of these drugs are chemically related to amphetamines, whereas others are not. In a general way, the stimulant effects of these drugs are roughly equivalent to those of caffeine, which has mild stimulant effects at low doses and profound stimulant effects at high doses, but which is not particularly euphoric.

Amphetamine analogues. The term *analogue* can describe drugs that are similar in function to another drug, even if the drugs originate from different sources or have different mechanisms of action. Most amphetamine analogues have effects on the central nervous system similar to those of the amphetamines, but produce less euphoria and are thought to be less abused than the amphetamines. The majority of these drugs are sold as appetite suppressants: benzphetamine (Didrex), fenfluramine (Pondimin), mazindol (Mazanor, Sanorex), phentermine (Fastin Capsules), phendimetrazine (Prelu-2, Trimstat, Trimtabs), phenmetrazine (Preludin), and diethylpropion (Tenuate).

Two additional amphetamine-like stimulants deserve special attention. The drugs pemoline (Cylert) and methylphenidate (Ritalin) are used in the treatment of attention-deficit hyperactivity disorder in children. The hallmark features of this disorder are impulsivity and inattention. In the average person, stimulants promote impulsivity, inattention, and hyperactivity. However, certain stimulants paradoxically help to calm children with attention-deficit hyperactivity disorder. This suggests that for these children, hyperactivity may result from "underarousal" of a part of the brain (the midbrain) that would normally inhibit hyperactivity. These stimulants appear to stimulate the midbrain, which in turn suppresses the hyperactivity. Young males who were diagnosed as having hyperactivity during childhood have higher-than-average rates of substance use problems, but they have far greater rates of attention-deficit disorder and antisocial disorders.[9] There is no substantial evidence that the use of stimulants to treat attention-deficit hyperactivity disorder leads to later use of stimulants or other drugs.

Methylphenidate is also used in the medical management of narcolepsy. Narcolepsy is a sleep disorder that is characterized by chronic, excessive daytime sleepiness, with several recurrent episodes of sleep daily. Methylphenidate is used to control drowsiness and sleep attacks.

Epinephrine and ephedrine. Epinephrine (adrenaline), a neurotransmitter that has also been synthesized, is used as a cardiac stimulant. It can be found in Bronkaid Mist and other asthmatic drugs because it is a vasoconstrictor and relaxes bronchioles—small airways of the breathing system from the bronchi to the lobes of the lung. The effects of ephedrine are less powerful but more prolonged than the effects of epinephrine. Epinephrine is most effective when injected or inhaled, whereas ephedrine is most effective when taken orally. Ephedrine produces more anxiety and less euphoria than the amphetamines. Ephedrine dilates the bronchial muscles, contracts the nasal mucosa, and increases blood pressure. It is chiefly used for its bronchodilator effects in patients with asthma and bronchitis and as a nasal decongestant in patients with hay fever. Ephedrine is found in Primatene P Formula, Bronkotabs, and Azma Aid.

Phenylpropanolamine. Phenylpropanolamine, a synthetic stimulant, replaced ephedrine in many over-the-counter cough and cold products because it acts as an effective decongestant with minimal effect on the central nervous system or the cardiovascular system.[10] Phenylpropanolamine has medical indications as a nasal decongestant, for bronchodilation, and for short-term use as an appetite suppressant. It can be found in Acutrim Appetite Suppressant, Allerest 12 Hour Caplets, various Contac decongestant/antihistamine formulas, Coricidin "D" Decongestant Tablets, various Dexatrim appetite suppressants, assorted Dimetapp elixirs, St. Joseph Cold Tablets for Children, various Triaminic tablets and syrups, and Tylenol Cold Medication Effervescent Tablets.

Caffeine.   Caffeine is the most widely used psychoactive drug in the world. Most North American adults drink either coffee or tea daily.[11] In addition to its use to combat drowsiness and mental fatigue, caffeine is used as partial treatment for migraine headaches. Despite the cultural approval of caffeine, it is a stimulant drug, and problems occur with overstimulation, dependence, and withdrawal.[12] Caffeine overstimulation effects include tremulousness, tinnitus, talkativeness, sweating, stomachache, and insomnia.[13] Caffeine withdrawal, characterized by symptoms of anxiety, depression, low vigor, high fatigue, and headache, has been identified among people who cease their regular consumption of 2.5 cups per day.[14]

Caffeine can be found in coffee, teas, prescribed medications, and various over-the-counter preparations. Caffeine-containing products include various Anacin analgesic tablets, Aspirin-Free Excedrin Analgesic Caplets, No Doz Fast Acting Alertness Aid Tablets, Vanquish Analgesic Caplets, and Vivarin Stimulant Tablets.

The collective group of amphetamine analogues—ephedrine, phenylpropanolamine, and caffeine—can be found in various combinations and marketed for various purposes. These drugs appear as ingredients in appetite suppressants, cold and cough preparations, over-the-counter stimulants, look-alike drugs, and drugs of deception.

Appetite suppressants.   Two classic side effects of stimulants are decreases in appetite and sleep. In fact, weight loss and insomnia are two of the signs of stimulant addiction. Because stimulants cause a temporary decrease in appetite, pharmaceutical companies produce appetite suppressants that are amphetamine-related. These include phentermine (Fastin Capsules, Obestin-30, and Wilpowr), phenmetrazine (Preludin), phendimetrazine (Appecon Capsules, Phendiet), and phenylpropanolamine (Dexatrim, Dex-A-Diet, Acutrim 16 Hour Steady Control Appetite Suppressant). Prescription appetite suppressants include benzphetamine (Didrex), diethylpropion (Tenuate), and phentermine (Adipex-P, Fastin, Obestin, Unifast).

Stimulant appetite suppressants are sold for the short-term management of obesity. Because users quickly develop tolerance to the appetite suppressant effects, they are useful only for a few weeks.

They are indicated for use only in conjunction with a regimen of weight reduction based on a restriction of calories, exercise, and behavior modification. In general, stimulant appetite suppressants have very limited usefulness.

Cold and cough medicine and decongestants. Some stimulants provide temporary symptomatic relief of local swelling and congestion of nasal mucous membranes. Thus, some stimulants appear in various cold and cough medications. In many cases, cold and cough preparations contain antihistamines (which often have a mild sedative effect), ephedrine or pseudoephedrine, phenylpropanolamine, and additional relatives of amphetamine found in appetite suppressants.

A few examples include various Actifed products, A.R.M. Maximum Strength Caplets, Allerest Children's Chewable Tablets, BC Cold Powder, various Contac products, CoAdvil Caplets, Comtrex, various Naldecon DX, CX, and EX products, assorted Sine-Aid products, several Sine-Off products, many Sudafed products, assorted Triaminic products, Tylenol Cold Medication, and numerous Vicks cold and cough products.

Over-the-counter stimulants. Although cold and cough medications and decongestants may contain stimulants, some over-the-counter preparations exist only for the purpose of stimulation. These products are marketed as providing increased energy and reducing the need for sleep.

Caffeine is generally the principal or only ingredient in over-the-counter stimulants. For all practical purposes, products like Caffedrine, No Doz, Quick Pep, and Vivarin Stimulant Tablets are the equivalent of a cup of coffee in pill or capsule form (both about 100 milligrams of caffeine). Some over-the-counter stimulants, such as Wake Ups, contain caffeine and theophylline, a stimulant similar to caffeine.

Look-alike stimulants. Look-alike drugs are legal, nonprescription psychoactive drugs that resemble more powerful controlled prescription drugs in appearance, effects, or name.[15] Thus, look-alike stimulants contain over-the-counter stimulants such as caffeine, ephedrine, and phenylpropanolamine. They are packaged in capsules or tablets that resemble more powerful stimulants such as methamphetamine. They are often marketed with names similar to those of prescription stimulants.

Look-alike drugs are legally sold through ads in magazines that are targeted to teenagers, with no attempt to deceive the readers into thinking that these are the more powerful stimulants. Because consumers legally purchase look-alike drugs through the mail, they often realize that these drugs are not the more powerful amphetamines. Thus, they often increase the dosage to create a stronger stimulant effect and experience toxic effects as a result. Nevertheless, the drugs normally found in look-alike stimulants have a relatively wide margin of safety in regard to overdose.[16]

Stimulant drugs of deception. In contrast to look-alike drugs, drugs of deception are counterfeits of more powerful controlled or prescription drugs. A drug of deception may contain legal over-the-counter drugs, may be a different prescription drug than it purports to be, may be a different illicit drug than it purports to be, or may be a combination of these. Stimulant drugs of deception may be created to mimic cocaine, street amphetamine, or prescription stimulants. For example, counterfeit cocaine might contain methamphetamine or milder amphetamine analogues. It might also contain a local anesthetic such as procaine to mimic the numbing sensation of cocaine.[17] Similarly, over-the-counter drugs such as caffeine, ephedrine, and phenylpropanolamine can be formed into tablets and capsules with the same markings as prescription stimulants, and deceptively sold as such.

Psychedelic amphetamines. Although most drugs can be described as stimulants, depressants, or psychedelics, a few have multiple qualities. In particular, some analogues of amphetamine have the properties of both stimulants and psychedelics. The most recent example is the drug methylenedioxymethamphetamine, more commonly called MDMA or "Ecstasy." The psychedelic amphetamines are more fully described in the chapter on psychedelic drugs.

■ Stimulant Use Patterns

Stimulant use ranges from low-dose to high-dose use and from infrequent, experimental use to chronic or binge patterns. The effect of the stimulant on the central nervous system will vary in relation to the frequency of drug use, the amount of other drugs being used, the amount of stimulant being consumed, and whether tolerance has developed to the stimulant effects.

Low-Dose Stimulant Effects

Low doses of stimulants cause a moderate increase in central nervous system activity, resulting in arousal and a heightened sense of well-being and pleasure. This general arousal can reduce fatigue and prolong physical endurance and mental concentration. People often feel less sleepy, more alert, more talkative than normal, less depressed, and somewhat more energetic. Some feel more confident and motivated.[18]

Medium-Dose Stimulant Effects

Somewhat higher doses cause a significant increase in central nervous system activity. Experiencing a strong sense of well-being and euphoria is likely. However, at this and higher levels of stimulant use, negative side effects also become more likely. Thus, sensations of increased energy may become stimulation; feelings of alertness may be replaced by nervousness; and feelings of confidence and motivation may be transformed into feelings of invincibility.

High-Dose Stimulant Effects

Large amounts of stimulants cause intense behavioral and mental stimulation, often with dramatic psychiatric signs and symptoms. General stimulation and arousal may increase to irritability and over-stimulation; nervousness may merge into agitation and anxiety; and excitability and talkativeness may be replaced by physical violence. High-dose stimulant use over an extended period of time, such as a stimulant binge lasting days or weeks, produces even more dramatic and dangerous psychiatric symptoms. Severe agitation, belligerence, and violence may occur, as may suspiciousness and paranoia. At the extreme, a stimulant psychosis may occur, which includes paranoid thinking, delusions (for example, of persecution), hallucinations, and repetitive, meaningless behavior. Stimulant psychosis is described in detail later in this chapter.

Nicotine

Tobacco smoking accounts for more sickness and death than all other psychoactive drugs combined. The predominant drug in tobacco is nicotine, which has complex effects on the body and is responsible for the addictive nature of tobacco. With regard to psychoactive properties, nicotine has stimulant effects as well as effects on the hormone systems that relate to opioids.[19] Nicotine is indeed a psychoactive drug, as evidenced by its euphoric effects and positive reinforcement patterns.[20]

After inhalation, the nicotine in the tobacco smoke rapidly passes into the bloodstream. Chewed tobacco is absorbed more slowly through the lining of the mouth. Once in the bloodstream, nicotine can affect the nervous system.

Acute effects. Nicotine acts primarily on the autonomic nervous system, which is the part of the nervous system that controls involuntary body processes such as heart rate. The effects of nicotine vary among individuals, often due to differences in dosage and tolerance.

Nicotine toxicity or poisoning includes nausea, salivation, abdominal pain, vomiting, diarrhea, headaches, dizziness, and cold sweat. Among people who do not have tolerance to nicotine, small amounts can slow the heart rate and cause nausea and vomiting.

Among chronic users, nicotine produces a calming, euphoric effect. This effect is more pronounced after a period of abstinence. Cigarette smokers report that the first cigarette of the day is the most satisfying.

Among people with tolerance, nicotine increases the heart rate and narrows the blood vessels, thus increasing blood pressure. Nicotine also stimulates the central nervous system, reducing fatigue, increasing alertness, and improving concentration temporarily.

Nicotine tolerance and withdrawal. Regular nicotine use causes tolerance to these effects, so that a higher intake is necessary to cause the same effects. However, the increase in intake is often slow and not readily detectable. Tolerance to nicotine can develop within 7–10 days.

Nicotine withdrawal effects develop gradually over 24–48 hours after cessation of use. The psychological symptoms of nicotine withdrawal include craving for cigarettes, irritability, anxiety, difficulty in concentrating, increased frustration, and restless anxiety.

The physical signs of nicotine withdrawal include decreased heart rate, increased eating, and increased sleep disturbance. Higher nicotine tolerance correlates with severity of withdrawal symptoms.

Adverse medical problems. In addition to nicotine, tobacco contains several chemicals that cause innumerable and severe medical problems such as lung and other cancers, bronchitis, and emphysema. The most significant harmful effect of smoking is coronary heart disease, which is the most common cause of death among middle-aged men in Western countries. Smoking seriously damages the arteries that supply blood to other parts of the body, such as the legs. Peripheral vascular disease often leads to amputation. Arteries of the brain can be damaged, leading to cerebrovascular accidents (strokes).

Smoking is associated with a higher incidence of peptic ulcer disease and exacerbates the symptoms of asthma. Smoking is extremely harmful during pregnancy. The babies of mothers who smoke are smaller and less likely to survive than babies of mothers who don't smoke. The children who survive are more likely to have asthma and other respiratory diseases.

■ The Stimulant Drug States

There are four main stimulant drug states: stimulant intoxication, stimulant delirium, stimulant psychosis, and stimulant withdrawal.

Stimulant Intoxication

Most people experience stimulant intoxication at moderate to high doses, although chronic users who have developed tolerance need increasingly larger amounts. Stimulant intoxication involves both physical and psychological symptoms and signs.

Psychological symptoms. Stimulants can change people's mood and emotional states; alter normal thinking, behavior, and decision making; distort normal sensory functioning; and temporarily affect personality. Stimulant intoxication may or may not include euphoria. During chronic use patterns, euphoria is less likely to occur. During the intoxication state, mood elevation will occur, followed by depression. Stimulant intoxication does not necessarily imply a pleasant or positive experience; rather, it describes an overstimulation experience that may or may not be pleasant.

Stimulant-intoxicated people often feel grandiose: they may develop an exaggerated opinion of their own knowledge, power, or importance. In extreme situations, grandiosity may become somewhat delusional; one delusion common to these users is that they have special talents and powers that others admire. Commonly, stimulant-intoxicated people engage in excessive behaviors such as overspending or illegal acts, believing that it is impossible for them to get in trouble.

The overstimulation often leads to an overload of sensory messages, such as sight, sound, and touch. People bombarded by this sensory input can become overly alert, hypervigilant, and agitated. They may become scared and want to flee, or they may become belligerent and physically violent.

They may experience visual or auditory hallucinations as well as *tactile hallucinations,* which are hallucinations that involve the sense of touch. They may feel the sensation of things crawling on top of or under the skin. The itching from so-called "coke bugs" often leads to intense scratching, cutting, and infection.

Some people experience personality changes during stimulant intoxication. Shy and cautious people may become assertive, aggressive, and pushy. Normally quiet people may become loud, obnox-

43

ious, and threatening. Many stimulant-intoxicated people will experience heightened sexual interest, or have interest in sexual activities that they do not normally consider when sober.

Physical and behavioral symptoms. Stimulant intoxication can cause elevated blood pressure, a more rapid heart rate, and a stronger pounding of the heart, as well as physical symptoms of panic attacks. Some individuals experience chills, perspiration, nausea, and vomiting, and the pupils of their eyes may dilate (become larger). Also, some people may experience a ringing in the ears, called tinnitus.

Stimulant intoxication causes behavioral and mental agitation called *psychomotor agitation*—uncontrolled or poorly controlled physical activity and mental tension and anxiety. Stimulant-intoxicated people generally talk extremely rapidly, have distortions in thinking, and have confusing and rambling speech. They may feel unable to sit still for more than a few seconds, perhaps vigorously tapping a foot or pacing around a room. They may feel very uncomfortable and restless when quiet and still, but may feel somewhat less tense when moving and talking. Some people experience episodes of muscle twitching.

Especially when combined with sedatives such as alcohol, stimulants can cause people to become socially and sexually disinhibited, leading to impulsive, impaired, and sometimes dangerous decisions. For example, people may have unprotected sex with strangers despite their normal tendency toward monogamy and the use of condoms. Stimulant-induced impulsiveness and impaired decision making frequently lead people into verbal and physical violence.

Stimulant Rage Reaction

The use of stimulants and combinations that involve stimulants can cause a syndrome that involves an impulsive reaction to environmental stressors.[21] A stimulant rage reaction generally involves a moderate- to high-dose stimulant binge. While intoxicated, the individual experiences environmental stimuli that would cause irritation, anxiety, agitation, or fear in the average person. Examples may include a baby crying, an uncomfortable situation, or an argument. Experiencing severe psychomotor agitation, the individual responds to the environmental stimuli in a way that is extremely out of proportion to the situation. The response is a spontaneous, reflexive, impulsive, unintentional, and unpremeditated attempt to silence the stimuli.

For example, in response to the crying of an infant, individuals may impulsively choke, shake, and kill the child. In response to an argument, individuals may impulsively stab, choke, or deliver fatal blows to a spouse. During the stimulant rage reaction, individuals lose control over their behavior and cannot stop stabbing, choking, or hitting. During the episode, they feel depersonalized or detached from their bodies. After the episode, they may have no memory of the incident or may gain memory of the incident slowly. A stimulant rage reaction is distinct from premeditated violence.

Stimulant Psychosis

During high-dose (especially during chronic high-dose) stimulant use patterns, people can experience a temporary break with reality called a stimulant psychosis. The hallmark features of stimulant psychosis are delusions, paranoid thinking, and stereotyped compulsive behaviors.

Delusions are false personal beliefs based on incorrect conclusions about reality. These beliefs are held despite evidence to the contrary and despite the fact that no one else has these beliefs. Stimulant-induced delusions are often persecutory or paranoid in nature.[22] For example, stimulant users may have the (incorrect) belief that they are being followed or that there is a plot to kill them.

A stimulant psychosis may also involve *ideas of reference,* which are incorrect beliefs that people, places, and events have specific significance to an individual, when in reality they are unrelated or coincidental. For example, a cocaine user may believe that late-night television talk-show host David Letterman's monologue contains secret, coded messages to the cocaine-user's mailman regarding a plot to haunt and threaten the cocaine user.

A stimulant psychosis may also involve hallucinations or

illusions. A *hallucination* is a false sensory perception without any stimulation of the sensory organ. For instance, people may "see," "hear," "smell," "taste," or "touch" something that does not exist. In contrast, an *illusion* is a misperception or misinterpretation of a sensory message. For instance, a bush moving in the wind at night may appear briefly as a moving person with a gun. Stimulant-induced delusions, hallucinations, and illusions can be severe or mild. Thus, people may be aware that a delusion or hallucination is in fact unreal. On the other hand, severe delusions and hallucinations may not be recognized as unreal until after the stimulant psychosis is over.

Stimulant psychosis may also include stereotyped compulsive behaviors, such as taking objects apart, sorting them into little piles, and then putting them back together again.[23] Similar behavior might include repetitiously analyzing objects for several hours. These stereotyped compulsive behaviors are often done without any specific goal in mind.

Stimulant Delirium

Some people experience a stimulant-induced episode of delirium, which is a state of mental confusion and excitement. People experiencing stimulant delirium do not necessarily lose complete touch with reality, but they are generally confused and experience difficulty thinking normally. They may be briefly disoriented as to time, place, and person: what day it is, where they are, and who they are.

They often have disorganized and fragmented thoughts, which may lead to disorganized and incoherent speech. Their ability to concentrate is made difficult by a tendency toward wandering attention and easy distraction. Thus, normal conversations are difficult, and questions may have to be repeated many times. Stimulant delirium may include disturbances in perception such as illusions, hallucinations, or misperceptions. These sensory problems may be associated with delusional beliefs.

Stimulant delirium may have various effects on emotional states. The range of emotional effects includes euphoria, anxiety, fear, and depression. Because the individual is mentally confused and excited, and because of the range of possible emotional states, the individual may be fearful and flee, become threatening and attack, feel depressed and cry, or become distraught and engage in self-destructive behavior.

Stimulant Withdrawal: Neurotransmitter Depletion

Stimulants produce what physicians call a biphasic effect on the central nervous system. *Biphasic* simply means two phases or stages. The first phase involves a temporary increase in neurotransmitters such as dopamine and norepinephrine, which causes emotional and behavioral stimulation. The second phase is a reduction of these neurotransmitters, which causes the opposite effect: depression, lethargy, and sadness. No matter which emotional mood state people are experiencing immediately before using a stimulant, the stimulant will elevate and then depress their mood.

For instance, consider Joe. Assume that he feels relatively normal before using a stimulant. After Joe takes the stimulant, his mood is elevated and he probably feels stimulated and maybe euphoric. In fact, Joe probably feels the most euphoric as the level of stimulant in his blood rises. However, as his blood stimulant level begins to plateau and then drop, he probably starts to experience drug hunger and wants to use more. In addition, the levels of dopamine and norepinephrine may become reduced or depleted. As these things occur, Joe begins to feel depressed. Because Joe instinctively knows that stimulants are (temporarily) effective for reducing depression, he wants more stimulant.

As illustrated in Figure 2–1, stimulant use causes initial stimulation followed by depression. Thus, continued stimulant use results in a downward spiral of increasing depression. Curve A on Figure 2–1 represents stimulant use by people who feel relatively normal.

Shortly after stimulant use, the stimulant-induced dopamine and norepinephrine increases cause stimulation and possible euphoria. However, this phase is followed by a period of depression and sadness. After the initial episode of stimulant use, people are slightly depressed and experience drug craving, and they are highly motivated to use more stimulant to stop the depression.

As curve B on Figure 2–1 shows, at this point the stimulant users are using a stimulant not to feel euphoric, but as an attempt to feel normal again. Stimulant use will indeed reduce the depression and allow the person to temporarily feel normal. However, this feeling of normalcy is followed by a period of depression that is even deeper than before.

Stimulant use is often in binge cycles measured in days and weeks. After a period of chronic use, stimulant users are extremely depressed and use stimulants in a hopeless attempt to reduce the depression. As curve C on Figure 2–1 suggests, stimulant use while feeling extremely depressed makes some people feel less depressed, but does not make them feel euphoric or even "normal." Rather, they continue to become progressively depressed.

Because some drugs, such as the amphetamines, are long acting

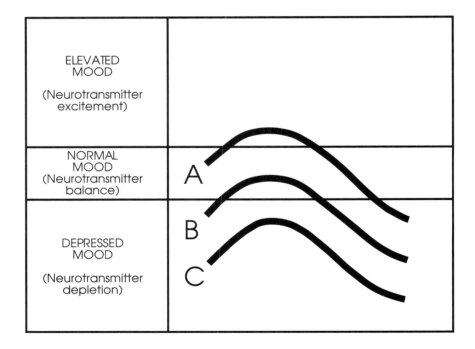

Figure 2–1. Stimulants, mood, and neurotransmitter balance.

compared with shorter-acting drugs such as cocaine and caffeine, the cycles of elevated and depressed mood differ in terms of time. Thus, some caffeine users experience many short and rapid elevated-depressed mood cycles each day. Cocaine users may experience more severe and slower cycles of elevated-depressed mood. Users of smokable amphetamine may experience longer cycles of extremely elevated and depressed mood.

■ Summary

Fluctuations in mood, anxiety, and mental and physical energy are a normal part of living. These fluctuations may be caused by internal or external events, but they are related to changes in the normal balance of neurotransmitters. Stimulants are able to alter people's mood and energy levels and can even cause psychiatric symptoms because of their impact on neurotransmitters.

Stimulants have a two-phase effect. The first phase (neurotransmitter increase) results in symptoms and signs ranging from alertness, arousal, euphoria, and excitement to agitation, anxiety, and stimulant psychosis. The second phase (neurotransmitter depletion)

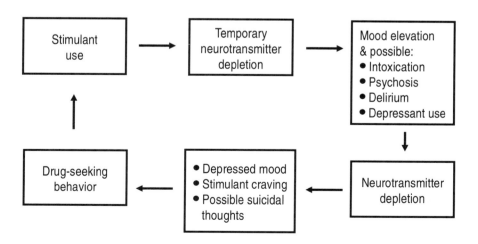

Figure 2–2. The cycle of stimulant use.

causes a longer-lasting episode that is essentially the opposite of the first phase. In the second phase, people often become depressed, agitated, and lethargic, and they experience stimulant drug hunger. This phase is particularly important because it is often a time of significant craving for stimulant drugs, leading to further use. This craving often leads to a cycle of stimulation–depression–self-medication and continued stimulation that may last for hours, days, or weeks.

Stimulants include cocaine and the amphetamines, which may be snorted, injected, swallowed, and smoked. Smoking cocaine and the amphetamines creates the most intense stimulant euphoria possible. Stimulants include amphetamine analogues, which are drugs that create symptoms similar to, but often weaker than, those created by the amphetamines. The majority of these drugs are appetite suppressants. Ephedrine, a stimulant that is similar to the neurotransmitter epinephrine, is chiefly used for its bronchodilator effects in asthma and bronchitis and as a nasal decongestant in hay fever. Phenylpropanolamine is a stimulant that is used as a nasal decongestant, a bronchodilator, and a short-term appetite suppressant. Caffeine is the most widely used psychoactive drug in the world; its stimulant effect is similar to that of many of the other stimulants, with the exceptions of cocaine and the amphetamines.

Amphetamine analogues, ephedrine, phenylpropanolamine, and caffeine can be found in numerous combinations and marketed for various purposes. These drugs appear as ingredients in appetite suppressants, cough and cold preparations, over-the-counter stimulants, look-alike drugs, and drugs of deception.

Stimulant use in low-dose, medium-dose, and high-dose patterns produces increasingly serious medical and psychiatric side effects. Stimulant use may produce a number of psychiatric states, including stimulant intoxication, stimulant delirium, stimulant psychosis, and stimulant withdrawal.

■ References

1. Gawin FH, Ellinwood EH: Cocaine and other stimulants: actions, abuse, and treatment. New England Journal of Medicine 318:1173–1182, 1988

2. Landry M: Update on cocaine dependence: crack and advances in diagnostics and treatment, in Treating Cocaine Dependency. Edited by Smith DE, Wesson DR. Center City, MN, Hazelden Foundation, 1988

3. Snyder CA, Wood RW, Graefe JF, et al: "Crack smoke" is a respirable aerosol of cocaine base. Pharmacology, Biochemistry and Behavior 29:93–95, 1988

4. Jaffe JH: Drug addiction and abuse, in The Pharmacological Basis of Therapeutics, 8th Edition. Edited by Gilman AG, Rall TW, Nies AS, et al. New York, Pergamon, 1990, pp 522–573

5. Landry MJ: An overview of cocaethylene, an alcohol-derived, psychoactive, cocaine metabolite. Journal of Psychoactive Drugs 24:273–276, 1992

6. Morgan JP, Wesson DR, Puder KS, et al: Duplicitous drugs: the history and recent status of look-alike drugs. Journal of Psychoactive Drugs 19:21–31, 1987

7. Ray O, Ksir C: Drugs, Society, and Human Behavior. St. Louis, MO, Times Mirror/Mosby College Publishing, 1987, pp 104–105

8. Tamura M: Japan: stimulant epidemics past and present. Bulletin on Narcotics 41:83–93, 1989

9. Mannuzza S, Klein RG, Bonagura N, et al: Hyperactive boys almost grown up. Archives of General Psychiatry 48:77–83, 1991

10. Silverman HI: A history of therapeutic uses of phenylpropanolamine in North America, in Phenylpropanolamine: Risks, Benefits, and Controversies. Edited by Morgan JP, Kagan DV, Brody JS. New York, Praeger, 1985

11. Gilbert RM: Caffeine as a drug of abuse, in Research Advances in Alcohol and Drug Problems, Vol 3. Edited by Gibbons RJ, Israel Y, Kalant H, et al. New York, Wiley, 1976, pp 49–176

12. Hughes JR, Higgins ST, Bickel WK, et al: Caffeine self-administration, withdrawal, and adverse effects among coffee drinkers. Archives of General Psychiatry 48:611–617, 1991

13. Greden JF: Caffeinism and caffeine withdrawal, in Substance Abuse: Clinical Problems and Perspectives. Edited by Lowinson JH, Reiz P. Baltimore, MD, Williams & Wilkins, 1981, pp 274–286

14. Silverman K, Evans SM, Strain EC, et al: Withdrawal syndrome after double-blind cessation of caffeine consumption. New England Journal of Medicine 327:1109–1114, 1992

15. Seymour R, Smith D, Inaba D, et al: The New Drugs: Look-Alike, Drugs of Deception and Designer Drugs. Minneapolis, MN, Hazelden Foundation, 1989

16. Morgan JP, Wesson DR, Puder KS, et al: Duplicitous drugs: the history and recent status of look-alike drugs. Journal of Psychoactive Drugs 19:21–31, 1987
17. Rehrig M: Cocaine look-alike. Critical Care Update 6:47–49, 1983
18. Addiction Research Foundation: Drugs and Drug Abuse: A Reference Text, 2nd Edition. Toronto, Canada, Addiction Research Foundation, 1987
19. National Institute on Drug Abuse: Drug Abuse and Drug Abuse Research: The Third Triennial Report to Congress. Rockville, MD, National Institute on Drug Abuse, 1991
20. Henningfield JE: Pharmacologic basis and treatment of cigarette smoking. Journal of Clinical Psychiatry 45:24–34, 1984
21. Landry MJ, Smith DE: Stimulant rage reaction: aggression dyscontrol. Unpublished manuscript, 1993
22. Satel SL, Southwick SM, Gawin FH: Clinical features of cocaine-induced paranoia. American Journal of Psychiatry 148:495–498, 1991
23. Snyder SH: A "model" schizophrenia mediated by catecholamines, in Amphetamine Use, Misuse and Abuse. Edited by Smith DE. Boston, MA, GK Hall, 1979, pp 189–204

Table 3–1. The depressant drugs

Type of depressant drug	Specific depressant drugs
Barbiturates	Amobarbital (Amytal); aprobarbital (Alurate); butabarbital (Buticaps); mephobarbital (Mebaral); metharbital (Gemonil); methohexital (Brevital); pentobarbital (Nembutal); phenobarbital (generic); secobarbital (Seconal); talbutal (Lotusate); thiamylal (Surital); thiopental (Pentothal); secobarbital and amobarbital (Tuinal)
Benzodiazepines	Alprazolam (Xanax); bromazepam (Lectopam); chlordiazepoxide (Libritabs, Librium); clonazepam (Klonopin); clorazepate (Tranxene); diazepam (Valium); estazolam (ProSom); flurazepam (Dalmane); halazepam (Paxipam); ketazolam (Loftran); lorazepam (Ativan); midazolam (Versed); nitrazepam (Mogadon); oxazepam (Serax); prazepam (Centrax); quazepam (Doral); temazepam (Restoril); triazolam (Halcion)
Nonbenzodiazepine, nonbarbiturate sedative-hypnotics	Alcohol (beer, wine, whiskey); chloral hydrate (Noctec, Somnos); ethchlorvynol (Placidyl); ethinamate (Valmid); glutethimide (Doriden); meprobamate (Miltown); methyprylon (Noludar); paraldehyde (Paral)
Opiates and semisynthetic opiates (opium-derived analgesics)	Codeine (Tylenol with Codeine No. 3 and No. 4); heroin; hydrocodone (Hycodan); hydromorphone (Dilaudid); morphine; opium (Paregoric); oxycodone (Percodan); oxymorphone (Numorphan)
Opioids (fully manmade, opiate-like analgesics)	Alfentanil (Alfenta); buprenorphine; butorphanol (Stadol); fentanyl (Sublimaze); L-acetyl-alpha-methadol (LAAM); levorphanol (Levo-Dromoran); meperidine (Demerol); methadone (Dolophine); 3-methylfentanyl ("China White"); nalbuphine (Nubain); pentazocine (Talwin); propoxyphene (Darvon); sufentanil (Sufenta)

Chapter 3

The Depressant Drugs

Depressant drugs, including alcohol and opiates, are among the oldest drugs known and used by man. Indeed, despite our extensive, modern pharmacopoeia, alcohol continues to be the most widely used and abused depressant drug in our society. Sedative-hypnotic drugs, appropriately prescribed, provide needed relief from debilitating anxiety and insomnia. Appropriately prescribed opiates ease the crippling effects of pain. Most people who need them respond well to them. Most physicians who prescribe them do so appropriately. But, influenced by genetic factors, environmental stressors, or inappropriate prescribing practices, a subgroup of patients experience a destructive compulsion when exposed to these critical drugs. The depressant drugs save the lives of many, and cause the destruction of others.

Joseph C. McCarthy, M.D.
Addiction Medicine Specialist
Private Practice
Newport Beach, California

■ Sedatives and Hypnotics

Many of the effects of the sedatives and hypnotics are roughly the opposite of the effects of stimulants. Although stimulants enhance mental and physical energy, the sedatives and hypnotics promote sedation and sleep. A *sedative* is a drug that promotes mental calmness; has a soothing, tranquilizing effect; reduces excessive anxiety; and may control dangerously aggressive behavior. Sedative drugs include most antianxiety drugs and some sleeping drugs. Certain antipsychotic and antidepressant medications have some sedative effect, but that is not their primary activity.

Sedation is a decrease in the individual's responsiveness to a constant level of stimulation, with a decrease in spontaneous mental and physical activity.[1] Stimulation may originate from the environment, such as sensory or social stimulation. Stimulation may be internal, such as excessive anxiety and worry. Thus, sedation describes a decrease in internal stimulation and a decreased response to external stimulation. That is exactly what happens when most people drink alcohol or take a prescribed sedative.

The term *hypnotic* is derived from the Greek word *hypnos,* meaning sleep. Thus, *hypnotics* are drugs that promote sleep or drowsiness. (The misnamed term *hypnotism* refers to a state of increased mental concentration, although the hypnotized individual may appear to be asleep.) A number of drugs promote a strong hypnotic effect, including alcohol, some benzodiazepines, and barbiturates. Certain antihistamine and antidepressant medications have a limited hypnotic effect. Hypnotics may be sedatives, analgesics, anesthetics, or intoxicants. People often drink alcohol, smoke marijuana, take an over-the-counter antihistamine, or take a prescribed sleeping pill for the hypnotic effect.

Sedation and hypnosis (sleep) are very closely related: they are at the same end of a spectrum of mental and behavioral excitement. As Figure 3–1 illustrates, the left half of this spectrum depicts mental and behavioral excitement. This excitement represents increased activity of the central nervous system by way of increases in the adrenalin-like neurotransmitters. These increases can be caused by the use of stimulant drugs, environmental stimulation (such as being robbed), or an anxiety disorder. The right side of Figure 3–1 depicts mental and behavioral depression, representing a slowing down of mental and behavioral processes caused by sedation of the central nervous system. As can be seen, sedation and hypnosis represent a range of mental and behavioral activity. In other words, hypnosis (sleep) is a progression of the sedative effect.

Indeed, drugs that depress the central nervous system and cause sedation at a low-dose level generally promote hypnotic effects at higher doses. Therefore, the term *sedative-hypnotic* can describe drugs that cause sedation or sleep and, with variations in dosage, can often do both.

Some drugs produce *anesthesia,* which is the partial or complete loss of normal sensation and awareness of pain and other stimuli. Anesthesia can occur over the entire body or in specific regions. *General anesthesia* involves unconsciousness, resulting in a total lack of sensation of pain and other stimuli. General anesthetics are usually inhaled as a gas or injected intravenously.

Stimulants produce a dose-dependent effect that ranges from mild stimulation to extreme overstimulation. Sedative-hypnotics also produce a range of dose-dependent sedation: from mild relief of anxiety to sleep, anesthesia, coma, and death.

A major problem with prescription sedative-hypnotics involves achieving the goal of sedation and hypnosis while minimizing excessive depression of the central nervous system. For instance, the ideal prescription sedative should decrease anxiety or promote calmness without significantly slowing down mental functioning and motor control behavior. Similarly, the ideal prescription hypnotic should

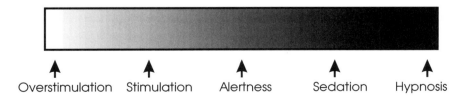

Figure 3–1. Mental and behavioral excitement and depression scale.

promote or prolong natural sleep without causing problems of its own.

The Barbiturates

During the 1960s, the barbiturates were among the most commonly prescribed drugs for anxiety, insomnia, and convulsant disorders. Although effective, barbiturates often promote a hangover or "drugged" feeling the day after use. Also, small increases in dose and the addition of other depressant drugs such as alcohol can easily cause toxicity and oversedation, with symptoms such as severe drowsiness, mental confusion, and motor incoordination.

The barbiturates are used to inhibit convulsions, for general anesthesia, and as sedative-hypnotics. Except for the ultra-short-acting barbiturates, most are useful in the short-term treatment of insomnia. However, after 2 weeks or less they lose the ability to promote and maintain sleep. Barbiturates reduce anxiety, apprehension, and tension, but they have been largely replaced by benzodiazepines, which are more effective and have fewer side effects.[2]

Phenobarbital is still highly recommended for medically managing the acute withdrawal from alcohol, benzodiazepines, and other sedative-hypnotics.[3] Phenobarbital's anticonvulsant properties, relatively lower dependence liability, longer duration of action, and lower street value compared with other barbiturates make it an ideal drug for managing acute sedative-hypnotic withdrawal, even for outpatient drug detoxification. Phenobarbital is still used in the treatment of epilepsy in combination with newer anticonvulsant drugs.[4]

Some barbiturates are used as preoperative medication to reduce anxiety and to facilitate anesthesia induction. Others are used as general anesthetics for short surgical procedures, for induction of general anesthesia, and as adjuncts to other anesthetic medications. Intravenous amobarbital and thiopental may be used for narcotherapy and narcoanalysis.

Barbiturate abuse. At low doses, the barbiturates decrease motor activity and produce sedation and drowsiness. Paradoxically, barbiturates may produce excitement, elation, and euphoria, called barbiturate intoxication. Additional symptoms and signs may include a disinhibition euphoria, slurred speech, staggering gait, confusion, slow heart rate, and general weakness.

At higher doses, the barbiturates further decrease cognitive ability, suppress motor activity, distort judgment, and provoke hypnosis. Barbiturate-induced sleep is quite different from normal sleep. Rapid eye movement (REM) or dreaming-stage sleep, necessary for restful overall sleep, is decreased. When the barbiturates are withdrawn, there is a rebound of REM sleep, often causing profound nightmares, dreams, and insomnia. Higher doses produce anesthesia.

The barbiturates generate the rapid development of tolerance. Because of this rapid tolerance and a corresponding increase in dosage, toxic barbiturate effects may emerge quickly, leading to overdose and death. Also, rapid withdrawal from chronic or high-dose barbiturate use causes severe withdrawal complications, including death.

The barbiturates create a potent dose-related depression of the respiratory and central nervous systems that is worsened with the addition of other depressants such as alcohol. As the dosage of barbiturates increases, the depression of the respiratory and central nervous systems can cause respiration problems, tachycardia (rapid heart rate), decreased body temperature, coma, and respiratory arrest.

In terms of lethality, the barbiturates are safe at controlled therapeutic-range doses. However, 10–15 times the daily therapeutic dosage is lethal (whereas some benzodiazepines may be used at dosages 100 times higher than the therapeutic range without death).[5] At one point during the 1970s, more than 15,000 deaths from barbiturate overdose were reported annually.

The Benzodiazepines

Benzodiazepines became a fixture in American medical practice in the early 1960s. They are one of the most widely prescribed medications in the world, replacing the barbiturates as the previous drug of choice for the management of anxiety and insomnia. They are less potent and far less lethal than the barbiturates. Some examples include diazepam (Valium), alprazolam (Xanax), chlordiazepoxide (Librium), and triazolam (Halcion).

The benzodiazepines are best known for the short-term treatment of anxiety and stress, with alprazolam and lorazepam being relatively popular treatments for mixed anxiety and depression. Benzodiazepines are used to reduce anticipated anxiety during surgical procedures, as adjuncts to anesthesia, for producing amnesia during surgery, and for the treatment of insomnia. Benzodiazepines are also used in the treatment of convulsive disorders and seizures, epilepsy, skeletal muscle spasm, and tremors. Some benzodiazepines are very useful in the short-term medical management of alcohol withdrawal.

The benzodiazepines are potent depressants of the central nervous system, producing a dose-dependent range of reactions from mild relaxation, sedation, and reduced muscle tension to hypnosis and general anesthesia. Compared with the barbiturates, benzodiazepines require greater dosage increases to produce progressive depression of the respiratory and central nervous systems; as a result, the benzodiazepines are toxicologically safe drugs.

At high doses, benzodiazepines cause symptoms that are similar to those caused by high doses of barbiturates and alcohol: slurred speech, incoordination, significant confusion, severe drowsiness, staggering gait, dizziness, unusually slow heartbeat, breathing difficulties, and severe weakness. In rare situations, a paradoxical intoxication resembling a stimulant intoxication may occur. Death by overdose (even with very high doses) is difficult unless the benzodiazepines are combined with other depressants such as barbiturates and alcohol.

Benzodiazepine abuse and addiction.   The benzodiazepines have proven to be effective and generally safe medications for most patients.[6] Although there is some debate regarding the magnitude of improper benzodiazepine use, investigators generally find that their use is appropriate to the prevalence of the medical and psychiatric conditions for which they are prescribed.[7,8]

Most medically unsupervised use of benzodiazepines involves the occasional or intermittent use of therapeutic doses for symptomatic relief. This pattern is not associated with dose escalation or high-dose recreational abuse.[9] Nevertheless, these are psychoactive and mood-altering drugs. They are subject to misuse and abuse, and they can be used in the context of addiction.[10]

As with alcohol, there can be different responses to the benzodiazepines. People who take benzodiazepines for medically prescribed and appropriate reasons do not generally experience dosage escalation or drug-related dysfunction. Studies have shown that benzodiazepine abuse and addiction are greater among alcoholic people than among the general population.[11,12] Benzodiazepines are rarely the primary drugs of choice.[13] Benzodiazepine abuse and addiction are generally but not entirely limited to patients involved in a polydrug use pattern.[14-17] Interestingly, the benzodiazepines appear to produce euphoric mood changes in alcoholic people that are not experienced by nonalcoholic people.[18] Even parental alcoholism is associated with benzodiazepine abuse and benzodiazepine-induced euphoric mood changes.[19]

In a review of the literature on benzodiazepine abuse and addiction, it was noted that 1) benzodiazepines have an abuse liability and can promote physical dependence; 2) the abuse liability is less than that for barbiturates, stimulants, and opioids; 3) benzodiazepine use for intoxication is infrequent; 4) benzodiazepines are not generally primary drugs of abuse; 5) some people are more susceptible than others to physical dependence on benzodiazepines; and 6) factors that predispose people to physical dependence include total lifetime use, use of other sedative-hypnotics, presence of severe psychiatric and medical problems, and severe, persisting stress.[20]

Second, the recreational abuse of benzodiazepines is uncommon. However, when abused, they are likely to be part of polydrug patterns.

Benzodiazepine dependence. When benzodiazepines are taken for long periods of time (especially if they are taken at moderate to high doses for months), benzodiazepine dependence may develop. In this book, *benzodiazepine dependence* refers to the development of physical dependence and adaptation and a subsequent withdrawal syndrome when drug use ceases.[21] In this context, benzodiazepine dependence is not equivalent to benzodiazepine addiction, which involves the development of compulsion, loss of control, and continued use despite adverse consequences. In fact, benzodiazepine dependence can occur in the context of addiction and abuse, but it can also occur in the context of appropriate, medically supervised prescription of the benzodiazepines. Research suggests that a subgroup of patients who take benzodiazepines chronically for therapeutic indications develop benzodiazepine dependences.[22–24]

Ideally, the benzodiazepines should be used for short periods of time, such as a few weeks. However, anxiety is most often a chronic problem. Thus, benzodiazepines are often prescribed for several episodes, each lasting a few weeks. Some people have severe anxiety disorders that seriously impair their ability to function normally. For instance, patients with severe agoraphobia are unable to leave their homes for months. Because the severity of their disorder is so great and because it is a chronic condition, some physicians will prescribe benzodiazepines for long periods of time. These patients may develop benzodiazepine dependence; those with a personal or family history of substance use problems are at higher risk for benzodiazepine addiction.

To be certain, the long-term use of psychoactive drugs like the benzodiazepines is not ideal psychiatric treatment. Rather, there are nondrug treatments and nonpsychoactive medications that may treat the anxiety without creating problems of their own.[25] However, psychiatrists and other physicians must find a balance between the potential risks and benefits of treatment. Benzodiazepine dependence is a severe risk for people at high risk for addiction. But benzodiazepines are a necessary and temporary benefit for other people. On the whole, benzodiazepine dependence in the general population is to be avoided whenever possible and endured whenever necessary to allow people to function.

Patients taking benzodiazepines for long periods of time should be evaluated by an addiction medicine specialist. If the medical decision is made to discontinue benzodiazepine treatment, the withdrawal and detoxification process can be carefully monitored. Under no circumstances should anyone abruptly stop taking benzodiazepines, or attempt to stop without the supervision of a physician. The withdrawal can be severe and life-threatening.

Nonbarbiturate, Nonbenzodiazepine Sedative-Hypnotics

For the medical management of insomnia and anxiety, physicians prescribed the bromides during the 1860s, chloral hydrate during the 1870s, paraldehyde during the 1880s, and barbital—a barbiturate—in the early 1900s. During the 1950s, various sedative-hypnotic drugs were introduced as alternatives to the barbiturates. These drugs include chloral hydrate, etchchlorvynol, ethinamate, glutethimide, meprobamate, methyprylon, and paraldehyde.

In fact, these drugs proved to be quite similar to the barbiturates in terms of efficacy; development of tolerance to the sedative, hypnotic, and euphoric qualities; narrow safety threshold; potential for abuse; disinhibition intoxication; physical dependence; complications associated with central nervous system depression; and overdose lethality. Abrupt withdrawal from these drugs may be life-threatening; withdrawal should be gradual and supervised by a physician. Even though the benzodiazepines have largely replaced these drugs and the barbiturates as drugs of choice for insomnia and anxiety, the sedative-hypnotics listed above are still prescribed and are still drugs of abuse.

Alcohol. Alcohol (wine, beer, whiskey) is a nonbarbiturate, nonbenzodiazepine sedative-hypnotic drug. It causes an overall, dose-related depression of the central nervous system, decreases anxiety, increases sedation, promotes sleep, and causes a disinhibition intoxication. High-dose use causes a hangover the next day, much as barbiturates do. Chronic use promotes tolerance to the sedative, hypnotic, and euphoric qualities of alcohol and causes the development of physical dependence and a severe and potentially life-threatening withdrawal.

Because alcohol is a popular legal drug, some people may not realize that it is indeed a drug, specifically a sedative-hypnotic drug. Like barbiturates, alcohol decreases the activity of the central nervous system, thereby reducing anxiety, tension, and inhibitions. Like the benzodiazepines, alcohol promotes relaxation, which may increase confidence during social and stressful events. Like other sed-

63

ative-hypnotics, alcohol reduces both physical and mental reaction time, thus impairing concentration, judgment, and awareness.

Low- to medium-dose alcohol effects. Alcohol enters the bloodstream from the stomach and colon, but is more rapidly absorbed from the small intestine. The absorption rate is less rapid when food is present in the stomach. Once alcohol has entered the bloodstream, the addition of food does nothing to slow down, minimize, or impede the sedative-hypnotic effects. Generally, alcohol is metabolized at the rate of 0.3 ounces of pure alcohol per hour, although there are wide variations depending on liver damage, liver size, and other medical conditions.

Because alcohol depresses the inhibitory and behavioral brain centers, an early symptom of alcohol use is often a behavioral and emotional disinhibition, commonly called intoxication. During this initial phase of alcohol use, people are often talkative, sociable, outgoing, relaxed, and more self-confident.

After this phase, thought processes, memory, and perception may become impaired. Thus, people may become slightly confused, have problems with short-term memory, and experience a misperception of time and distance. Reaction times are slower, physical dexterity is impaired, and speech may be slurred. The personality of intoxicated people is often an exaggeration or the opposite of their normal personality. Assertive people may become aggressive, or shy people may become outgoing. People may engage in inappropriate sexual or aggressive behaviors.

High-dose alcohol effects. At low to moderate doses of alcohol, people often experience a positive, upbeat, and even hyperactive episode. However, higher doses of alcohol often make people feel and appear depressed, sad, withdrawn, and lethargic. Also, some people may have abrupt mood swings and lower levels of frustration tolerance. The ability to think and communicate with others becomes significantly impaired, especially if speech becomes slurred. Thinking and judgment deteriorate, making poor decisions likely, especially those involving safety. Motor control is obviously impaired to the point of severe incoordination. At progressively higher doses,

Table 3–2. Relationship between blood-alcohol percentage and behavior

Approximate % alcohol in the blood	Approximate No. drinks in past hour—by body weight				Effect on behavior and function
	100 lb	140 lb	180 lb	220 lb	
0.02	1	1	2	2	Alterations in mood, personality, and behavior. People may become disinhibited, more animated, and cheerful. Thinking and motor control become impaired.
0.05–0.09	2–3	3–4	3–4	4–5	Unless tolerant to alcohol, many people become intoxicated at this level. They experience mental impairment, physical incoordination, and slower reaction time. Driving is impaired.
0.10–0.15	4–5	5–7	6–9	7–11	Unmistakably intoxicated. Most people have slurred speech, serious physical incoordination, and poor impulse control, and they make serious mistakes in thinking and behavior. A blood-alcohol concentration of 0.10% is the legal definition of intoxication in most states.
0.30	9	13	16	21	Nausea and vomiting, severe incoordination, double vision, and amnesia. Dangerously low body temperature, shallow and slow breathing, faint and slow heart rate. In a stupor. Death possible.
0.40+	12	18	24	30	Severe depression of the brain's respiratory center. Person is likely unconscious. Coma, respiratory failure, and death likely.

Note. One drink equals one 12-ounce bottle of beer (or a 3-ounce glass of wine or 1 ounce of 86-proof liquor). All figures are averages and approximations. People vary with regard to tolerance. Signs of intoxication are more apparent when blood-alcohol levels are rising than when they are falling. Food in the stomach slows the rate of alcohol absorption but does not diminish the eventual intoxication.

alcohol causes progressively stronger depression of the central nervous system, resulting in sleep, stupor, and coma. At these higher doses, barbiturate-like hangover effects are likely the next day. The symptoms of hangover—a brief withdrawal syndrome—may include headache, nausea, vomiting, nervousness, and uneasiness.

■ Opiates and Opioids

An opiate is any drug that contains or is derived from opium. Opium is the dried milky sap from the unripe capsules of the poppy *Papaver somniferum L.* It contains a number of organic compounds such as morphine and codeine. Thus, natural opium compounds such as morphine and codeine are called opiates. Medications such as hydromorphone and hydrocodone are derived from opium, but are further synthesized in the laboratory. Because they are ultimately derived from opium, they are called semisynthetic opiates.

Some opiate-like drugs are fully manmade. They are technically called *opioids,* which means opiate-like. The use of the term "opioid" has gradually come to include opiates, semisynthetic opiates, and synthetic opiates. Opioid also describes the type of activity that is produced by opiates. In this book, the term "opioid" is used to describe any drug or chemical that has opiate-like activity. For example, the body produces naturally occurring neurotransmitters called endorphins, which act as opioids.

In much the same way that sedative-hypnotic drugs function to reduce anxiety and promote sedation and hypnosis, the opioids reduce or eliminate pain. Some sedative-hypnotics manage pain by causing general anesthesia: the loss of normal sensation and awareness of stimuli, including pain. During general anesthesia, the central nervous system is severely depressed, causing loss of consciousness and thus lack of awareness of pain. General anesthetics are usually inhaled as a gas or injected intravenously. General anesthesia is on a continuum of sedation–hypnosis–general anesthesia–coma. Anesthesia literally means the absence of sensation or feeling.

Thus, sedative-hypnotics affect pain recognition by causing an overall depression of the central nervous system. In contrast, opioids reduce or eliminate pain by direct interaction with nerve pathways that specifically relate to pain. Opioid analgesics depress the region of the brain responsible for respiration. Thus, death from opioid overdose invariably involves respiratory arrest. Opioids reduce pain awareness through analgesia, which is the loss of pain sensation while remaining fully conscious.

Although all opioids exert analgesic effects, they vary with regard to potency of effect. Medications such as codeine (Tylenol With Codeine) and propoxyphene (Darvon) are used for mild to moderate pain. Meperidine (Demerol) has a more potent analgesic effect and is prescribed for moderately severe pain. Among the most potent opioid analgesics are heroin, hydromorphone (Dilaudid), and oxymorphone (Numorphan). These drugs are prescribed only for severe pain.

Many opioid analgesics are also potent cough suppressants. Thus, codeine, hydrocodone, and hydromorphone are used in cough-control medications. However, these medications also produce significant euphoria. Accordingly, there has been considerable research to develop noneuphoric opioid cough suppressants such as dextromethorphan (Benylin DM, Sucrets Cough Control Formula). Dextromethorphan has cough-suppressant activity roughly equivalent to that of codeine but does not have euphoric or analgesic properties and does not cause dependence.

Perhaps the most commonly known opioid in the street drug culture is heroin, which can be heated and inhaled, injected, or snorted intranasally. In fact, perhaps half of the people addicted to heroin entering treatment began by snorting heroin intranasally.[26] Clandestine chemists have synthesized an extremely potent "designer drug" opioid named 3-methylfentanyl, an analogue of the opioid fentanyl. Heroin addicts using this drug may suffer respiratory failure and die, not realizing that it is about 1,000 times as potent as morphine.[27] A similar clandestinely made analogue of meperidine (Demerol) called MPPP (1-methyl-4-phenyl-4-propionoxy-piperidine) has been responsible for causing immediate and irreversible parkinsonism.[28]

Morphine-Related Opioids

Several medications can induce analgesia and cause other effects similar to those caused by morphine, which is the standard against which analgesics are measured. Some of these medications include heroin (diacetylmorphine), hydromorphone (Dilaudid), oxymorphone (Numorphan), levorphanol (Levo-Dromoran), hydrocodone (Hycodan), and codeine, which is often combined with aspirin or other medications.

The morphine-related opioids produce several effects on the nervous system, including analgesia without loss of consciousness, mood changes, mental clouding and drowsiness, and respiratory depression. In people free from pain, these medications can cause nausea and vomiting, euphoria, a sense of apathy, decreased physical activity, and difficulty thinking. The morphine-related opioids depress respiration, which is discernible even with doses that are too small to disturb consciousness. These drugs slow down the passage of food through the stomach and intestines and often cause constipation.

Meperidine-Related Opioids

Meperidine (Demerol) produces effects that are similar but not identical to those produced by morphine. Meperidine-related opioids include medications that are used for very different purposes, depending on what specific properties of the drugs are targeted. For instance, meperidine is administered orally or through intramuscular or subcutaneous injection for the relief of moderate to severe pain. Diphenoxylate (Lomotil) and loperamide (Imodium) are opioids that slow down gastrointestinal activity and have potent constipating effects. They are used for the treatment of diarrhea. At therapeutic doses, these two medications produce few or no morphine-like subjective effects such as euphoria. The medications fentanyl (Sublimaze), sufentanil (Sufenta), and alfentanil (Alfenta) are synthetic opioids that are far more potent than morphine with regard to analgesia, and they are used as analgesic supplements to general anesthesia. They are also used as primary agents for the induction of anesthesia in patients undergoing general surgery. They are rapidly acting, short-acting drugs[29] and cause a brief, intense euphoria in pain-free people.

Methadone-Related Opioids

Methadone has pharmacologic properties that are qualitatively similar to those of morphine. Methadone is known for its potent analgesic abilities, its efficacy when administered orally, and its ability to suppress opioid withdrawal symptoms for prolonged periods of time. It can produce these effects despite repeated administration. Methadone is cross-tolerant to opioids of abuse and has prolonged activity. Thus, it can be used to prevent or relieve acute opioid withdrawal symptoms, and it can be used in the detoxification of patients dependent on opioids. The withdrawal of methadone itself produces symptoms that are less intense but more prolonged than those of heroin or morphine. Methadone and the related medication LAAM (L-acetyl-alpha-methadol) are also used in opioid maintenance programs wherein patients receive daily (or less frequent) doses of prescribed medication rather than illicit opioids. The basis for opioid maintenance is to alleviate opioid withdrawal symptoms and block heroin-induced euphoria in order to decrease the need for obtaining illicit opioids.[30] The medication propoxyphene (Darvon) is chemically related to methadone and is used orally to relieve mild to moderate pain. Its analgesic efficacy is less than that of other opioids.

Opioid Antagonists and Agonist-Antagonists

The classic opioids such as morphine and heroin are called *opioid agonists,* meaning that their primary activity is strongly opioid in nature. Opioids occupy the sites in the brain that trigger opioid activity. Similarly, *opioid antagonists* also occupy these receptor sites, actually displacing opioids if they are already there and stopping opioids from occupying the sites. As a result, opioid antagonists in sufficient doses prevent opioids from producing their effects.[31]

The drugs naloxone (Narcan) and naltrexone (Trexan) are examples of antagonists. Naloxone displaces opioids and causes a reversal of opioid symptoms; thus, it is used to reverse opioid overdose symptoms seen in emergency rooms. Whereas naloxone is short-acting, naltrexone has longer-lasting effects and is used by people in recovery from opioid addiction to stop impulsive opioid use. While a person is taking naltrexone, opioids have virtually no effect, including euphoria or pain relief.[32]

Some drugs have both agonist and antagonist activity. Although a discussion of opioid receptor sites is beyond the scope of this book, it is useful to know that there are several types of sites, each with slightly different activities. Drugs that have mixed agonist-antagonist activity often have different effects on these different receptor sites. Some of the mixed agonist-antagonists include pentazocine (Talwin), which was synthesized for the intentional purpose of producing an effective analgesic with little or no abuse potential. However, it produces essentially morphine-like effects and is a drug of abuse.

Additional agonist-antagonists include nalbuphine (Nubain), butorphanol (Stadol), and buprenorphine (Buprenex). Pentazocine, butorphanol, and buprenorphine can be used as analgesics, and nalbuphine is used to produce analgesia. Buprenorphine appears to be useful as a maintenance drug for opioid-dependent patients. Pentazocine, butorphanol, and nalbuphine produce morphine-like effects in low doses and, to varying degrees, dysphoric effects as the dose is increased. Buprenorphine produces morphine-like effects at lower doses and antagonist effects with minimal or no dysphoria as the dose is increased. Overall, the agonist-antagonist opioids are clinically effective analgesics with a generally low potential for abuse.[33] Also, because these opioids have antagonist activity, opioid withdrawal symptoms can occur when they are administered to people who are physically dependent on morphine-related opioids.[34]

■ Depressant Drug States

Central nervous system depressants cause a variety of drug states, depending on the amount of drug used, the length of time it is used, the presence or absence of tolerance to effects, and the total combination of drugs used.

Sedative-Hypnotic Intoxication

Sedative-hypnotic intoxication involves a disinhibition euphoria of varying intensity. Intensity levels are a function of dose, how fast the drug is metabolized, the specific pharmacology of the drug, and host variables such as tolerance. The effects are behavioral, cognitive, and emotional. Behavioral signs include slurred speech, unsteady gait, incoordination, and clumsiness. Cognitive impairment may include impaired judgment and memory. Frequently, there is a disinhibition of sexual and aggressive impulses. In general, the ability to fulfill normal social and occupational responsibilities is impaired.

Idiosyncratic Sedative-Hypnotic Intoxication

Alcohol and other sedative-hypnotics have been known to produce an idiosyncratic intoxication that paradoxically involves excitation and agitation. While in this state, people may become aggressive, agitated, assaultive, and violent.

This paradoxical stimulation may occur shortly after drug consumption and represents a departure from the individual's previous behavioral and mood state and a departure from or an exaggeration of the individual's normal personality characteristics. When caused by alcohol, the disorder may occur rapidly and disappear as the alcohol is metabolized. Amnesia to the episode may occur. People with brain trauma may be predisposed to such severe reactions to small amounts of sedative-hypnotics.

Sedative-Hypnotic Amnestic Disorder

In general, amnestic syndrome is an impairment in short-term and long-term memory due to a specific physical cause such as sedative-hypnotic drug use. Typically, people are able to remember past events better than recent events. They may have gaps of memory loss, which may cause confusion and a tendency to "create" a memory unconsciously. Other people may be aware of the memory loss but fail to see it as a problem. There may be significant social and occupational impairment, depending on the severity of the syndrome.

Amnesia is routinely induced through the use of intravenous benzodiazepines during surgery.[35] However, oral ingestion of the benzodiazepines can also have various effects on memory, including *anterograde amnesia*,[36,37] which is the loss of memory of events from a specific point on. Anterograde amnesia also can be induced by clinical administration of benzodiazepines.[38] In addition, various memory problems can develop in response to benzodiazepine withdrawal.

Alcoholic amnestic disorder appears to be related to thiamine and vitamin B_{12} deficiency caused by chronic, high-dose alcohol consumption. The first stage of this process is called Wernicke's disease, which often causes associated signs and symptoms of confusion, ataxia (failure of muscle coordination), and abnormalities in eye movements. If not treated by high doses of B_{12} and thiamine, memory impairment may become permanent (Wernicke's psychosis). Wernicke's encephalopathy is swelling of the brain due to thiamine deficiency.

The alcoholic blackout. The alcoholic blackout shares some characteristics with alcoholic amnestic disorder. Both involve anterograde amnesia. However, the alcoholic blackout may be pharmacologic in nature, perhaps related to rising levels of alcohol rather than severe trauma to the brain. The intoxicated person may appear oriented and rational to others, but have no memory of events from the time of the increase in blood alcohol levels through stabilization or decrease in blood alcohol levels.[39] Alcoholic blackouts can be induced clinically.[40]

It may be wise to think of amnesia and memory problems on a continuum of severity, rather than as all-or-nothing events. Patients frequently talk about sedative-hypnotic "brownouts," referring to periods about which memory is foggy and incomplete.

Sedative-Hypnotic Withdrawal

Drug withdrawal is usually understood as a period of time that follows both physical dependence and cessation (or reduction) of use of a psychoactive substance. Sedative-hypnotic withdrawal consists of two phases: acute and prolonged withdrawal. Acute sedative-hypnotic withdrawal symptoms begin within hours of cessation or reduction of drug use and may last up to 2 weeks. In contrast, prolonged sedative-hypnotic withdrawal symptoms may begin shortly or many weeks or months after the last drug use.

Acute Sedative-Hypnotic Withdrawal

Once physical dependence and tolerance have developed, the elimination or reduction of sedative-hypnotic use produces a range of characteristic signs and symptoms of withdrawal that invariably include anxiety and insomnia. Different sedative-hypnotic drugs may produce essentially identical clusters of withdrawal symptoms with respect to type, although there may be differences in terms of severity, speed of onset, duration of the syndrome, and even patients' personal reactions to the syndrome. Variables may include the specific drug of choice, the drug's duration of action, the chronicity of drug use, the daily dosage, the level of tolerance, and the total number of drug combinations used. As a rule, the higher the dosage and the longer the period of use, the more severe the withdrawal.

In general, a drug's withdrawal symptoms are the opposite of its acute effects. Thus, stopping or reducing depressant consumption causes emotional and behavioral stimulation and anxiety. The autonomic nervous system is stimulated, prompting "fight or flight" responses such as increased heart rate, elevated blood pressure, and disruption in smooth muscle activity. Drugs that have longer half-lives tend to have a later onset of withdrawal symptoms than their short-half-life counterparts.[41] Thus, the withdrawal from alcohol and short-acting benzodiazepines begins before the withdrawal from long-acting benzodiazepines.

Minor sedative-hypnotic withdrawal signs and symptoms occur first. These may include elevated pulse and respiration rates, tachycardia, muscular pain, weakness, and postural hypotension, which is a decrease in blood pressure and faint feelings on assuming an upright posture. Other signs and symptoms include anxiety, apprehension, insomnia, nightmares, anorexia, and profuse sweating. Additional symptoms may include agitation, irritability, nausea, vomiting, and a tremor of the hands, eyelids, and tongue.

Acute sedative-hypnotic withdrawal begins shortly after cessation of use and increases in intensity within a few days (Figure 3–2). Symptoms may begin 1–2 days after stopping short-acting benzodiazepines, 2–4 days after stopping long-acting benzodiazepines, and 24–36 hours after the last dose of secobarbital or pentobarbital.[3]

Severe withdrawal symptoms may include an unusually high fever, delirium, grand mal seizures, psychosis, and possibly death. Psychosis may appear on the fourth to seventh drug-free day, and it is characterized by paranoia with visual and auditory hallucinations.

Seizures occur in about 80% of nonmedicated patients withdrawing from short-acting barbiturates, and they can occur during withdrawal from other sedative-hypnotics, including alcohol.[42] Because of the availability of effective drugs such as the benzodiazepines, barbiturates, and propranolol, no patient should endure sedative-hypnotic withdrawal without medical management. As Figure 3–2 depicts, one of the medical techniques used during sedative-hypnotic withdrawal is to temporarily substitute another sedative-hypnotic for the duration of the withdrawal syndrome.[3] In this example, the long-acting barbiturate phenobarbital is provided dur-

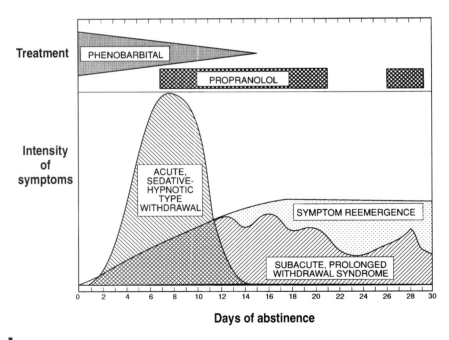

Figure 3–2. Sedative-hypnotic withdrawal syndromes. *Source.* Adapted with permission from Smith DE, Wesson DR: "Benzodiazepine Dependency Syndromes." *Journal of Psychoactive Drugs* 15:85–95, 1983.

ing the entire course of the acute sedative-hypnotic withdrawal. Figure 3–2 also depicts the use of the drug propranolol during the peak of symptom intensity and for the next 2 weeks. Propranolol is a nonpsychoactive drug that is used to treat irregular heart rhythms such as tachycardia and high blood pressure. Used during a sedative-hypnotic withdrawal, it can help to reduce some of physical symptoms of withdrawal and anxiety.

Benzodiazepine and barbiturate withdrawal should be slow and gradual—at least 3 to 4 weeks—depending on the typical daily dosage, the length of time the patient used sedative-hypnotics, and the degree of tolerance. The sedative-hypnotic withdrawal syndrome will begin to decrease in intensity a few days after the peak in symptom intensity (Figure 3–2).

Subacute Sedative-Hypnotic Withdrawal

People can experience depressant withdrawal symptoms after the acute withdrawal period. Subacute withdrawal, sometimes called prolonged or protracted withdrawal, has been documented for opiates, alcohol, and the benzodiazepines.[3,43–45] For example, prolonged benzodiazepine withdrawal typically consists of a small cluster of symptoms such as anxiety, insomnia, possible muscle spasms, and paresthesias (unusual tingling, prickling, or numbness).

Symptoms of prolonged sedative-hypnotic withdrawal may suddenly appear and fade a few or numerous times within 1 year of abstinence. The prolonged withdrawal syndrome may peak and fall repeatedly, but generally it diminishes over time, in contrast to re-emergence of psychiatric symptoms, which would increase in severity and remain relatively constant (Figure 3–2). Patients should be informed that this syndrome will fade over time. Indeed, as Figure 3–2 notes, the prolonged withdrawal syndrome can be called "subacute," which means between acute (short-term) and chronic (long-term). Indeed, Figure 3–2 depicts the use of propranolol during a 3-day burst of symptoms. This represents the safe use of a non-psychoactive drug to medicate a brief period of intense anxiety, insomnia, and drug craving that otherwise might lead to a relapse.

Disorder Reemergence

Sedatives and hypnotics are prescribed for anxiety and sleep disorders, respectively. Alcohol is frequently used to self-medicate anxiety and insomnia. Some people begin their sedative-hypnotic drug use to medicate anxiety and sleep disorders. Therefore, these people may experience a return of their original disorder after the acute withdrawal.

Figure 3–2 depicts the reemergence of the symptoms of an original anxiety disorder. Note that the symptom intensity does not fluctuate but rather levels off, remaining constant. In this example, the constant intensity of an anxiety disorder can be contrasted with the fluctuating intensity of a prolonged withdrawal syndrome.

For instance, the benzodiazepines or alcohol may have been used to medicate anxiety, panic, and social phobias. After the acute sedative-hypnotic withdrawal, the anxiety, panic, or social phobias may reemerge with the same intensity as before. In fact, they may reemerge with more intensity. Either way, serious efforts must be made to find nonpsychoactive treatment alternatives for the anxiety disorders of these dually diagnosed people.

Withdrawal Symptom Interpretation

When people medicate their psychiatric problems with long-term, psychoactive drug use, they also medicate ordinary feelings such as "normal" anxieties. Thus, people who have been using prescribed benzodiazepines or drinking alcohol for an extended period of time may become confused and frightened about their returning feelings. In particular, people may overinterpret their symptoms.[3] Symptom overinterpretation involves misdescribing normal aches and pains as withdrawal symptoms and anxiously desiring treatment for fear of supposed additional, severe withdrawal symptoms. Similarly, if some time has passed since the last onset of the anxiety disorder, the symptom reemergence may prompt the patient to misinterpret the present symptom severity as being worse than it was in the past. On the other hand, it is possible for a psychiatric problem to progress despite the fact that symptoms have been treated. Thus, some people may accurately describe their reemerging anxiety disorder as being more intense than it was before it was medicated.

Sedative-Hypnotic Withdrawal Delirium

The mental process of cognition involves awareness, perception, reasoning, judgment, intuition, and memory. The withdrawal from sedative-hypnotic drugs can cause a psychiatric condition called delirium, which is a fairly global impairment of cognition. Delirium describes the impaired ability to sustain appropriate mental attention to environmental stimuli and to shift to new stimuli when necessary. Thinking is disorganized, with associated incoherent or rambling communication. There is often some memory impairment, such as the inability to learn or retrieve recent information. The individual may have a disturbance of the sleep-waking cycle and may not be oriented as to place or time. In some cases, the individual may experience disturbances of perception, possibly including hallucinations.

Alcohol Hallucinosis

During acute withdrawal from chronic, high-dose alcohol use, a patient may experience an organic hallucinosis consisting of auditory and visual hallucinations. The hallucinosis may occur after a period of abstinence lasting a few hours to a few weeks, but it usually occurs within 2 days of the last drink. It may also occur while the patient is actively drinking, perhaps during a reduction in intake. It improves spontaneously within a few days or perhaps weeks, but the hallucinations may last for months. The content of the hallucinations (such as threats) and the associated mental states (such as anxiety) may vary. The hallucinations may be transient and intermittent and often are more frequent in the evening. The individual is often aware that they are, in fact, hallucinations.

Opioid Intoxication

Opioid intoxication superficially resembles sedative-hypnotic intoxication in that both drug groups cause central nervous system depression. However, opioid intoxication differs because of the presence of analgesia and the quality of euphoria. At doses that are intoxicating, opioid analgesia involves an alteration of both perception of and reaction to pain. There is an increased pain threshold as well as an indifference to pain and other stimuli. The euphoric aspects of opioid intoxication involve a greatly exaggerated state of well-being and seemingly total freedom from anxiety and distress. People intoxicated with opioids generally experience a pleasurable, floating, and tranquil sensation, often with a feeling of drowsiness.[46]

Opioid intoxication generally consists of two phases: a brief euphoric episode followed by a longer period of apathy. The euphoric episode may last a few minutes to a half hour. The longer period of apathy may last a few hours, depending on the drug, the amount, and the person's tolerance. During the period of apathy, people have impaired and typically slower reactions and may have slurred speech and appear sleepy and drowsy. Frequently, they "nod out," or appear to fall asleep during conversations. In contrast to people with alcohol and other sedative-hypnotic intoxication, opioid-intoxicated people do not generally experience a period of disinhibition stimulation or psychomotor agitation, although it can occur.

Opioid Withdrawal

After the cessation or reduction of moderate to heavy prolonged opioid use, an opioid withdrawal syndrome will occur. Withdrawal symptoms from long-acting opioids such as methadone will occur within a day or two of the last use. Withdrawal symptoms from short-acting opioids such as heroin or morphine will emerge within 6–10 hours. Opioid withdrawal symptoms are nearly identical to symptoms of influenza (the flu).

People invariably feel dysphoric and agitated, with a sustained craving for an opioid or even a sedative-hypnotic to provide sedation. They frequently feel nauseous and may have periods of vomiting. Muscle aches and pains are common. People often have watery eyes, runny noses, sweating, fever, and diarrhea. Insomnia and yawning are common features of opioid withdrawal.

■ Summary

Central nervous system depressants include the sedative-hypnotics and the opioid analgesics. Both sedative-hypnotics and opioid analgesics reduce central nervous system activity, resulting in increased sedation and pain relief, respectively. Sedation is a decrease in the individual's responsiveness to a constant level of stimulation, with a decrease in spontaneous activity and ideation. Thus, a sedative is a drug that promotes mental calmness, has a soothing, tranquilizing effect, reduces excessive anxiety, and may control dangerously aggressive behavior. Hypnotics are drugs that promote sleep or drowsiness. Sedative-hypnotics are those drugs that can cause sedation or sleep, and with variations in dosage, can often do both. The sedative-hypnotics include barbiturates, benzodiazepines, and nonbarbiturate, nonbenzodiazepine sedative-hypnotics such as chloral hydrate, glutethimide, and alcohol.

During the 1960s, the barbiturates were widely prescribed for anxiety and insomnia. Although effective, they can easily cause overdose when they are mixed with other sedative-hypnotics such as alcohol. Barbiturates rapidly cause physical dependence and tolerance. Withdrawal from barbiturates is often difficult and dangerous. They have been largely replaced by the safer and less potent benzodiazepines for the treatment of anxiety and insomnia. Like the barbiturates, the benzodiazepines produce a dose-dependent range of central nervous system depression from relaxation, sedation, and muscle relaxation to hypnosis and general anesthesia. Benzodiazepines are not generally a primary drug of abuse or addiction. Rather, benzodiazepine abuse and addiction are most frequent in people with polydrug use patterns who are at high risk for alcoholism. Prolonged use of benzodiazepines may cause physical dependence in some, but not all, people. Benzodiazepine withdrawal should never be abrupt, but rather slow, gradual, and under a physician's direction.

A number of sedative-hypnotic drugs are neither barbiturates nor benzodiazepines: alcohol, chloral hydrate, ethchlorvynol, ethinamate, glutethimide, meprobamate, methyprylon, and paraldehyde. Except for alcohol, they were introduced as alternatives to the barbiturates, but in fact cause roughly the same symptoms and signs that barbiturates and alcohol do.

The sedative-hypnotics can alter pain by causing overall sedation of the central nervous system, resulting in a loss of consciousness and thus unawareness of pain. In contrast, opioids alter the perception of pain by inhibiting the nerves that carry the pain messages. Opioids reduce pain through analgesia, which is the loss of pain awareness while remaining fully conscious. Opioid analgesics depress the region of the brain responsible for respiration. Thus, death from opioid overdose invariably involves respiratory arrest.

The morphine-related opioids produce analgesia without loss of consciousness, mood changes, mental clouding and drowsiness, and respiratory depression. They can cause nausea and vomiting, euphoria, apathy, decreased physical activity, and difficulty thinking. These drugs often cause constipation.

Meperidine produces effects that are similar but not identical to those produced by morphine. Meperidine-related opioids include medications that are used for very different purposes. For example, meperidine is administered for the relief of moderate to severe pain. Diphenoxylate and loperamide slow down gastrointestinal activity and are used for the treatment of diarrhea. Fentanyl, sufentanil, and alfentanil are used as analgesic supplements to general anesthesia and for induction of anesthesia.

Methadone is known for its potent analgesic abilities, its efficacy when administered orally, and its ability to suppress opioid withdrawal symptoms for prolonged periods of time. It is useful for opioid detoxification. Methadone and the related medication LAAM (L-acetyl-alpha-methadol) are also used in opioid maintenance programs. The medication propoxyphene (Darvon) is chemically related to methadone and is used orally to relieve mild to moderate pain. Its analgesic efficacy is less than that of other opioids.

Naloxone and naltrexone are opioid antagonists. Naloxone reverses opioid overdose symptoms by displacing the opioids from their receptor sites. Naltrexone produces longer-lasting effects than naloxone, and it is used by people in recovery from opioid addiction to stop impulsive opioid use.

The mixed agonist-antagonists include pentazocine, which produces essentially morphine-like effects. Additional agonist-antagonists include nalbuphine, butorphanol, and buprenorphine, which produce morphine-like effects at low doses and, to varying degrees, dysphoric effects as the dose is increased. Buprenorphine produces morphine-like effects at lower doses and antagonist effects with minimal or no dysphoria as the dose is increased. Overall, the agonist-antagonist opioids are clinically effective analgesics with a generally low potential for abuse.

Depressant drugs cause a number of drug states. They include sedative-hypnotic intoxication, idiosyncratic sedative-hypnotic intoxication, sedative-hypnotic amnestic disorder, alcoholic blackout, acute and prolonged sedative-hypnotic withdrawal, sedative-hypnotic withdrawal delirium, alcohol hallucinosis, opioid intoxication, and opioid withdrawal. In addition, anxiety disorders that may have been hidden during prolonged periods of sedative-hypnotic use may reemerge after cessation of drug use.

■ References

1. Trevor AJ, Way WL: Drugs used for anxiety states and sleep problems, in Review of General Psychiatry, 2nd Edition. Edited by Goldman HH. Norwalk, CT, Appleton & Lange, 1988
2. Lader M: Introduction to Psychopharmacology. Kalamazoo, MI, The Upjohn Company, 1983
3. Smith DE, Wesson DR: Benzodiazepine dependency syndromes. Journal of Psychoactive Drugs 15:85–95, 1983
4. Cox RC, Jacobs MR, LeBlanc AE, et al: Drugs and Drug Abuse: A Reference Text. Toronto, Canada, Addiction Research Foundation, 1987
5. Wesson DR, Smith DE: Barbiturates: Their Use, Misuse and Abuse. New York, Human Sciences Press, 1977
6. DuPont RL (ed): Abuse of benzodiazepines: the problems and the solutions: a report of a committee of the Institute for Behavior and Health, Inc. American Journal of Drug and Alcohol Abuse 14 (suppl 1):1–69, 1988
7. Mellinger GD, Balter MB, Uhlenhuth EH: Antianxiety agents: duration of use and characteristics of users in the U.S.A. Current Medical Research and Opinion 8 (suppl 4):21–36, 1984

8. Woods JH, Katz JL, Winger G: Use and abuse of benzodiazepines. Journal of the American Medical Association 260:3476–3480, 1988

9. American Psychiatric Association: Benzodiazepine Dependence, Toxicity, and Abuse: A Task Force Report of the American Psychiatric Association. Washington, DC, American Psychiatric Association, 1990

10. Cole JO, Chiarello RJ: The benzodiazepines as drugs of abuse. Journal of Psychiatric Research 24 (suppl 2):135–144, 1991

11. Ciraulo DA, Sands BF, Shader RI: Critical review of liability for benzodiazepine abuse among alcoholics. American Journal of Psychiatry 145:1501–1506, 1988

12. Woods JH, Katz JL, Winger G: Use and abuse of benzodiazepines: issues relevant to prescribing. Journal of the American Medical Association 260:3476–3480, 1988

13. Smith DE, Landry MJ: Benzodiazepine dependency discontinuation: focus on the chemical dependency detoxification setting and benzodiazepine-polydrug abuse. Journal of Psychiatric Research 24 (suppl 2):145–156, 1990

14. Farnsworth MG: Benzodiazepine abuse and dependence: misconceptions and facts. Journal of Family Practice 31:393–400, 1990

15. Smith DE, Wesson DR, Camber S, et al: Perceptions of benzodiazepine and cocaine abuse by U.S. addiction medicine specialists, in Prevention and Control/Realities and Aspirations: Proceedings of the 35th International Congress on Alcoholism and Drug Dependence, July 31–August 6, 1988, Vol 4. Norway, National Directorate for the Prevention of Alcohol and Drug Problems, 1989, pp 371–390

16. Marks J: The Benzodiazepines: Use, Overuse, Misuse, Abuse, 2nd Edition. Lancaster, England, MTP Press, 1986

17. Chan AWK: Effects of combined alcohol and benzodiazepine: a review. Drug and Alcohol Dependence 13:315–341, 1984

18. Ciraulo DA, Barnhill JG, Greenblatt DJ, et al: Abuse liability and clinical pharmacokinetics of alprazolam in alcoholic men. Journal of Clinical Psychiatry 49:333–337, 1988

19. Ciraulo DA, Barnhill JG, Ciraulo AM, et al: Parental alcoholism as a risk factor in benzodiazepine abuse: a pilot study. American Journal of Psychiatry 146:1333–1335, 1989

20. Senay EC: Addictive behaviors and benzodiazepines: abuse liability and physical dependence. Advances in Alcohol and Substance Use 8:107–124, 1989

21. Landry MJ, Smith DE, McDuff DR, et al: Benzodiazepine dependence and withdrawal: identification and medical management. Journal of the American Board of Family Practice 5:1–9, 1992

22. Marks J: The Benzodiazepines: Use, Overuse, Misuse and Abuse. Lancaster, England, MTP Press, 1978

23. Marks J: The benzodiazepines—for good or evil. Neuropsychobiology 10:115–126, 1983

24. Lader M: Dependence on benzodiazepines. Journal of Clinical Psychiatry 44:121–127, 1983

25. Landry MJ, Smith DE, McDuff DR, et al: Anxiety and substance use disorders: the treatment of high-risk patients. Journal of the American Board of Family Practice 4:447–456, 1991

26. Casriel C, Rockwell R, Stepherson B: Heroin sniffers: between two worlds. Journal of Psychoactive Drugs 20:437–440, 1988

27. Hibbs J, Perper J, Winek CL: An outbreak of designer drug–related deaths in Pennsylvania. Journal of the American Medical Association 265:1011–1013, 1991

28. Seymour R, Smith D, Inaba D, et al: The New Drugs: Look-Alikes, Drugs of Deception and Designer Drugs. Center City, MN, Hazelden Foundation, 1989

29. Monk JP, Beresford R, Ward A: Sufentanil: a review of its pharmacological properties and therapeutic use. Drugs 36:286–313, 1988

30. Jaffe JH, Epstein S, Ciraulo DA: Opioids, in Clinical Manual of Chemical Dependence. Edited by Ciraulo DA, Shader RI. Washington, DC, American Psychiatric Press, 1991, pp 95–133

31. Jacobs MR, Fehr K O'B: Drugs and Drug Abuse: A Reference Text. Toronto, Canada, Addiction Research Foundation, 1987

32. Gonzalez JP, Brogden RN: Naltrexone: a review of its pharmacodynamic and pharmacokinetic properties and therapeutic efficacy in the management of opioid dependence. Drugs 35:192–213, 1988

33. Peachey JE: Clinical observations of agonist-antagonist analgesic dependence. Drug and Alcohol Dependence 20:346–365, 1987

34. Rosow CE: The clinical usefulness of agonist-antagonist analgesics in acute pain. Drug and Alcohol Dependence 20:329–337, 1987

35. Dundee JW, Pandit SK: Anterograde amnesic effects of pethidine, hyoscine and diazepam in adults. British Journal of Pharmacology 44:140–144, 1972

36. Scharf MB, Saskin P, Fletcher K: Benzodiazepine-induced amnesia: clinical and laboratory findings. Journal of Clinical Psychiatry Monograph 5:14–17, 1987

37. Lister T: The amnesic action of benzodiazepines in man. Neuroscience and Biobehavioral Review 9:87–94, 1985

38. Wolkowitz OM, Weingartner H, Thompson K, et al: Diazepam-induced amnesia: a neuropharmacological model of an "organic amnestic syndrome." American Journal of Psychiatry 1441:25–29, 1987

39. Butz RH: Intoxication and withdrawal, in Alcoholism: Development, Consequences and Interventions, 2nd Edition. Edited by Estes NJ, Heinemann ME. St. Louis, MO, CV Mosby, 1982

40. Goodwin DW: The phenomena of alcoholic blackouts. Presented at the Workshop on Alcoholic Blackouts, sponsored by the National Institute of Alcohol Abuse and Alcoholism, St. Thomas, U.S. Virgin Islands, March 23–24, 1972

41. Bernstein JG: Handbook of Drug Therapy in Psychiatry. Littleton, MA, Wright-PSG, 1983

42. Kanas N: Psychoactive substance use disorders: alcohol, in Review of General Psychiatry, 2nd Edition. Edited by Goldman HH. Norwalk, CT, Appleton & Lange, 1988, pp 286–298

43. Carlson KR, Cooper DO: Morphine dependence and protracted abstinence: regional alterations in CNS radioligand binding. Pharmacology, Biochemistry and Behavior 23:1059–1063, 1985

44. Meyer RE: Anxiolytics and the alcoholic patient. Journal of Studies on Alcohol 47:269–273, 1986

45. Mossberg D, Liljeberg P, Borg S: Clinical conditions in alcoholics during long-term abstinence: a descriptive, longitudinal treatment study. Alcohol 2:551–553, 1985

46. Ling W, Wesson DR: Drugs of abuse—opiates. Western Journal of Medicine 152:565–572, 1990

Table 4–1. The psychedelic drugs

Psychedelic drug type	Specific psychedelic drugs
LSD and related psychedelics	LSD (D-lysergic acid diethylamide, acid)
	DET (*N,N*-diethyltryptamine)
	DMT (*N,N*-dimethyltryptamine)
	Psilocybin mushrooms (dimethyl-4-phosphoryl-tryptamine)
Psychedelic amphetamines	2CB (4-bromo-2,5-dimethoxyphenethylamine)
	DOB (2,5-dimethoxy-4-bromoamphetamine)
	Euphoria (4-methyl-aminorex)
	STP/DOM (4-methyl-2,5-dimethoxyamphetamine)
	MDA (3,4-methylenedioxyamphetamine, "The Love Drug")
	MDE (3,4-methylenedioxyethamphetamine, "Eve")
	MDMA (3,4-methylenedioxymethamphetamine, "Ecstasy," "Adam")
	MMDA (3-methoxy-4,5-methylenedioxyamphetamine)
	Mescaline (peyote cactus) (3,4,5-trimethoxy-phenylethylamine)
Dissociative anesthetics	PCP (phencyclidine, "Angel Dust")
	Ketamine (Ketalar)
	PCE (*N*-ethyl-1-phencyclohexalamine)
	TCP (1-[1-2-thienyl-cyclohexyl]piperidine)
	PHP (1-[1-phencyclohexyl]pyrrolidine)
	PCC (1-piperidinocyclohexane carbonitrile)
Cannabis	Tetrahydrocannabinol (THC), marijuana, hashish

Chapter 4

The Psychedelic Drugs

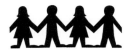

The controversial nature of the diverse substances found in the catchall category called "psychedelic drugs" is illustrated by disagreements over how best to describe their actions. Drugs such as LSD, MDMA, PCP, and marijuana have obvious differences. They are not identical in action or effect. However, there are commonalities and shared effects among these drugs. Less predictable than the classic stimulants or depressants, the psychedelic drugs are characterized by their wide-ranging psychological effects. Contextual factors such as set (expectations) and setting, different motivations and expectations, together with environmental influences and psychological stability, greatly modify the perceived benefits and problems associated with their use.

Jerome Beck, Dr.P.H.
Co-Principal Investigator
Institute for Scientific Analysis
Berkeley, California

■ The Psychedelic Experience

No other drugs are as misunderstood and controversial as the psychedelic drugs, in part because they do not form as cohesive a drug group as the stimulants or the depressants. Indeed, the group of psychedelic drugs includes several different drugs with dissimilar mechanisms of action, each with a range of psychological, emotional, and behavioral effects. Despite these differences, there are common features that define them all as psychedelic drugs.

Psychedelic drugs are used by different groups of people, for different purposes, with different expectations, in different settings, and with different results. They are used in the context of polydrug addiction,[1] in infrequent social situations, for rare experimental purposes,[2] in the supervised context of psychotherapy,[3] and for spiritual and religious purposes.[4,5] Addiction experts treat psychedelic drug abuse, whereas a few psychotherapists describe the usefulness of psychedelic drugs as an aid to psychotherapy.[6]

Definitions and Terms

Some confusion about psychedelic and hallucinogenic drugs relates to terminology. A *hallucination* is a sensory perception without basis in reality and without stimulation of the sensory organ(s) in question. It is the result of the stimulation of certain sensory activities such as vision, hearing, taste, and touch, but without stimulation of the sensory organs. People may "hear," "see," "smell," or "feel" things that do not exist. Sometimes people are aware that hallucinations are drug induced (pseudohallucinations); sometimes they believe that their hallucinations are, in fact, reality.

The literal definition of the term *hallucinogen* is a drug that causes hallucinations. However, some drugs that are casually called hallucinogens do not cause hallucinations. Conversely, some drugs cause hallucinations under special conditions, but the hallucinations are side effects rather than the primary effects or regular effects of the drugs. For example, stimulants can cause hallucinations with chronic, high-dose use, but hallucinations are not the primary effect of stimulants. Thus, the term "hallucinogen" is too restrictive to use as a general description of psychedelic drugs.

The term *psychedelic* means "mind-manifesting" or "mind-revealing" and was coined by psychiatrist Humphrey Osmond in 1956 because it is a neutral and less misleading term than "hallucinogen" to describe the variety and range of effects that these drugs can produce.[7] Thus, the phrase *psychedelic drugs* is used in this book to describe those drugs that characteristically and consistently produce some combination of distortions of thinking, feeling, and perception, collectively known as the psychedelic experience.

Elements of the Psychedelic Experience

People who have never used them often ask, "What do psychedelic drugs do?" Describing the subjective effects of these drugs involves some discussion of emotional, psychodynamic, spiritual, and metaphysical concepts, which are the playing field of psychedelic drugs. Indeed, some aspects of psychedelic drug experiences are similar to religious ecstatic experiences, spiritual awakenings, dream states, and several psychiatric states. Psychedelic drugs do far more than merely stimulate or depress behavior and emotions. Rather, they seem to act as keys that unlock parts of the mind that are normally inaccessible. This explains some people's positive interpretations of increased self-awareness and others' reports of frightening experiences and psychiatric problems.

Although a specified blood-alcohol level will produce similar reactions among people, psychedelic experiences are mercurial. Psychedelic experiences vary even when subjective and environmental factors are identical. Some of these factors include dosage amount, expectations, previous psychedelic experiences, current mood, immediate environment, the mood of others, and sensory stimuli. Slight changes in these factors can cause dramatic differences among psychedelic drug experiences.

The elements of the psychedelic experience may include distortions of perception, emotion, thinking, and self-perception, as well as changes in spiritual and psychological perception (Table 4–2).[8] A given psychedelic experience may include some combination of these elements.

Perceptual distortions. Often, one of the first and most conspicuous effects is distortion of sensory perception, such as perceiving colorful, vibrant geometric patterns while one's eyes are closed. More intense, moving images and shapes may be perceived with open eyes, with a prolonged afterimage. Pseudohallucinations may occur, and hallucinations are likely with high doses. *Synesthesia* is a sensory crossover effect during which people "see" sounds, "hear" bright lights, or "taste" colors. For example, a loud guitar note may be visually perceived as a blue bolt of lightning. Additional distortions of perception may include distortions of time, such as the impression that time is standing still.

Table 4–2. Elements of the psychedelic experience

Element	Description
Perceptual distortions	*Alteration of sensory perception:* vibrant geometric visual imagery; heightened auditory perceptions; pseudohallucinations; synesthesia; distortions of time perception; true hallucinations
Emotional distortions	*Alteration of mood and emotions:* possible apprehension, anxiety, and panic; possible ecstasy and calm; possible mood shifts from sadness to joy; possible anger and rage
Thought distortions	*Alteration of normal thinking:* creative problem solving; fantasy thoughts; pseudoprofound thoughts; preoccupation with thinking itself; loosening of associations; possible paranoia, grandiosity, and delusions
Ego boundary distortions	*Alteration of the sense of self:* loss of boundary between self and others; possible loss of boundary between self and external world; possible depersonalization; distorted body image
Spirituality and insight	*Various philosophical, spiritual, and psychodynamic perceptions:* concern with meaning of life; heightened perception of spiritual importance; enhanced empathy, intimacy, and communication; loosening of defenses; enhanced personal insight

Emotional distortions. The psychedelic experience invariably involves intense moods and emotions, which may be perceived as enjoyable or overwhelming. Some people experience a state of ecstasy or complete relaxation. Others may become fearful of the perceptual distortions (such as visual distortions) and become anxious and panic-stricken.

Emotions can repeatedly alternate between joy and sadness or pleasure and depression. These emotions can progressively intensify to a peak and then become less intense until the predrug emotions return. Under some circumstances, such as very high doses and high levels of internal or external stress, social withdrawal and paranoid rage reactions may occur.

Thought distortions. Thinking becomes distorted during the psychedelic experience. People may become preoccupied with the actual process of thinking and thought. Although thinking and problem solving may become genuinely creative and unusually insightful,[9] people may also have "profound thoughts" that do not seem profound after the drug wears off.

There may be a loosening of associations—a type of thinking in which ideas shift from one topic to another. Although the topics may be completely unrelated or only obscurely related, the individual does not show any awareness that the topics are unconnected. Thinking may become nonlogical and fantastic in nature. Paranoia, grandiosity, and delusions may occur.

Ego boundary distortions. The term "ego" can describe a conscious awareness of the self. The phrase "ego boundaries" can describe the perception that there are differences between the self and others, or between the self and internal images or external reality. Because the psychedelic experience often involves a distortion of normal ego boundaries, the perception of the self may become distorted.[10] There may be a lack of distinction between the self and others, between the self and internal images, or among memories, images, and events.

Ego boundary distortions may include depersonalization, an alteration of the perception of the self to the point that one's own reality is temporarily lost. This sense of unreality may include the perception of watching oneself from a distance or from above (an "out of body" experience). Similarly, one's body image may become distorted, with the entire body or parts of the body seemingly increasing or decreasing in size or perhaps disappearing.

Spirituality. To the mother of an adolescent who uses psychedelic drugs in the context of polydrug abuse, descriptions of the role these drugs can play in achieving personal insight or spiritual growth may seem pointless. However, their abuse does not diminish the unusual ability of some psychedelic drugs to tap into areas of human experience that relate to spirituality, conscious awareness, and emotional growth. These descriptions can provide a deeper understanding of the psychedelic drug experience and why some people use these drugs.[11]

The use of cultivated plants for magical, religious, and other mystical purposes is ancient.[12] The Aztecs incorporated psychedelic experiences into culturally sanctioned practices, while frowning on alcohol intoxication and psychedelic drug use for personal pleasure.[13] Psychedelic drug use during the late 1950s through the mid-1960s was associated with a specific cultural context within a subculture. At that time, the primary motivation for using psychedelic drugs was related to spiritual, personal, and interpersonal awareness, not "recreation." Proponents of psychedelic drugs, writing in underground newspapers such as *The San Francisco Oracle,* described the use of these drugs for spiritual awakenings.[14] They described a specific context of promoting insight, peace, harmony, and understanding. But by the time of the 1967 "Summer of Love," psychedelic drugs were associated with a "turn on, tune in, and drop out" context and were used for "recreation" and abuse, as well as insight.

In a series of medical studies during the 1950s and 1960s, LSD* was administered to alcoholic individuals in the belief that large doses of LSD would mimic alcoholic delirium tremens (DTs), a serious and sometimes fatal psychotic reaction to abrupt withdrawal of

---

*Please see Table 4–1 for spelled-out versions of drug abbreviations.

alcohol in chronically alcoholic individuals. The researchers believed that the alcoholic individuals would be discouraged from further drinking after the noxious experience.[15–17] Instead, the researchers found that some of the patients reported mystical experiences through which they gained new insight into the meaning of life and found the experience beneficial.

During the psychedelic experience, some people become more aware of the perspective of their companion or experience being "one with the universe." After the experience, they may retain insight about their role in society and acknowledge a newly discovered respect for cooperation rather than competition, harmony rather than aggression, and interdependence rather than independence. It is plausible that distortion of the ego boundary causes spiritual and insightful experiences for some individuals and traumatic psychological crises for others.

Insight and therapy. There is a long, if clandestine, history of use of psychedelic drugs in psychotherapy. Before LSD was banned by U.S. federal law in 1966, LSD-assisted psychotherapy was a vibrant area of psychiatric research.[18–20] Several studies described the beneficial effects of MDA as an adjunct to psychotherapy.[21–23] Psychedelic drug-assisted psychotherapy continues today in clandestine fashion because of the illegal status of these drugs.[*] Overall, the tight government control over psychedelic drug–assisted psychotherapy has been based primarily on political, not medical, concerns.[20] The Food and Drug Administration has approved the protocols for a few studies that will examine the physiological and neurological effects of psychedelic drugs and the possible role of these drugs in the treatment of substance use and psychiatric disorders.

What are the psychedelic drug effects that may be of value to psychotherapy? Some psychedelic drugs appear to promote empathy and enhanced communication.[24] Some of them are so well known

---

[*]Personal communication with several psychiatrists and psychotherapists who currently use MDMA and other psychedelic drugs as an adjunct to psychotherapy on a limited basis, for some patients, for certain psychological problems.

for this effect that they are described in those terms: MDA has been called "The Love Drug,"[25] and MDMA and related drugs have been described as "empathogens" (promoting empathy), and "entactogens" ("producing a touching within").[26] For some users, drugs such as MDMA and LSD can facilitate insights, memories, and fantasies and enhance the therapeutic alliance by inviting self-disclosure and trust.[6,27] They sometimes facilitate communication and intimacy between people involved in emotional relationships, enhance understanding of another's viewpoint, bring unconscious information to conscious awareness, and enhance personal insight.[22,28,29]

Phases of the Psychedelic Drug Experience

A specific psychedelic drug experience may include several psychedelic elements or just a few. Depending on the specific drug, dosage, set, setting, and individual characteristics, psychedelic drugs such as LSD can produce three consecutive, but significantly overlapping, phases.[30]

Sensory phase. The first phase of the psychedelic experience is characterized by alterations of sensory perceptions. During this phase, the individual may experience perceptual distortions of normal vision, touch, hearing, smell, taste, and kinesthesia (the sensation of position, movement, and tension of the body). The sensory phase may begin shortly after ingestion and continue for as long as 5 hours for some drugs.

Symbolic and recollective phase. A second phase may include vivid visual imagery in vibrant colors. The imagery may become remarkably intense, perhaps progressing to illusions, hallucinations, and pseudohallucinations. Alterations in mood and emotions may occur at this time, perhaps including moody reflections on past experiences, both positive and negative. This phase may last from hours 2–8.

Heightened sensibility phase. A third phase of the experience centers around changes in philosophical and personal perception.

94

During this phase, people may become intensely concerned about personal philosophy, religious and spiritual issues, and the meaning of life. Some may have enhanced psychological perceptions and insights that result in meaningful life changes. Many will not experience profound perceptions or insights. During this phase, people may display exaggerations of their normal character traits (positive or negative) and may more readily perceive psychodynamic conflicts.

Adverse Psychedelic Experiences

Psychedelic drugs can cause disturbing episodes resembling schizophrenic psychoses; delirium; mania; depressive episodes; other distortions of thinking, emotion, and perception; and panic attacks.[31] They are loosely described as "bad trips." Because psychedelic experiences involve distortions of thinking, perception, and emotion, the difference between a "good trip" and a "bad trip" is likely caused by environmental, psychiatric, and emotional factors. Several causes for negative psychedelic drug experiences have been described: preexisting character structure, setting, insecurity, set, negative experience, problems of reentry, dose, frequency of use, current mood and stress level, and insufficient preparation.[32]

Some people are vulnerable to adverse psychedelic experiences because of preexisting psychiatric problems or low stress tolerance.[33] The setting of psychedelic drug use may influence the experience because of the heightened suggestibility of the user and because of sensory stimuli. Because psychedelic drugs temporarily reduce people's defenses and increase emotional vulnerability, using these drugs while feeling insecure or with someone who instills insecurity may cause problems. Also, the drug user's negative set and anticipation may result in fulfilled negative expectations. Psychedelic drug use while depressed or anxious may lead to an exacerbation of those problems.

Adverse responses such as panic may lead to further emotional deterioration during the drug experience. Some people have a difficult time leaving the experience and coming back to reality. Others fear being "stuck" in the psychedelic experience. Higher doses tend to cause more intense, longer-lasting, and more dissociative experiences, feared by some and sought after by others. Mild confusion, memory impairment, and motivation loss may result with frequent use. People who are emotionally and psychologically unprepared for distortions of perception, thinking, and feelings are likely to have an adverse experience.

Tolerance to the psychedelic experience develops rapidly, and users who want to repeat the experience with any intensity must often wait days or weeks between experiences. Also, the psychedelics do not promote euphoria as much as sensory distortions. There is no evidence for the development of physical tolerance or withdrawal for most psychedelic drugs. Thus, psychedelic drugs such as LSD and MDMA are among the least likely drugs to promote patterns of frequent compulsive use.

Patterns of Drug Use

Drugs can be used in a variety of patterns: experimental, social-recreational, circumstantial-situational, intensified, and compulsive use.[34] *Experimental use* is the short-term use of a drug, generally with friends, often motivated by curiosity and a desire to experience the anticipated effect. *Social-recreational use* describes drug use by people who have previously had the drug experience and wish to share this experience with others in a social setting. The motivation is primarily social and the use is voluntary, not the result of compulsion. *Circumstantial-situational drug use* describes self-limited use, with variable patterns, intensity, and duration. Users are motivated to enhance a specific condition or situation, such as performance enhancement or pleasure enhancement. *Intensified drug use* describes a pattern of chronic drug use, often motivated by a perceived need or desire to obtain relief from a stressful situation or persistent problem. *Compulsive drug use* is characterized by frequent or intense use of a drug for long durations or in binges. The motivation is often intense drug cravings or avoidance of withdrawal.

The psychedelic drugs related to LSD and the psychedelic amphetamines are often used experimentally: for example, a psychedelic drug may be used infrequently in a therapeutic setting by a person dying of AIDS to enhance communication with his angry father. LSD and the psychedelic amphetamines are most often used in social-recreational situations. These include rock concerts and the recent fad of "rave dance parties" during which many or most participants consume MDMA, abstain from alcohol, and dance for several hours.

Among psychedelic drugs, marijuana and PCP are the most likely to be used in a compulsive, addictive pattern. But drugs such as marijuana and the psychedelic amphetamines have dual properties: marijuana has both psychedelic and depressant properties, whereas psychedelic amphetamines have both psychedelic and stimulant properties. It is likely that marijuana is used in abuse patterns not because of the psychedelic properties, but because of the depressant properties. The chronic use of marijuana (and the psychedelic amphetamines) reduces the potential for the psychedelic experience.

Table 4–3 demonstrates how psychedelic drugs tend to be used in nonchronic patterns. For example, over 80% of people in the survey of U.S. households have used alcohol at least once, 66% drank alcohol within the past year, and slightly over half of the population drank some alcohol within the past month. In comparison, only 7.6% of the population have ever used a psychedelic drug. Barely over 1% of the population used a psychedelic drug within the past year, and

Table 4–3. Prevalence of drug use in U.S. households: psychedelic drugs and alcohol

Drug	% U.S. households		
	Ever used	Used past year	Used last month
Hallucinogens (includes PCP)	7.6	1.1	0.3
PCP	3.0	0.2	NA
Marijuana	33.1	10.2	5.1
Alcohol	83.2	66.0	51.2

Note. NA = not available; PCP = phencyclidine.
Source. Adapted from the National Institute on Drug Abuse: *National Household Survey on Drug Abuse: Population Estimates 1990.* Washington, DC, U.S. Department of Health and Human Services, 1991.

fewer than one-half of 1% (0.3%) used psychedelics within the past month. Thus, psychedelics are generally used infrequently rather than continuously.

■ LSD and Related Psychedelics

LSD is the prototype psychedelic drug because it can cause the most elements of the psychedelic experience. It is one of a group of drugs that act on the neurotransmitter tryptamine. These drugs include LSD, psilocybin ("magic") mushrooms, and the less popular DMT and DET. They are normally consumed orally and absorbed from the gastrointestinal tract, causing drug effects in about an hour. The effects of LSD may last 8–24 hours, whereas the effects from psilocybin, DET, and DMT may last 2–6 hours.

The LSD-related drugs are potent psychedelics, capable of causing distortions in sensory perception, emotions, thinking, and ego boundaries. They can also promote spiritual experiences and psychotherapeutic effects. They are notorious for robust alteration of sensory perception, especially visual and auditory distortions. Pseudohallucinations and synesthesias are common; hallucinations are less frequent. Emotional experiences may become unusually intense and may change frequently and suddenly.

Just as sensory reality is greatly altered, reality itself seems altered. Thus, people may experience great shifts regarding religious, philosophical, and personal matters, often including insights that may be important, personally significant, and lasting for some, but may only have the appearance of profundity for others.[35,36] Also, the sense of the self may be greatly changed during the experience; for example, there may be distortions of ego boundary and body image.

■ Psychedelic Amphetamines

The psychedelic amphetamines include certain members of the amphetamine family such as MDA (methylenedioxyamphetamine) that have both stimulant and psychedelic properties. This group includes

MDMA ("Ecstasy," "Adam"), MDE ("Eve"), STP, and mescaline, which is derived from the peyote cactus. Low doses cause a psychedelic effect, and high doses cause stimulant effects, although these effects are generally less powerful than those of amphetamine and methamphetamine.

Compared with LSD, psychedelic amphetamines cause a narrow range of psychedelic effects. They do not cause severe impairment of visual sensory perception such as hallucinations or pseudo-hallucinations—except at high doses. Generally, they cause subtle visualization of dream-like images when the eyes are closed, which disappear when the eyes are open. More prominently, they intensify feeling, whether pleasure, sadness, or anxiety.[37] They are noted for the facilitation of insight and empathy.[16,38–40] They can promote introspection, heightened self-awareness, and greater intuitiveness[24] and can facilitate intimacy with others.[41] They appear to temporarily decrease psychological defense mechanisms, resulting in enhanced communication and a greater willingness to look at personal problems.[42] For these reasons, the psychedelic amphetamines have been used and suggested for use as adjuncts to psychotherapy.[22] A recent study noted that most users reported altered time perception, increased ability to interact with others, decreased defensiveness, decreased fear, decreased sense of separation or alienation from others, changes in visual perception, increased awareness of emotions, and decreased aggression.[43]

The differences among the psychedelic amphetamines include the length of time the psychedelic effect will last. The primary intensity of MMDA can last between 2 and 3 hours, that of MDMA can last between 3 and 5 hours, and that of MDA can last 8–12 hours. The drug DOB has extremely long-lived effects, with peak effects in 3–4 hours and a gradual descent of intensity between 24 and 36 hours.[44] Currently, the most common psychedelic amphetamine is MDMA.

MDMA Use: Adverse Consequences

The following model of the adverse consequences of MDMA use is based on interviews with psychotherapists who have used MDMA in clinical settings, interviews with over 100 people who have used MDMA, and a self-report questionnaire administered to users.

Acute MDMA toxicity. At lower dosages, some people will experience a paradoxical effect of relaxation and calm.[45] Others will develop dry mouth and throat, mild anxiety, agitation, mild apprehension, sweating, temporarily blurred vision, muscle tension in the lower jaw, and teeth grinding.[46] Because people frequently use MDMA for personally important reasons, apprehension about the event may merge with the drug-induced symptoms of anxiety, sometimes causing panic.

At somewhat higher doses, people may experience subtle visual distortions such as afterimages, vibrant geometric shapes with the eyes closed, or visual embellishments such as perceiving something as being shimmering or jittering. Some people may have a compelling need to talk more than normal. People's mood may shift from an empathic understanding of others to a noticeable depression, perhaps shifting a number of times. Some people experience significant anxiety, psychomotor agitation, and tachycardia.

Large doses of MDMA may cause stimulant intoxication, promoting severe symptoms of anxiety such as panic, tachycardia, and mental and behavioral agitation. Symptoms may escalate to hypervigilance, suspiciousness, paranoia, and violence.

Prolonged MDMA toxicity. Some people may take MDMA daily for a week or more on one or more occasions. The first day of MDMA use causes the expected psychedelic effects. The second day of MDMA use causes caffeine-like anxiety symptoms such as restlessness, talkativeness, and agitation. After the second day, tolerance to the anxiety symptoms develops and the symptoms disappear. However, prolonged MDMA use decreases mental clarity, increases mental confusion, and causes periods of memory impairment. Also, there can be mild disorientation and lack of normal motivation. Appetite suppression and insomnia may occur. In general, prolonged use of MDMA decreases the "positive" effects of the drug and increases the negative effects.[41]

MDMA-induced psychopathology. Many people are motivated to use psychedelic drugs to help solve personal problems. Thus, people in the middle of a crisis and people who want to solve long-standing problems may take these drugs as a "quick fix." Although the psychedelic drugs LSD and MDMA are able to bring to conscious awareness information that has been suppressed, they do not help the user to resolve and appropriately deal with these issues. Accordingly, people may become more aware of their problems and realize the depth and complexity of these problems. Thus, psychedelic drugs may cause people to be overwhelmed by the problems they had previously handled to some degree.

During interviews with people who used MDMA for "self-therapy," some individuals with anxiety and depressive disorders reported experiencing an exacerbation of these problems after MDMA use. In general, they described an increase in symptom frequency or an increase in symptom severity, or both. In addition, some people developed psychological problems only after the MDMA experience, primarily describing symptoms of anxiety, panic, and depression.

Finally, one additional MDMA-induced problem should be mentioned. People who use MDMA for nontherapeutic purposes, such as before a rock concert or during a party, sometimes become flooded with intense emotions and long-repressed thoughts and feelings. Some people are able to process the intense experience with friends who provide nonprofessional emotional support. On the other hand, some are overwhelmed by the experience and become deeply depressed, anxious, or both.

■ Drugs With Psychedelic Properties: PCP and Marijuana

Although the primary effects of drugs such as LSD are psychedelic, some drugs have secondary psychedelic effects. These include prescription drugs such as the antiparkinsonian drugs trihexyphenidyl (Artane) and benztropine (Cogentin). Although abuse is rare, at high doses they can cause an anticholinergic intoxication, including visual hallucinations and distortions of body image.[47] Somewhat more commonly used drugs that cause a similar intoxication include the herbs deadly nightshade (*Atropa belladonna*) and jimsonweed (*Datura stramonium*). Intoxication from these drugs can include hallucinations and a state of delirium (agitated mental confusion and disorientation).[48] Far more common drugs of abuse that have psychedelic effects are PCP and marijuana.

Dissociative Anesthetics: PCP and Related Drugs

In many ways, PCP represents the dark side of psychedelic drugs. Although the psychedelic amphetamines can promote empathy and intimacy, PCP is capable of unleashing a volatile, demonic, frenzied rage of violent behavior and psychosis. At worst, PCP can cause temporary madness that results in unbelievable horror and destruction. Oddly, PCP enjoys the quaint name of "Angel Dust" and was known as the "PeaCe Pill" during the late 1960s. PCP and the closely related PCE, TCP, PHP, and PCC are manufactured easily from simple materials.

Between 1963 and 1965, PCP was used for surgical anesthesia. General anesthesia normally involves the complete lack of sensation of pain as a result of unconsciousness. In contrast, PCP causes general anesthesia not by making people unconscious, but by dissociating the mind from the body. Patients retain a level of consciousness but are unconcerned about the surgery. Thus, PCP is called a "dissociative anesthetic."

Although PCP can be considered the prototype dissociative anesthetic, the drug ketamine (Ketalar) is a legal prescription dissociative anesthetic with effects that are nearly identical to those of PCP but that are of shorter duration. It is an analogue or derivative of PCP. In a recent study to document the effects, ketamine was administered to subjects on multiple occasions.[49] Although the psychedelic experiences varied, all subjects experienced most of the following phenomena: a sensation of light throughout the body, distortions of the physical makeup of the self, distortions of body image, perception of floating in space, an experience of leaving the body, visual distortions and visions, distortions of time such as experiencing virtual timelessness, sudden insight into the existence of the self, emotional distortions, and ego boundary distortions. Some subjects noted a sense of empathy that lasted beyond the psychedelic experience.

PCP intoxication. The sought-after effects of PCP intoxication include increased sensitivity to external stimuli, stimulation of mood and behavior, and a sense of intoxication. PCP intoxication invariably involves distortions of sensory perceptions, such as visual distortions, illusions, pseudohallucinations, and hallucinations. PCP intoxication often involves ego boundary distortions, especially a dissociation of the mind from the body and "out of body" experiences.

PCP is fickle because the dosage range between intoxication and toxic effects is narrow. In addition to the desired effects of PCP, a number of possible adverse reactions can occur. These include acute PCP toxicity during PCP intoxication, prolonged toxic psychosis associated with chronic PCP abuse, PCP-precipitated psychotic episodes, and PCP-induced depression.[50]

Acute PCP toxicity. People may have severe reactions within moments or hours of ingestion, lasting from 3 hours to 3 days. Lower doses of PCP may cause episodes of combativeness: people may rapidly become hostile, aggressive, belligerent, and antisocial and may experience severe mental and behavioral agitation. They may have symptoms of disordered thinking, paranoia, negativism, preoccupation with death, depersonalization, and grossly altered body image.[51]

People using low doses of PCP can also experience an episode of catatonia, characterized by extreme muscle rigidity, blank stare, and shallow respiration. At high doses, the analgesia effects become more pronounced, resulting in general anesthesia, stupor, or coma. Still higher doses may result in a prolonged coma, muscle rigidity, and convulsions.[52]

PCP toxic psychosis. After acute PCP toxicity, users—especially chronic users—may develop PCP toxic psychosis. PCP toxic psychosis is characterized by impaired judgment, paranoid delusions, agitation, and both auditory and visual hallucinations. These users may be a danger to themselves or others and may engage in extreme and often bizarre violence. The PCP toxic psychosis is temporary, lasting from 2 days to a week or more.

PCP-precipitated psychotic episodes. Some PCP users will experience psychotic reactions similar to schizophrenia. In contrast to the shorter PCP toxic psychosis, PCP-precipitated psychotic episodes last from a week to a month or more. In effect, a PCP-precipitated psychotic episode represents the use of PCP as a catalyst to prompt the development of an ongoing psychotic episode.

PCP-induced depression. Some PCP users, especially those who have experienced a PCP toxic psychosis or a PCP-precipitated psychosis, may experience severe depression. The depression may be accompanied by temporary memory impairment. The PCP-induced depression may last from 1 day to a month.

Marijuana

Marijuana is the dried leaves and flowering tops of *Cannabis sativa,* a plant containing numerous chemicals, some of which are psychoactive. The most well known of these chemicals is tetrahydrocannabinol (THC). THC is likely the primary psychoactive chemical in marijuana and hashish. Marijuana can be prepared and eaten in foods (such as brownies), but it is generally smoked. Certain potent marijuana strains (for example, sensemilla) have been developed.

Marijuana is the most widely used illicit drug in America. A 1990 survey by the National Institute on Drug Abuse indicated that about one-third of the population has used marijuana at least once, about 10% used marijuana within the past year, and about 5% used marijuana within the past month (Table 4–3). Also, 2.7% of the population reported using marijuana once a week or more.[53]

Marijuana can be described as a depressant drug with psychedelic properties. For instance, marijuana is partially cross-tolerant with alcohol. Thus, people addicted to alcohol and marijuana often increase the consumption of one drug during periods of abstinence from the other, and some people alternate between alcohol and marijuana for the self-medication of insomnia. The psychedelic effects are most noticeable when used in nonchronic patterns by nontolerant users.

Marijuana intoxication. The effects of marijuana are complex and varied, depending on the frequency, the dosage, and variables such as personality characteristics, set, and setting. For the occasional user who has not developed tolerance to the psychedelic effects, marijuana intoxication can have a significant psychedelic effect: peaceful relaxation, a feeling of time slowing down, fantasy thoughts and images, and a self-conscious preoccupation with the process of thinking. Marijuana can affect sensory perceptions, especially visual and auditory stimuli. Because sensory experiences are intensified, marijuana is frequently used during rock music concerts to enhance the music and visual effects. Some people experience a dream-like marijuana euphoria, sometimes with a floating sensation. Mood elevation, laughter, inappropriate laughter, gregariousness, increased appetite, and conjunctival injection ("red eyes") are common. Symptoms and signs begin within a few minutes of smoking and may last 2–4 hours, depending on the dosage and potency.

Acute marijuana toxicity. High doses of marijuana or use of potent marijuana by nontolerant people can result in a variety of intense and largely negative experiences. Marijuana intoxication generally includes an increase in heart rate, although tolerance develops to this effect with chronic use. Reaction to tachycardia and palpitations may include apprehension, anxiety, and fear, culminating in a panic episode. Mood may shift from pleasure to dysphoria and depression, and the depression may be rather morbid. Social gregariousness may be replaced by social withdrawal. Some ego boundary distortions may occur, resulting in depersonalization or body image distortion. Thinking may become distorted, sometimes with a suspicious quality, perhaps leading to a marijuana delusional disorder.

Marijuana delusional disorder. Occasionally, the use of marijuana causes severe but temporary disordering of thinking, including the development of paranoid and persecutory thoughts. Delusions of persecution may be accompanied by anxiety, depression, or depersonalization. This syndrome may last for 4–6 hours. Because marijuana delusional disorder occurs during marijuana intoxication, other symptoms and signs of marijuana intoxication are likely to be present.

Chronic marijuana toxicity. Chronic marijuana use leads to tolerance of the psychedelic effects. Thus, the desired pleasurable effects may diminish, whereas undesirable effects remain unchanged or perhaps increase with chronic use.[54] Daily or prolonged use of marijuana may produce a chronic marijuana toxicity state, commonly called an "amotivational syndrome."[55]

Chronic marijuana use can cause loss of energy and interest in social and occupational areas. Chronic users may become passive, apathetic, and unconcerned about productivity and ambition. They may have poor frustration tolerance, moodiness, and some degree of depression and agitation. Chronic marijuana use impairs intellectual functioning in terms of concentration, the processing of new material, short-term memory, comprehension, judgment, and recalling information. Psychomotor problems include impaired coordination and driving skills.[56]

■ Summary

Psychedelic drugs can cause combinations of an assortment of distortions of thought, feeling, and perception called the psychedelic experience. Elements of the psychedelic experience may include perceptual distortion, emotional distortion, alteration of normal thinking, distortions about the self, and changes in spiritual and psychological perception. Perceptual distortions include alterations in the perception of sight, sound, touch, taste, and smell.

Emotional distortions include increased intensity of mood and emotions, ranging from ecstasy to fear, anxiety, and panic. Mood may alternate between pleasure and depression. Thinking becomes altered: people may become preoccupied with thinking, problem solving may become creative, or a loosening of associations may occur, in which ideas shift from one subject to another. Paranoia, grandiosity, and delusions may occur. The perception of the self may be changed greatly during psychedelic drug use, including ego boundary distortions, depersonalization, and body image distortions. The psychedelic drug experience may also include increased self-awareness; spiritual insights; and enhanced empathy, communication, and trust. Adverse consequences of psychedelic drug use are strongly influenced by preexisting character structure, setting, insecurity, set, negative experience, problems of reentry, dose, frequency of use, and current mood and stress level.

LSD is one of a group of drugs that includes LSD, psilocybin mushrooms, DMT, and DET. They can cause distortions in sensory perception, emotions, thinking, and ego boundaries. They can also promote spiritual experiences and psychotherapeutic effects. Pseudohallucinations and synesthesias are common; hallucinations are less frequent. Emotional experiences may become unusually intense and may change frequently and suddenly.

Psychedelic drug experiences often include three phases. The first phase is characterized by alterations in sensory perceptions. The second phase may include vivid visual imagery in vibrant colors, perhaps progressing to illusions, pseudohallucinations, and hallucinations. Alterations in mood and emotions may occur, perhaps including moody reflections on past experiences, both positive and negative. A third phase of the psychedelic experience centers around changes in philosophical and personal perception. People may become intensely concerned about their personal philosophy, religious and spiritual issues, and the meaning of life. Some people have enhanced psychological perception and insight that result in meaningful life changes. In contrast, some people have apparently profound thoughts that later seem unimportant.

The psychedelic amphetamines have both stimulant and psychedelic properties. They include members of the amphetamine family such as MDA, MDMA, MDE, STP, and mescaline, which comes from the peyote cactus. High doses cause stimulant effects, and low doses cause a narrow range of psychedelic effects, including an intensification of feelings, whether pleasure, sadness, or anxiety. These drugs can facilitate insight and heightened empathy; promote introspection, heightened self-awareness, and greater intuitiveness; and facilitate intimacy with others.

The dissociative anesthetic drugs PCP and ketamine can temporarily dissociate consciousness from the body and cause distortions of body image, visual distortions, illusions, hallucinations, emotional distortions, and ego boundary distortions. PCP toxicity may include combative hostility, paranoia, depersonalization, and violence as well as extreme muscle rigidity and coma. PCP can cause a brief toxic psychosis that may include delusions of persecution, hallucinations, and violence. PCP can also precipitate a psychotic state that may last for a month or more, as well as a severe depression.

Marijuana has depressant and psychedelic properties. Infrequent use can cause psychedelic effects such as peaceful relaxation, fantasy thoughts, distortions of time, and sensory alterations, especially of vision and hearing. Acute marijuana toxicity may include apprehension, anxiety, panic, alternating periods of pleasure and depression, and distorted ego boundaries and body image. Marijuana can cause a delusional disorder, usually a paranoid delusion of being persecuted. Chronic marijuana use may cause a prolonged toxicity characterized by lack of motivation, passivity, poor frustration tolerance, moodiness, and some degree of agitation and depression.

■ References

1. Hemsley DR, Ward ES: Individual differences in reaction to the abuse of LSD. Personality and Individual Differences 6:515–517, 1985
2. Siegal RK: MDMA: nonmedical use and intoxication: the MDMA Conference. Journal of Psychoactive Drugs 18:349–354, 1986
3. Grof S: The use of LSD in psychotherapy. Journal of Psychedelic Drugs 3:52–62, 1970
4. Leary T: The religious experience: its production and interpretation. Journal of Psychedelic Drugs 3:76–86, 1970
5. Pahnke WN, Richards WA: Implications of LSD and experimental mysticism. Journal of Psychedelic Drugs 3:92–108, 1970
6. Grinspoon L, Bakalar JB: Can drugs be used to enhance the psychotherapeutic process? American Journal of Psychotherapy 40:393–404, 1986
7. Grinspoon L, Bakalar JB: Psychedelics and arylcyclohexylamines, in Psychiatric Update: American Psychiatric Association Annual Review, Vol 5. Edited by Frances AJ, Hales RE. Washington, DC, American Psychiatric Association, 1986, pp 213–225

8. Cohen S: The hallucinogens, in Treatments of Psychiatric Disorders: A Task Force Report of the American Psychiatric Association. Washington, DC, American Psychiatric Association, 1989, pp 1203–1209

9. Krippner S: Psychedelic drugs and creativity. Journal of Psychoactive Drugs 17:235–245, 1985

10. Twemlow SW, Bowen WT: Psychedelic drug-induced psychological crises: attitudes of the "crisis therapist." Journal of Psychedelic Drugs 11:331–335, 1979

11. Watson L, Beck J: New Age seekers: MDMA used as an adjunct to spiritual pursuit. Journal of Psychoactive Drugs 23:261–270, 1991

12. de Candolle A: Origin of Cultivated Plants. New York, Hafner Publishing, 1959

13. Elferink JGR: Some little-known hallucinogenic plants of the Aztecs. Journal of Psychoactive Drugs 20:427–435, 1988

14. Timothy Leary press conference. The San Francisco Oracle, December 16, 1966, pp 1–8

15. Hoffer A, Osmond H: The Hallucinogens. New York, Academic Press, 1967

16. Osmond H: A review of the clinical effects of psychotomimetic agents. Annals of the New York Academy of Sciences 66:418–434, 1957

17. Osmond H: On being mad. Saskatchewan Psychiatric Services Journal 1:63–70, 1952

18. Crockett R, Sandison RA, Walk A (eds): Hallucinogenic Drugs and Their Psychotherapeutic Use. London, HK Lewis, 1963

19. Freedman DX: On the use and abuse of LSD. Archives of General Psychiatry 18:330–347, 1968

20. Neill JR: "More than medical significance": LSD and American psychiatry 1953 to 1966. Journal of Psychoactive Drugs 19:39–45, 1987

21. Naranjo C: The Healing Journey—New Approaches to Consciousness. New York, Random House, 1973

22. Turek IS, Soskin RA, Kurland AA: Methylenedioxyamphetamine (MDA) subjective effects. Journal of Psychedelic Drugs 6:7–13, 1974

23. Yensen R, Dileo FB, Rhead JC, et al: MDA-assisted psychotherapy with neurotic outpatients: a pilot study. Journal of Nervous and Mental Disease 163:233–245, 1976

24. Greer G, Tolbert R: Subjective reports of the effects of MDMA in a clinical setting. Journal of Psychoactive Drugs 18:319–327, 1986

25. Thiessen PN, Cook DA: The properties of 3,4-methylenedioxyamphetamine (MDA), II: studies of acute toxicity in the mouse and protection by various agents. Clinical Toxicology 6:193–199, 1973

26. Nichols DE: Differences between the mechanism of action of MDMA, MBDB, and the classic hallucinogens: identification of a new therapeutic class: entactogens. Journal of Psychoactive Drugs 18:305–313, 1986

27. Greer G: Using MDMA in psychotherapy. Advances 2:57–59, 1985

28. Nichols DE, Glennon RA: Medicinal chemistry and structure-activity relationships of hallucinogens, in Hallucinogens: Neurochemical, Behavioral, and Clinical Perspectives. Edited by Jacobs BL. New York, Raven, 1984

29. Smith DE, Wesson DR, Buffum J: MDMA: "Ecstasy" as an adjunct to psychotherapy and a street drug of abuse. California Society for the Treatment of Alcohol and Other Drug Dependencies News 12:1–3, 1985

30. Smith DE, Landry MJ: Psychoactive substance use disorders: drugs and alcohol, in Review of General Psychiatry, 2nd Edition. Edited by Goldman HH. Norwalk, CT, Appleton & Lange, 1988, pp 266–285

31. Smith DE, Seymour RB: Dream becomes nightmare: adverse reactions to LSD. Journal of Psychoactive Drugs 17:297–303, 1985

32. Cohen S: LSD: The varieties of psychotic experience. Journal of Psychoactive Drugs 17:291–296, 1985

33. Bowers MB, Swigar ME: Vulnerability to psychosis associated with hallucinogen use. Psychiatry Research 9:91–97, 1983

34. National Commission on Marijuana and Drug Abuse: Drug Use in America, Problem and Perspective. Washington, DC, U.S. Government Printing Office, 1973

35. Stafford P: Re-creational uses of LSD. Journal of Psychoactive Drugs 17:219–228, 1985

36. Krippner S: Psychedelic drugs and creativity. Journal of Psychoactive Drugs 17:235–245, 1985

37. Shulgin AT: Profiles of Psychedelic Drugs: MDMA. Journal of Psychedelic Drugs 8:331, 1976

38. Naranjo C, Shulgin AT, Sargent T: Evaluation of 3,4-methylenedioxyamphetamine (MDA) as an adjunct to psychotherapy. Medical and Pharmacologic Experiments 17:359–364, 1967

39. Greer G: MDMA: a new psychotropic compound and its effects in humans. Unpublished manuscript, 1983

40. Greer G: Written testimony submitted on behalf of Drs. Grinspoon and Greer, Professors Bakalar and Roberts, United States Department of Justice, Drug Enforcement Administration Hearings, Docket No 84-48, April 22, 1985

41. Peroutka SJ, Newman H, Harris H: Subjective effects of 3,4-methylenedioxymethamphetamine in recreational users. Neuropsychopharmacology 1:273–277, 1988

42. Seymour RB: MDMA. San Francisco, CA, Richard B. Seymour, 1986
43. Liester MB, Grob CS, Bravo GL, et al: Phenomenology and sequelae of 3,4-methylenedioxymethamphetamine use. Journal of Nervous and Mental Disease 180:345–352, 1992
44. Shulgin AT: Profiles of psychedelic drugs: DOB. Journal of Psychoactive Drugs 13:99, 1981
45. Beck J: The popularization and resultant implications of a recently controlled psychoactive substance. Contemporary Drug Problems 13(1):23–63, 1986
46. Riedlinger JE: The scheduling of MDMA: a pharmacist's perspective. Journal of Psychoactive Drugs 17:169–171, 1985
47. Tacke U, Ebert MH: Hallucinogens, in Clinical Manual of Chemical Dependence. Edited by Ciraulo DA, Shader RI. Washington, DC, American Psychiatric Press, 1991, pp 259–278
48. Weil A, Rosen W: Chocolate to Morphine: Understanding Mind-Active Drugs. Boston, MA, Houghton Mifflin, 1983
49. Hansen G, Jensen SB, Chandresh L, et al: The psychotropic effect of ketamine. Journal of Psychoactive Drugs 20:419–425, 1988
50. Smith DE, Wesson DR: PCP abuse: diagnostic and psychopharmacological treatment approaches, in PCP: Problems and Prevention. Edited by Smith DE, Wesson DR, Buxton ME, et al. Dubuque, IA, Kendall/Hunt, 1982, pp 102–108
51. Daghestani AN, Schnoll SH: Phencyclidine abuse and dependence, in Treatments of Psychiatric Disorders: A Task Force Report of the American Psychiatric Association. Washington, DC, American Psychiatric Association, 1989, pp 1209–1218
52. Aniline O, Pitts FN Jr: Phencyclidine (PCP): a review and perspectives. CRC Critical Review of Toxicology 10:145–177, 1982
53. National Institute on Drug Abuse: National Household Survey on Drug Abuse: Population Estimates 1990. Rockville, MD, U.S. Department of Health and Human Services, 1990
54. Weller RA, Halikas JA: Change in effects from marijuana: a five- to six-year study. Journal of Clinical Psychiatry 43:362–365, 1983
55. Smith DE: The acute and chronic toxicity of marijuana. Journal of Psychedelic Drugs 2:37–47, 1968
56. Nicholi AM: The college student and marijuana: research findings concerning adverse biological and psychological effects. Journal of American College Health 32:73–77, 1983

Table 5–1. The inhalants

Type of inhalant	Specific inhalants
Aliphatic nitrites	Amyl nitrite, butyl nitrite, isobutyl nitrite
Aliphatic and aromatic hydrocarbons	Gasoline, petroleum distillates, benzene, hexane, naphtha, toluene, xylene, butane
Halogenated hydrocarbons	Chloroform, methylchloroform, halothane, ethylene dichloride, methylene chloride, trichloroethylene
Fluorinated hydrocarbons (Freons)	Cryofluorane, dichlorodifluoromethane, dichlorotetrafluoromethane, trichlorofluoromethane
Ketones	Acetone, cyclohexanone, methyl ethyl ketone, methyl isobutyl ketone, methyl butyl ketone, methyl amyl ketone
Alcohols and glycols	Methyl alcohol, isopropyl alcohol, ethylene glycol, methylcellulose
Inhalation anesthetics	Diethyl ether, nitrous oxide, enflurane, halothane, isoflurane, methoxyflurane

Chapter 5

The Inhalants

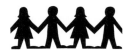

"Getting high" can be cheap, legal—and deadly. Children as young as 9 years old have died from intentional Freon inhalation. Every year, teenagers die from inhaling butane lighter fluid fumes. Others die from deliberately breathing typewriter correction fluid, fabric protector sprays, aerosol propellants, paints, paint thinners, and gasoline. "Sudden sniffing death syndrome" describes the rapid onset of an irregular heartbeat and death in an otherwise healthy individual. Most inhalant abusers don't die, but it is impossible to predict who will suffer fatal consequences. Inhalant abuse can be difficult to detect. The euphoric effects of deliberate inhalation are relatively short-lived, and inhalants are not detected by typical drug screens. Parents, teachers, counselors, and health care professionals must know which inhalants are abused locally, and have some knowledge of the typical behaviors associated with inhalant abuse.

Rose Ann G. Soloway, R.N., M.S.Ed., C.S.P.I.
Education and Communications Coordinator
National Capital Poison Center
Georgetown University Hospital
Washington, D.C.

■ What Are Inhalants?

The inhalants are a group of diverse chemicals that either create fumes or vapors or can be obtained in a gas state and may be inhaled for intoxicating effects. There are three types of inhalants: volatile solvents, volatile nitrites, and anesthetic gases.

Most of the commonly abused inhalants are called *volatile solvents*. The word *volatile* describes chemicals that evaporate or cause fumes when exposed to air. At room temperature these liquid or semiliquid chemicals will create psychoactive vapors and fumes that can be inhaled.

The word solvent describes chemicals such as paint thinners or spot removers that help to dissolve other substances. Volatile solvents are generally produced from petroleum and natural gas.

Volatile solvents are found in various industrial, automotive, and household products such as paints, paint thinners, glues, cleaning fluids, and automotive fuels. Some have been used as pressured propellants in aerosol spray cans.

The *volatile nitrites* are a second type of commonly abused inhalants. Volatile nitrites include amyl nitrite, butyl nitrite, and isobutyl nitrite. These drugs are called vasodilators, meaning that they dilate or widen blood vessels, allowing more blood to flow in the vessels. The volatile nitrites are generally found in a liquid form and create a psychoactive vapor when exposed to air. They cause a mild euphoria.

In addition to the volatile solvents and volatile nitrites, certain *inhalation anesthetics* are also abused. In particular, ether and nitrous oxide are available as gases. They produce a range of reactions from euphoria to anesthesia and can be used during surgical procedures.

■ Volatile Solvents

Where Are They Found?

As mentioned earlier, volatile solvents are found in a variety of household and industrial products. These products include paints, paint thinners, paint and varnish removers, correction fluids and thinners, nonstick cooking sprays, and spot removers.

For instance, nail polish remover may contain acetone or aliphatic acetates and previously contained benzene. Gasoline contains a number of solvents such as naphtha and toluene. Plastic styrene cements and lacquer thinners may contain acetone, aliphatic acetates, toluene, and trichloroethylene. Model or airplane cements may include acetone and toluene. Household cements may include acetone, methyl ethyl ketone, methyl isobutyl ketone, and toluene.

Some household cleaning fluids and spot removers contain trichloroethane, trichloroethylene, and naphtha. One example includes the well-known fabric protector Scotchgard. It was reported that the manufacturer was aware that more than 20 deaths in a 2-year period were directly related to inhaling Scotchgard.[1] Scotchgard contains trichloroethane and Freon as a propellant.

In addition to consumer products that contain solvents as an ingredient, Freon and butane can be purchased directly. For instance, butane can be inhaled directly from disposable lighters or from refill tanks. Similarly, refills of Freon refrigerant can be purchased for just a few dollars. Some people tap into car and home air-conditioner systems and refrigerators to inhale Freon.[2]

Route of Administration

As the name implies, inhalants are generally inhaled through the mouth or nose by using a variety of techniques.[3] Inhalants are generally in a liquid, thick, semiliquid, or vapor state. Thus, the route of administration will vary according to the state.

Inhalants in a liquid form can be inhaled directly from the bottle or receptacle in which they were purchased or stored. For example, butyl and isobutyl nitrite are generally inhaled directly from the bottles in which they are purchased. Inhalant users may inhale chemicals from jars or bottles that they use to store the liquid chemicals. Liquids can be soaked into a cloth and placed on or near the mouth and nose.

Liquids and thicker semiliquid products can be placed into a plastic bag, which is then placed over the mouth and nose. The user then breathes the fumes in the bag. Inhalants can be placed into large bags such as garbage bags, allowing users to cover their entire head with the bag. They may tie the bag around their neck.

In some cases, aerosol sprays may be inhaled directly from the bottle, such as inhaling butane from disposable lighters or Freon from refill bottles. Alternatively, they may be sprayed into a plastic bag, allowing the user to inhale from the bag.

Users often describe the process of inhaling a cloth soaked with a volatile solvent as "huffing," although others may use the term to describe solvent inhalation in general.

Solvent Intoxication

Although the subjective effects vary somewhat, solvent intoxication resembles the intoxication effects of sedatives and hypnotics, but is far more pronounced than alcohol intoxication.[4] The initial sensation may be a brief stimulation and reduction of inhibitions. During this brief disinhibitory phase, users may become impulsive, belligerent, assaultive, or sexually impulsive. However, the predominant reaction is an alcohol-like, depressant intoxication. Symptoms may include slurred speech, unsteady gait, and drowsiness. Solvent users may become lethargic, have slowed reflexes, and possibly feel euphoric.

Solvents may also cause short-term distortions of sensory perception. Users may experience sensations of numbness, weightlessness, and depersonalization. They may experience distortions in time and visual perception. Visual and auditory pseudohallucinations and hallucinations may occur.

The intoxicating effects of toluene and butane may include elevation of mood, hallucinations, and delusions of the ability to fly; toluene can promote slower thoughts, a sensation of time passing quickly, and tactile hallucinations.[5]

Solvent use may cause brief delusions, such as that of invincibility, leading to risky behavior. Impulsivity and violence may occur. While using inhalants, users may have a flushed face and appear intoxicated. They may also display personality changes and appear nervous and moody.

The effects of butane and Freon are generally the same as those of the volatile solvents, except that the Freons have greater cardiac toxicity.

In general, solvent intoxication occurs rapidly, within minutes of inhalation. Symptoms from a single episode of inhalant use may last about an hour.

Acute Solvent Toxicity

As with alcohol, high doses of solvents over a short period of time produce severe symptoms and signs of central nervous system depression. Thus, higher solvent doses and episodes of intense and prolonged inhalation may cause the person to become noticeably incoordinated, have sluggish reactions, and become physically weak. Solvent users often experience headaches, nausea, vomiting, dizziness, confusion, and stupor. Still higher doses may cause sleep, anesthesia, coma, and death.

Single episodes of solvent use may cause serious medical problems, including death. Solvent use may cause a severe depression of the central nervous system, including the brain's respiratory center. This depression can lead to the sudden cessation of breathing, failure of oxygen to reach tissues, cardiac arrest, brain damage, coma, and death.

Similarly, suffocation can occur if a user loses consciousness while solvent-rich cloth is next to the mouth and nose, or if a user asphyxiates while a plastic bag covers the face or entire head.

Solvents can cause extremely rapid, irregular, ineffective, and uncoordinated contractions of the heart, called ventricular fibrillation. As a result, the heart ceases to pump blood effectively, causing death.

Inhalants may also cause damage to the lungs and airway. For instance, Freon inhalation may cause freezing of the airway and lungs as a result of rapid vaporization. During use, aerosols may replace oxygen and prevent it from being absorbed in the lungs. Thus, prolonged use of aerosols may cause brain damage because of insufficient oxygen circulating in the blood.

Chronic Solvent Toxicity

Because inhalants such as solvents are essentially poisons, they can cause severe damage to living tissue. Thus, chronic solvent use may cause damage to the mucous membranes lining the nose and throat.

Inhalants can cause severe or fatal damage to the airway or lungs with chronic use; severe lung inflammation may occur. Inhaling gases directly from high-pressure tanks can cause immediate damage to the lungs.

Solvents may also cause damage to the tissues of the kidney, liver, and brain. Chronic use of volatile solvents is associated with deterioration of neurological, psychiatric, and intellectual dysfunction.[6] Serious psychiatric consequences of solvent inhalation—especially toluene-based solvents—include paranoid psychosis that may persist, temporal lobe epilepsy, and decreased IQ. Furthermore, studies suggest that these effects are serious and potentially irreversible.[7]

For instance, prolonged use of toluene is known to cause atrophy or shrinking of the brain, profound impairment of motor control, and impairment of some intellectual and memory capacities.[8-11] These impairments and neurological abnormalities are persistent if not permanent.[12]

Long-term exposure to solvents may cause aplastic anemia, a medical problem in which the bone marrow can no longer make red blood cells. Because red blood cells carry oxygen, their decreased numbers cause reduction of oxygen-rich blood and lack of oxygen in body tissue. The chronic inhalation of gasoline may result in toxic levels of lead.

Many of the volatile solvents are extremely flammable. Users risk experiencing explosions and burns when they use these agents near flames.

■ Volatile Nitrites

What Are "Poppers"?

The volatile nitrites include amyl, butyl, and isobutyl nitrite. These chemicals have been used medically as vasodilators—drugs used to dilate or open narrow blood vessels.

For example, amyl nitrite is a prescription medication that can be used to treat angina pectoris. Angina pectoris is the name for chest pain caused by an inadequate supply of blood to the heart muscle, often because the cardiac blood vessels are clogged or too narrow.

Amyl nitrite can dilate or widen these cardiac blood vessels and increase the amount of oxygen-rich blood flowing to the heart muscle, thus avoiding heart muscle death.

Amyl nitrite is prepared for medical use in a very thin glass ampule that is covered in a gauze material. The drug is administered by breaking the glass ampule, allowing the drug to soak the gauze, and having the patient inhale the vapors. The name "poppers" was derived from the fact that the glass ampule must be "popped" to be used. In current usage, the term "poppers" also describes butyl and isobutyl nitrite even though they are not sold in glass ampules.

Unlike amyl nitrite, butyl and isobutyl nitrite are not prescription drugs. For some reason, they are not federally regulated. Most people have seen these drugs, but did not know that they were, in fact, drugs.

Butyl nitrite and isobutyl nitrite are commonly sold in convenience stores, poster shops, drug paraphernalia shops, and certain gay-oriented bookstores and shops. They are marketed deceptively as "room odorizers," with names such as "Locker Room," "Rush," "Kick," and "Bolt," in very small screw-top glass containers.[13]

The Effects of Nitrite Inhalants

The initial effect of the nitrite inhalers is a "head rush," or a sensation of fullness in the head. This effect is likely due to the dilation or enlargement of blood vessels in the brain. After this brief experience, users typically experience a mild euphoria that begins a few seconds after inhalation and lasts for perhaps a minute.

During this brief euphoria, users experience a sudden drop in blood pressure, which causes a state of consciousness that may resemble becoming faint or going under general anesthesia. Symptoms often include a feeling of warmth and flushing of the skin, lightheadedness, and dizziness.[14] The euphoria often includes a distorted perception of time, generally that time is being slowed down.

During the 1980s, the nitrite inhalers gained popularity as aphrodisiacs. They were thought to enhance libido and to intensify and prolong orgasm. During the 1960s through the 1970s, the nitrite inhalers were in particularly wide use among certain gay male groups. They were commonly used in gay bars, gay bath houses, and at gay dances. Nitrite inhalant use among gay men began declining during the 1980s, while it remained constant among nongay drug users.[15]

One of the known effects of the nitrite inhalers is relaxation of the rectal sphincter tone. Although the use of nitrite inhalers during the 1980s was significant in the gay male community, it is not known whether the predominant motivation was the euphoric or the physiological effects.[16]

One of the reasons for the decline in inhalant use by gay men relates to the apparent relationship between nitrite inhalant use and acquired immunodeficiency syndrome (AIDS). Indeed, nitrite inhalant use seems to be related to suppression of immune function,[17] although the use of nitrite inhalants is likely one of many factors necessary for the development of cancers and AIDS.

The nitrite inhalants also cause problems with the respiratory system. These chemical fumes are irritating to the respiratory system and can cause a bronchitis-like syndrome. In addition, the nitrites hamper red blood cell activity, reducing the amount of oxygen delivered to body tissue and perhaps promoting additional respiratory problems.

■ Inhalation Anesthetics

Ether and Nitrous Oxide

Ether was the first general anesthetic, commonly used for surgery until the 1930s. As a general anesthetic, it suppresses pain and other sensations by depressing brain activity to the point of unconsciousness. This depression of central nervous system activity is very strong and occurs within seconds of inhalation.

Ether causes complete loss of consciousness. The patient will remain unconscious as long as ether is administered and for a short while afterward. Because ether has powerful depressant activity, it can cause death by stopping the respiration center of the brain.

At doses lower than those needed for general anesthesia, ether causes a sedative-hypnotic type of intoxication resembling alcohol intoxication. Some people experience mystical revelations and profound insights during ether use.

For use as a general anesthetic, ether is soaked into a gauze mask placed over the patient's nose and mouth. The ether fumes cause pain relief, profound muscle relaxation, and a state of unconsciousness. It is among the safest of anesthetics. However, it is particularly flammable. Even small amounts of static electricity can cause ether to explode. Thus, ether has been replaced by safer general anesthetics in North America but continues to be used in less developed countries.

Nitrous oxide is a somewhat weaker drug than ether and other general anesthetics. Nitrous oxide does not produce complete loss of consciousness or anesthesia deep enough for major surgery.

Also, because nitrous oxide does not significantly depress respiration, it is safer than some other general anesthetics. Often, nitrous oxide is used to make surgical patients relaxed and semiconscious before giving them stronger general anesthetics.

Nitrous oxide can be abused in a variety of ways. Large tanks of the gas are common in dentists' offices, and they can be easily ordered by a physician, clinic, or hospital. These tanks can be diverted for personal use or for use at parties. In a medical setting, nitrous oxide and oxygen are usually inhaled simultaneously through a mask.

In a nonmedical setting, nitrous oxide is inhaled by attaching a rubber hose to the tank or by filling balloons and breathing the gas. Nitrous oxide can be used as a propellant for products such as whipped cream, and it is often inhaled directly from the nozzle of unshaken, upright cans of whipped cream.

The intoxication from nitrous oxide is a complex experience that resembles a combination of intoxication from sedative-hypnotic drugs and intoxication from psychedelic drugs.[18] Most users experience a positive mood that is calm, pleasant, and perhaps euphoric. Some users have a mild to moderate psychedelic experience, including introspection and transcendence. Nitrous oxide intoxication causes impairment in cognition, time perception, and psychomotor activity.

■ Summary

The inhalants are a group of diverse chemicals that either create fumes or vapors or can be obtained in a gas state and may be inhaled for intoxicating effects. There are three broad types of inhalants: volatile solvents, volatile nitrites, and anesthetic gases.

Most of the commonly abused inhalants are volatile solvents. They are described as volatile because they are liquids or semiliquids that evaporate or cause fumes when exposed to air. Products such as paint thinners, nail polish removers, and spot removers are called solvents because they help to dissolve other substances. Volatile solvents are found in paints, paint thinners, glues, cleaning fluids, and automotive fuels. Related chemicals include butane and Freon, which are commonly found in a gas form. Because volatile solvents are often volatile liquids, users can inhale the fumes directly from a container, pour the liquid into plastic bags for inhalation, or soak a cloth with the substance and inhale the vapors.

Volatile-solvent intoxication resembles sedative-hypnotic intoxication, but it is more intense and often more severe. Users may experience a period of disinhibition stimulation, which may provoke aggressive and violent behavior. After that brief phase, inhalant intoxication predominantly resembles the central nervous system depression caused by alcohol, with users experiencing lethargy, slowed reflexes, and sensory distortions. Volatile solvents may cause depression of the respiration center and death. Chronic solvent use may cause severe psychiatric and neurological problems and cause damage to the airways, lungs, kidneys, liver, and brain.

Volatile nitrites include amyl nitrite, butyl nitrite, and isobutyl nitrite. These vasodilators have been used to treat poor blood flow in cardiac blood vessels. Amyl nitrite is a prescription drug used for this purpose, whereas butyl and isobutyl nitrite are generally sold deceptively as "room odorizers." These drugs cause a "head rush," or a sensation of fullness in the head, and cause a sudden drop in blood pressure (which may be experienced as becoming faint or undergoing anesthesia), a feeling of warmth and flushing of the skin, lightheadedness, dizziness, and possible distortions in perception.

Inhalation anesthetics such as ether and nitrous oxide are also abused. They produce a range of reactions from euphoria to anesthesia. They cause general anesthesia by depressing the activity of the brain. Ether is more potent and causes total loss of consciousness, whereas nitrous oxide produces a less deep state of anesthesia. Nitrous oxide intoxication is a complex experience that resembles a combination of intoxication from sedative-hypnotic drugs and intoxication from psychedelic drugs. Most users experience a positive mood that is calm, pleasant, and perhaps euphoric. Some users have a mild to moderate psychedelic experience, including introspection and transcendence. Nitrous oxide intoxication causes impairment in cognition, time perception, and psychomotor activity.

Among the inhalants, the volatile solvents are particularly dangerous because even casual use of these agents can cause sudden death. Equally important is the fact that the volatile solvents are used in a vast number of industrial and household products. They are often rather inexpensive and can be obtained by the very young and the very poor.

■ References

1. Hiaasen R: Newest deadly high among youths: inhaling Scotchgard. The Virginian-Pilot, April 8, 1991, p B4
2. Holmberg M: Freon, butane are "cool" but can be deadly. Richmond Times-Dispatch, September 11, 1990, pp 1–2
3. Barnes GE: Solvent abuse: a review. International Journal of the Addictions 14:1–26, 1979
4. Addiction Research Foundation: Drugs and Drug Abuse, A Reference Text. Toronto, Canada, Addiction Research Foundation, 1987
5. Evans AC, Raistrick D: Phenomenology of intoxication with toluene-based adhesives and butane gas. British Journal of Psychiatry 150:769–773, 1987
6. Ron MA: Volatile substance abuse: a review of possible long-term neurological, intellectual and psychiatric sequelae. British Journal of Psychiatry 148:235–246, 1986
7. Byrne A, Kirby B, Zibin T, et al: Psychiatric and neurologic effects of chronic solvent abuse. Canadian Journal of Psychiatry 36:735–738, 1991
8. Fornazzari L, Wilkinson DA, Kapur BM, et al: Cerebellar, cortical, and functional impairment in toluene abusers. Acta Neurologica Scandinavica 67:319–329, 1983
9. Schikler KN, Seitz K, Rice JF, et al: Solvent abuse associated cortical atrophy. Journal of Adolescent Health Care 3:37–39, 1982

10. Allison WM, Jerrom DW: Glue sniffing: a pilot study of the cognitive effects of long-term use. International Journal of the Addictions 19:453–458, 1984
11. Spencer PS, Schaumburg HH: Organic solvent neurotoxicity: facts and research needs. Scandinavian Journal of Work, Environment and Health 11 (suppl 1):53–60, 1985
12. Hormes JT, Filley CM, Rosenberg NL: Neurologic sequelae of chronic solvent vapor abuse. Neurology 36:698–702, 1986
13. Inaba DS, Cohen WE: Uppers, Downers, All Arounders. Ashland, OR, Cinemed, 1989
14. Schwartz RH, Peary P: Abuse of isobutyl nitrite inhalation (Rush) by adolescents. Clinical Pediatrics 25:308–310, 1986
15. Lange W, Dax EM, Haertzen CA: Nitrite inhalants: contemporary patterns of abuse, in National Institute on Drug Abuse Research Monograph Series No 83. Rockville, MD, U.S. Department of Health and Human Services, 1988, pp 86–95
16. Schuckit MA: The nitrite inhalants. Drug Abuse and Alcoholism Newsletter 19(10):1–4, 1990
17. Dax EM, Nagel JE, Lange WR, et al: Effects of nitrites on the immune system of humans, in National Institute on Drug Abuse Research Monograph Series No 83. Rockville, MD, U.S. Department of Health and Human Services, 1988, pp 75–80
18. Atkinson RM, Green JD, Chenoweth DE, et al: Subjective effects of nitrous oxide: cognitive, emotional, perceptual and transcendental experiences. Journal of Psychoactive Drugs 11:317–330, 1979

Treating Addiction: From Intervention to Recovery

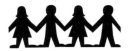

■ Introduction

The second half of this book describes the mechanisms by which family members and health care professionals can intervene, arrest the addiction, and allow the treatment and recovery processes to begin. Chapter 6 provides an overview of the treatment process, including the different levels of care and the variety of treatment settings. The chapter also contains a description of the phases and critical components of the treatment process.

Chapter 7 contains an explanation of the process, phases, and elements of recovery. Also described are frequently seen characteristics of good recovery and the relationship between recovery and relapse. Recommendations about appropriate family responses to relapse are included.

Critical to understanding addiction is an understanding of unconscious defense mechanisms that help to sustain the addiction and distort the addicted person's perception of reality. Thus, Chapter 8 contains descriptions of unconscious defense mechanisms such as denial, minimization, rationalization, intellectualization, projection, regression, and physical isolation. Also described is the relationship of blackouts and euphoric recall to defense mechanisms. In addition, the chapter covers defense mechanisms frequently seen in family members, including enabling and codependence.

The process of arresting the addiction at least long enough to initiate treatment is called addiction intervention. Chapter 9 contains a description of the intervention process, including data gathering, team building, education, planning, and implementation.

In Chapter 10, special issues that relate to adolescents who are addicted are identified. This chapter was written in collaboration with adolescent addiction specialist and psychiatrist Martha A. Morrison, M.D., Medical Director of Young Adult Services for Talbott Recovery System and Anchor Hospital, Atlanta, Georgia. This chapter contains descriptions of important developmental tasks of adolescents, as well as an explanation of how psychoactive drugs may be used to deal with these tasks. Various triggers for adolescent problems and the different course of addiction for adolescents are also described.

The relationships between psychoactive drugs and psychiatric problems are described in Chapter 11, including the problem of dual disorders (the coexistence of psychiatric and substance use disorders). This chapter contains a review of some of the problems that relate to people with dual disorders, including treatment approaches, conflicts with medications, use of medication and self-help groups, and the related issues of double treatment and double recovery.

The appropriate use of medications during the treatment and recovery processes is described in Chapter 12. Included is a review of the use of medications during the detoxification phase and for treatment of prolonged withdrawal, as well as the use of disulfiram (Antabuse) and naltrexone. In addition, the chapter contains a discussion of the role of methadone for both detoxification and maintenance of opioid addiction.

Chapter 13 contains an overview of the research on alcoholism. In part because alcohol is far more widely used than all other illicit drugs combined, there has been far more research on the process of addiction to alcohol than to other drugs. In particular, biopsychosocial risk factors for developing addiction to alcohol are described, and the various genetic studies—including twin, adoption, and animal studies—are reviewed.

■ Themes and Perspectives

Several assertions and themes that make it easier to understand the processes of addiction, treatment, and recovery run throughout this book. In many ways, these themes help to create a unitary theory of addiction rather than an understanding based on fragmentary knowledge.

■ **The word *drug* means all psychoactive, mood-altering chemicals.** In the popular culture, people often make unnatural distinctions between alcohol and other drugs. These distinctions are political, legal, or cultural. Alcohol is indeed a drug—a legal drug—whereas some drugs are controlled by prescription, and others are illegal for personal use.

In relation to the diagnosis, treatment, and recovery from addiction, the distinction between legal and illegal drugs is artificial. In this book, drugs are described in terms of their effects on people's behavior, emotions, and thinking, not in terms of their political, legal, or cultural status.

Accordingly, the word *drug* or *psychoactive drug* is used to describe all psychoactive, mood-altering chemicals, including alcohol.

■ **Addiction, not the drug, is the focus.** Just as popular culture creates an artificial distinction between alcohol and other drugs, so it often creates a distinction between people addicted to alcohol and people addicted to other drugs. In terms of addiction, treatment, recovery, and relapse, this distinction is artificial.

An underlying theme in this book is the fact that addiction is a process that involves multiple influences, including biological factors, environmental factors, psychological factors, social factors, and pharmacologic issues. Regardless of the drug of choice, the development and progression of addiction, as well as the processes of treatment, recovery, and relapse, are far more similar than they are different.

Therefore, the phrase "addicted people" describes all people who have developed the disease of addiction. That includes people addicted to any psychoactive drug, including alcohol, prescription drugs, marijuana, and even Freon. The focus of the term *addiction* is on the presence and process of the addiction, not on the specific drug of choice, which often changes and is often used in combination with other drugs.

■ **Addiction is a primary biopsychosocial disease.** Throughout this book, addiction is described as a biopsychosocial disease. This term implies the presence of two separate principles. First, the initiation, development, and progression of addiction are influenced by biological, psychological, and social factors.[1] In turn, the addiction process strongly influences people's biological, psychological, and social lives.

Addiction is accurately described as a medical disease because it has characteristic symptoms and signs and a reliable prognosis or course of action if left untreated and it requires appropriate medical treatment. Addiction does not occur because of poor willpower or because some people lack good sense. Addiction is not the secondary symptom of an underlying psychiatric disorder. Rather, addiction is a primary disorder in its own right, and it demands a sobriety-oriented biopsychosocial treatment and recovery process.

■ **Addiction, treatment, recovery, and relapse are all processes.** One of the most important ideas presented in this book is that addiction, treatment, recovery, and relapse are all processes with identifiable stages. Because they are all processes, they can be described in terms of characteristic symptoms and signs.

As a result, these processes can be identified in terms of early or late stage and can be described in terms of the quality of the process. For instance, addiction can be severe or moderate, treatment can be optimal or minimal, recovery can be full or partial, and relapse can be early or full.

Using cocaine as the example, Figure I–1 depicts the progression of addiction from experimental use to compulsive and dysfunctional use. As the cocaine user becomes progressively more

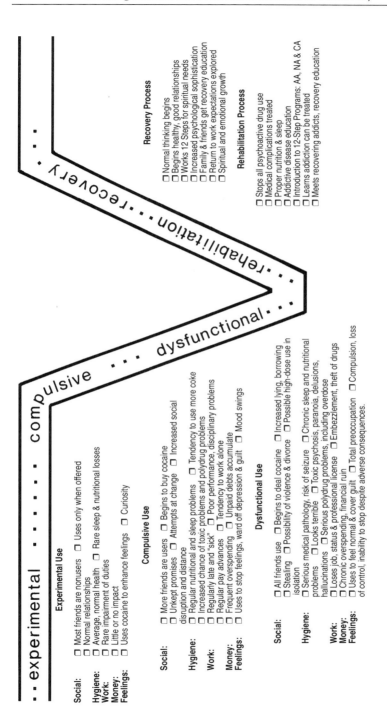

Experimental Use

Social:
- Most friends are nonusers ☐ Uses only when offered
- Normal relationships

Hygiene: Average, normal health ☐ Rare sleep & nutritional losses
Work: Rare impairment of duties
Money: Little or no impact
Feelings: Uses cocaine to enhance feelings ☐ Curiosity

Compulsive Use

Social:
- More friends are users ☐ Begins to buy cocaine
- Unkept promises ☐ Attempts at change ☐ Increased social disruption and distance

Hygiene: Regular nutritional and sleep problems ☐ Tendency to use more coke
☐ Increased chance of toxic problems and polydrug problems
Work: Regularly late and "sick" ☐ Poor performance, disciplinary problems
☐ Regular pay advances ☐ Tendency to work alone
Money: Frequent overspending ☐ Unpaid debts accumulate
Feelings: Uses to stop feelings; ward off depression & guilt ☐ Mood swings

Dysfunctional Use

Social:
- All friends use ☐ Begins to deal cocaine ☐ Increased lying, borrowing
- ☐ Stealing ☐ Possibility of violence & divorce ☐ Possible high-dose use in isolation

Hygiene: Serious medical pathology, risk of seizure ☐ Chronic sleep and nutritional problems ☐ Looks terrible ☐ Toxic psychosis, paranoia, delusions, hallucinations ☐ Serious polydrug problems, including overdose
Work: Loses job, status & professional license ☐ Embezzlement, theft of drugs
Money: Chronic overspending, financial ruin
Feelings: Uses to feel normal & cover guilt ☐ Total preoccupation ☐ Compulsion, loss of control, inability to stop despite adverse consequences.

Recovery Process

- Normal thinking begins
- Begins healthy, good relationships
- Works 12 Steps for spiritual needs
- Increased psychological sophistication
- Family & friends get recovery education
- Return to work expectations explored
- Spiritual and emotional growth

Rehabilitation Process

- Stops all psychoactive drug use
- Medical complications treated
- Proper nutrition & sleep
- Addictive disease education
- Introduction to 12-Step Programs: AA, NA & CA
- Learns addiction can be treated
- Meets recovering addicts, recovery education

Figure I–1. Cocaine abuse: progression and recovery. *Source.* Reprinted with permission from Smith DE: "Cocaine-Alcohol Abuse: Epidemiological, Diagnostic and Treatment Considerations." *Journal of Psychoactive Drugs* 18(2):119, 1988. Figure by Mim Landry.

addicted, a number of critical areas of life become impaired. In this example, cocaine-addicted people experience progressive deterioration with respect to their social life, their physical and psychological hygiene, and problems related to work, finances, feelings, and emotions.

After intervention and arrest of the addiction, rehabilitation begins the process of reversing addiction-induced impairment. The recovery process involves further reversal of addiction-related impairment, and it characterizes the addicted person's emotional, social, and spiritual growth beyond predrug use.

■ Reference

1. Donovan DM: Assessment of addictive behaviors: implications of an emerging biopsychosocial model, in Assessment of Addictive Behaviors. Edited by Donovan DM, Marlatt GA. New York, Guilford, 1988, pp 3–48

Chapter 6

The Treatment Process

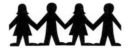

Addiction treatment requires a holistic and systemic approach to address the physical, psychological, social, and spiritual consequences of addiction, not only for patients, but also for their family and significant others. Therapy for drug addiction may include didactic and experiential learning; group, family, and individual counseling; and participation in the Twelve-Step groups such as Alcoholics Anonymous. Treatment can include addiction education, legal counseling, vocational training, parenting skills, recreation therapy, and relapse prevention training. Many aspects of treatment should be individually tailored to meet the specific needs of individual patients and family members. A stepped approach—succeeding from more to less structured treatment—is often required, with increased intensity during episodes of stress or relapse.

Lori D. Karan, M.D.
Medical Director, Inpatient Services
Assistant Professor of Medicine and Psychiatry
Division of Substance Abuse Medicine
The Medical College of Virginia
Richmond, Virginia

What Is Addiction Treatment?

Addiction is far from the mere use of drugs on a frequent basis; rather, it is a process that involves progressive impairment in addicted people's physical, cognitive, psychological, emotional, social, and spiritual lives. A shortcut to describing this multidimensional process is to describe addiction as a biopsychosocial disease.

Because addiction can cause impairment in several areas of life, addiction treatment must address all these areas. Although the process of addiction is remarkably similar (even among people addicted to different drugs), the specific areas in which addiction causes damage and impairment differ among people. For example, one person may have intense physical dependence on alcohol and require detoxification; someone else may feel suicidal during cocaine withdrawal and require antidepressant medication and short-term observation; someone else may have no drug-free friends; another may need housing and a job. These are examples of treatment needs.

Not only do different people have different treatment needs, but treatment needs also change over time: as some treatment needs get met, other treatment needs become apparent. As a result, addiction treatment must be flexible and must involve a wide range of strategies and services that can address each patient's individual biopsychosocial treatment needs. Thus, *addiction treatment* is a biopsychosocial therapeutic strategy designed to address the specific treatment needs of people who are addicted.

Addiction Treatment: Levels of Care

The spectrum of addiction treatment services ranges from basic addiction education and counseling to intense medical and psychiatric care. Treatment services can be described or grouped in progressively intense levels of care: 1) outpatient, 2) intensive outpatient, and 3) inpatient addiction treatment. These levels of care differ with regard to the types of treatment services that are available, the intensity of treatment, and the range of treatment options. Each level of care itself encompasses a range of treatment services and intensity.

Outpatient Treatment

Outpatient addiction treatment is the least intense level of care. Because it involves few treatment services at one time, it consists of only a few hours of treatment per week. Thus, outpatient treatment is appropriate for patients who do not have intense treatment needs. Treatment services may include as little as one individual or group session per week or as many as 8 hours per week of some combination of services (for example, medical examinations, medical detoxification, psychiatric evaluations, educational components, individual therapy, group therapy, and family therapy). Many outpatient treatment programs only offer individual or group therapy. Some provide treatment for addiction-related problems, such as relapse prevention, codependence, spouse abuse, incest, and violence.

The people who are appropriate for this level of care are often employed, have stable and supportive social and family environments, recognize the existence of the problem, and desire help.[1] Outpatient treatment programs may or may not provide medical and psychiatric evaluation and management. Thus, outpatient treatment programs differ in their ability to provide treatment for medical and psychiatric crises and detoxification.

Outpatient addiction treatment can be provided in a variety of different settings: community-based, nonprofit treatment programs; public- and community-sector programs; private outpatient treatment programs; and satellite therapy programs affiliated with hospitals. Outpatient treatment services also include the aftercare or continuing-care phase that follows more intensive treatment.

Intensive Outpatient Treatment

Intensive outpatient addiction treatment describes a moderate to intensive level of care. Because several treatment services are provided, there may be from 9 to more than 60 hours of treatment each week. Intensive outpatient treatment can be provided in several ways. Some programs provide a few hours of treatment on weekday evenings and several hours each weekend (an evening program). Other programs provide as many as 8 hours of treatment each day

(day programs). Patients may participate in intensive outpatient treatment for 6–12 weeks or more.

Compared with outpatient treatment, intensive outpatient treatment offers more structure and more hours of treatment per week; it also can provide multiple treatment components in the same setting. For instance, an intensive outpatient treatment program has more time for educational classes, including daily education groups on medical aspects of addiction, relapse prevention, stress management, relationships, assertiveness, nutrition, and emotional well-being. This level of care allows greater access to family, group, and individual therapy; therapeutic exercises; and drug-free recreational activities.

Intensive outpatient treatment also allows for increased bonding among peers in treatment, which may facilitate a drug-free social network of friends who have sobriety as a central focus. The frequent contact with treatment providers and other patients is a more intensive exposure to addiction treatment. It also allows treatment providers to observe subtle changes in patients and intervene on small problems as they emerge, before the problems progress.

Partial hospitalization or day treatment. Partial hospitalization is a form of intensive outpatient treatment that resembles inpatient treatment but that is not 24 hours per day.[2] Patients may participate for 8 hours daily for 5, 6, or 7 days per week for several months.

Because patients attend treatment during the day but return home each evening, the costs are far lower than those for inpatient hospitalization. These programs may provide limited medical and nursing care, which further lowers the treatment costs. However, they often provide a thorough physical examination on admission and weekly or periodic medical examinations during the stay. Except for the lack of structure in the evenings, partial hospitalization can provide the same type of psychosocial rehabilitation as residential and inpatient hospitalization.

Residential treatment. Residential addiction treatment can describe a variety of programs that involve living on the premises with other people in treatment. They include long-term therapeutic communities; short-term, nonmedical ("social model") detoxification residences; and halfway houses. Some of these programs combine partial hospitalization with a residential setting.

In this model, patients attend a partial-hospitalization program during the day and return to the residence after the treatment day. The residence may be a house or an apartment that is used exclusively for these patients. Ideally, a health care professional or paraprofessional works as a residence manager to provide some level of supervision and crisis management.

In residential treatment, patients are often responsible for normal activities of daily living. Many programs are designed so that patients are responsible for obtaining and preparing their own meals, doing their own laundry, keeping the residence clean, and keeping house rules. Thus, residential treatment forces patients to communicate with one other, learn to compromise, become interdependent, and learn to be responsible for their own behavior. Simple projects such as deciding what to cook for meals become therapeutic exercises in communication, compromise, and cooperation.

The intensity of living with other addicted people can be significant. Naturally, there will be episodes of anger, disagreement, and distrust. These problems will be addressed in group therapy sessions if they are not resolved appropriately within the residence. Patients learn that experiencing problems is not unhealthy, as long as the problems are resolved and worked through. They learn that avoiding problems, stuffing emotions, and pretending that nothing is wrong is unhealthy.

Residential treatment is designed to mimic the natural, healthy family. It is also an opportunity to establish healthy habits, such as attending Twelve-Step programs such as Alcoholics Anonymous (AA), Narcotics Anonymous, and Cocaine Anonymous. Typically, residential programs have on-site Twelve-Step meetings, and residents attend outside meetings as well.

Inpatient Hospitalization

During the 1980s, inpatient hospitalization increased significantly, in part because of public awareness of cocaine addiction. During that time, 30-day inpatient treatment programs became the norm. Today, treatment often occurs in a combination of inpatient, residential treatment, day treatment, intensive outpatient, and outpatient treatment settings.

Inpatient settings can offer substantially more intensive medical, psychiatric, and nursing intervention. Thus, inpatient hospitalization is particularly valuable for medical and psychiatric evaluations, medical management of detoxification, management of medical problems related and unrelated to the addiction, and psychiatric crises.

Because of the accessibility to medical and psychiatric care, the inpatient setting is often the site for intensive medical, psychiatric, and psychosocial evaluations. These evaluations are particularly valuable when there is a question about whether or not an individual is addicted.

Some hospitals provide multiple levels of treatment. For instance, a program may have a detoxification and psychiatric unit to medically manage drug detoxification and psychiatric crises. This program will likely have a rehabilitation unit for patients who no longer need intensive medical, psychiatric, and nursing supervision and intervention. Many programs will also offer residential treatment or day treatment in a different area of the hospital or perhaps off the premises. Some programs offer one or more components of treatment and cooperate with other programs and agencies to help provide a continuum of care.

Selecting Appropriate Treatment

The selection of a treatment program can be bewildering to a family in the middle of a crisis. Nonprofit programs such as local chapters of the National Council on Alcoholism and Other Drug Dependencies and various community programs can provide a summary of local treatment resources. In addition, these programs can often suggest levels of care based on interviews with family members and the addicted family member. However, a more precise recommendation should be made only after the patient has been assessed by health care professionals. Many treatment programs provide free assessments and make recommendations about the level of treatment.

However, for-profit treatment programs are competitive businesses and are profit-driven. They make greater profits when patients are treated in inpatient settings. Recommendations about treatment selection should be based on a variety of objective factors, some of which are described in Table 6–1.

The selection of a treatment program and an appropriate level of care should be based on the specific treatment needs of the patient. The American Society for Addiction Medicine has described a system for placing patients in the appropriate level of care that involves evaluation of six dimensions.[3] Increased risks for problems in these dimensions suggest more intensive levels of care. These dimensions can be described as follows:

- What is the patient's risk for withdrawal?
- What is the patient's risk for medical complications?
- What are the patient's risks for emotional and behavioral conditions?
- What is the patient's level of treatment acceptance or resistance?
- What is the patient's potential for relapse?

Table 6–1. Suggested guidelines for treatment setting

Suggests intense levels of care	Suggests less intense levels of care
Serious medical problems	No medical crises
Severe withdrawal syndrome	No or minor withdrawal
Severe psychiatric crises	No psychiatric crises
Severe denial of addiction	States awareness of problem
Intensely avoiding treatment	Requests help for problem
Appears to be a flight risk	Resigned to treatment
Long-term severe addiction	Mild, recent addiction
Chronic psychiatric problems	Overall good mental health
Other efforts unsuccessful	Completed previous treatment phase
Lack of family or social support	Family cooperation and support
Family members are addicted	Family attends Al-Anon
Thinks others are the problem	Willing to work for recovery

■ Does the patient's environment support recovery? Does the patient have the skills or supports to handle an unsupportive environment?

■ Phases and Components of Treatment

The phases of addiction treatment include evaluation and assessment, treatment planning, medical and psychiatric management, psychosocial rehabilitation, and continuing care.

Evaluation and Assessment

Many treatment programs provide free addiction screenings. An *addiction screening* is a brief evaluation that helps to determine whether an individual has a substance use disorder and whether further evaluation is recommended. Local chapters of the National Council on Alcoholism and Other Drug Dependencies perform free screenings, provide basic addiction education, and explore local treatment options.

When a screening suggests that an individual requires further evaluation, a diagnostic evaluation is performed. Whereas an addiction screening can suggest that an individual probably has a substance use disorder, a *diagnostic evaluation* documents the presence of a substance use disorder and specifically describes that disorder. Based on the diagnosis, health care professionals have a general idea of the nature of an individual's problem.

But because the goal of addiction treatment is to provide therapeutic services that directly address the individual treatment needs of each patient, the treatment needs must be identified. This is done through a series of assessments. The more intensive the level of care, the wider the variety and intensity of the assessments.

Intake evaluation. An intake evaluation may include an addiction screening and a diagnostic assessment, as well as a comprehensive history of the patient's substance use disorders. When performed by medical or nursing staff, the intake evaluation documents the patient's medical condition and medical history and includes an analysis of the patient's current neurological and psychological concerns.

The intake evaluation is often the basis for a decision to admit the patient or to make a referral to a more appropriate emergency or specialized medical or psychiatric program rather than, or before, admission for addiction treatment.[4] It is a clinical snapshot of the individual on arrival to the program.

Medical assessments. In most treatment settings, patients receive a medical assessment that helps to determine whether they have a current or imminent medical problem that needs attention. These can include addiction-related problems such as withdrawal, acquired immunodeficiency syndrome (AIDS), or hepatitis, or medical problems unrelated to the addiction (and perhaps ignored for several years). The medical assessment generally includes a physical examination, a thorough drug history, and various tests: chest X ray, electrocardiogram, liver function tests, urine and blood tests, and drug screening tests.[5]

Nursing assessment. Especially during detoxification in inpatient settings, nursing staff can provide daily assessments of the patients' response to drug cessation, response to medication, interactions with other patients and staff, and early response to treatment.

Psychiatric assessment. Psychiatrists and psychologists may conduct various psychological tests during the initial assessment phase of treatment and at various points later in treatment. Some tests are used to confirm and assess the presence and severity of substance use disorders. These are generally question-and-answer, self-report tests and structured interviews. Some examples include the Michigan Alcoholism Screening Test,[6] the Alcohol Dependence Scale,[7] the Alcohol Use Inventory,[8] and the Addiction Severity Index.[9]

Psychological testing may include the use of personality tests such as the Minnesota Multiphasic Personality Inventory to assess substance use problems as well as various personality traits and disorders.[10] Various tests assess the presence of psychiatric and emotional problems that may need special attention during the treatment process. Overall, testing provides information that counselors can use to plan treatment strategies and that generally helps to provide optimum treatment.[11]

Nutritional assessment.   During active addiction, nutritional needs are often unmet. For instance, stimulants such as cocaine and the amphetamines decrease appetite significantly, often leading to insufficient nutritional intake. Similarly, chronic alcohol use is associated with various nutritional deficiencies. In fact, malnutrition is common in alcoholic people who receive most or all of their caloric intake from alcohol.[12,13]

Thus, some patients may have significant nutritional deficits that may need to be corrected shortly after admission to treatment. Nutritionists and other health care professionals may use structured interviews and laboratory tests to determine the presence and severity of nutritional problems and then make recommendations for solving those problems.

Family assessment.   Family therapy specialists may interview the patient and other family members to obtain a clearer understanding of the individual's family dynamics, the effect of the addiction on the function of the family, and the effect of the family structure on the individual's addiction. The family assessment provides information on the expected level of support for the individual's treatment and recovery and on the family's understanding of addiction, treatment, and recovery.

Social and emotional assessment.   Various social and emotional problems may have played a role in people's initial drug use, as well as in their continued drug use. Identification of these issues can be important for relapse prevention. Also, people differ with regard to social and emotional strengths and weaknesses. Treatment should involve enhancing poor skills and encouraging the use of existing skills for personal growth. Problems with trust, fear, and self-esteem may require therapeutic attention.

Recreation, stress, and leisure assessment.   Recreation is participation in an activity, pastime, or exercise that provides pleasure to the participant. It includes sports, exercise, hobbies, and various games. Leisure is pleasurable activity that has no specific goal except for leisure. Thus, taking a walk at the beach, talking with friends, and reading a book are healthy leisure activities. During addiction, people often stop participating in recreational and leisure activities.

A recreation and leisure assessment can help to determine an individual's level of stress, level of social skills, ability to trust others, healthy interests, ability to cooperate with others, general level of physical activity and exercise, and previous drug-free experiences of having healthy fun.

Legal assessment.　Several legal problems can occur as a result of addiction. For instance, being arrested for drug possession may have been the factor that initiated treatment. Some people have legal problems that are associated with illegally selling or using prescription drugs. People often steal items or embezzle money to support their addiction.

While under the influence of drugs, people often make poor decisions, such as not paying taxes or alimony. Others may ignore small financial or legal problems, which become more serious over time. Such problems might include credit card debts, back rent, and lawsuits.

Thus, people often need to address certain legal problems such as court appearances immediately. Some problems need to be addressed, but can be postponed. Legal problems can become a potent area of stress and anxiety, and they can be identified as subjects for discussion in a therapeutic setting.

Vocational assessment.　Some people in treatment have a stable job situation, and they are participating in treatment at the recommendation of the company's employee assistance program. As these people leave treatment, they may return to their job and be monitored for ongoing recovery. In contrast, some people may have jeopardized their job situation, perhaps even losing their job while in treatment. Obviously, these people have vocational needs that should be addressed during treatment. Similarly, many people have already lost their job and could benefit from an evaluation of their vocational interests and skills, as well as an overview of their vocational opportunities.

The vocational assessment is an evaluation of the individual's skills, interests, job history, and addiction-related occupational problems. This assessment can pinpoint areas that need to be addressed during treatment.

Treatment Planning

The assessments document information about an individual's treatment needs, as well as the strengths and resources that can be used to meet those treatment needs. Using these assessments, counselors create a master treatment plan for each patient. The treatment plan describes an individual's specific treatment needs as well as identifying specific objectives for meeting those needs. It describes how those objectives will be met and provides an estimated time line for meeting them.

The goal of addiction treatment is to achieve the objectives described in the treatment plan. Ideally, patients remain in treatment as long as the majority of their treatment goals are unmet. They are released or moved to a lower level of care when all or most of the treatment goals are met.

Medical and Psychiatric Management

On entering treatment, patients may have various medical and psychiatric crises that need immediate attention. For example, many patients will be experiencing acute withdrawal, which can be life threatening. Some patients will experience subacute or prolonged withdrawal symptoms that can be treated with nonpsychoactive medications. Similarly, some patients will have psychiatric crises such as suicidal depression resulting from stimulant withdrawal. The treatment needs of some patients include medical problems that relate to addiction, such as hepatitis or infections. Also, some patients have medical problems that are unrelated to the addiction, such as asthma or high blood pressure. These treatment needs should be addressed through regular physical examinations, medical management as required, and regular medical follow-ups.

Psychosocial Rehabilitation

Psychosocial rehabilitation describes the process of putting the treatment plan recommendations into active operation. Patients attend lectures, classes, groups, activities, games, and therapy sessions during treatment, as well as participate in the Twelve-Step self-help groups.

Group therapy. The group is the primary setting for addiction treatment activities such as educational lectures, community meetings, therapeutic games, recreational activities, and therapy. In many ways, group therapy is the core component of addiction treatment.

Group therapy generally involves 6–12 patients and 1 or 2 therapists. In many settings, newly arriving patients join existing groups. This allows patients in very early treatment to observe a progressive mental clearing in other patients in later stages of treatment. In other settings, all patients join the group at the same time.

Because many patients have medicated their feelings with drugs for several years, group therapy may put some people in touch with their feelings for the first time in a long time. One of the goals of group therapy is to have patients articulate their feelings, including anger, peacefulness, depression, joy, resentment, and happiness. Patients learn to identify their feelings, to communicate these feelings to others, and to listen to needs of others.

Addicted people often believe that they are "special," "different," and not like the other patients. For example, people addicted to alcohol may believe that their addiction is dramatically different from that of people addicted to cocaine; a sophisticated businessman may think that his addiction bears little resemblance to a blue-collar worker's addiction. As addiction-related struggles are articulated in group therapy, patients may begin to identify with each other and recognize their common addiction and struggles.

During active addiction, people develop defense systems that help to protect them from the reality of their addiction. As they progress through group therapy, they learn to identify these defense mechanisms in themselves and in others. Thus, group therapy becomes a setting for peers to confront each other about the honesty of their statements. Insights, criticisms, and confrontations are often more readily accepted from peers in treatment than from authority figures. For example, one patient may confront another who claims not to be disturbed about losing his wife because of addiction.

The group therapist typically gives the group members various assignments, which are often discussed in the group therapy session. Group therapy is an opportunity to discuss emotionally charged issues in a confidential and psychologically safe environment.

Education. Addiction treatment involves education in the form of didactic lectures, interactive classes, videos, and reading assignments. Educational activities can be provided by physicians, nurses, therapists, nutritionists, family therapists, and even paraprofessionals in long-term recovery.

Most educational activities are done in a group setting. At a minimum, educational activities should address the process of addiction, the effects of drugs of abuse, medical and psychiatric aspects of addiction, the Twelve-Step programs, social and family issues related to addiction, signs and symptoms of relapse, spirituality, stress management, and AIDS.

Twelve-Step group education and participation. If group therapy is the core of addiction treatment, then participation in the Twelve-Step self-help groups is the core of the recovery process, which merely begins during treatment. During treatment, patients are exposed to educational classes, videos, lectures, and written material about the Twelve-Step programs, as well as participating in the Twelve-Step groups themselves.

These programs are casually referred to as the Twelve-Step programs because they are based on twelve steps or suggestions for the initiation and maintenance of sobriety and personal growth. These steps are further described in Chapter 7.

Participation in the Twelve-Step programs is generally expected during all phases of treatment. An important criterion for selecting a treatment program should be whether it supports participation in the Twelve-Step programs. For instance, many treatment programs have in-house Twelve-Step meetings, provide Twelve-Step education, and encourage participation in outside meetings.

The unwavering focus of the Twelve-Step programs is on abstinence from all psychoactive drugs. These programs are not analytical, and they do not place great priority on figuring out why people become addicted. Rather, they are remarkably focused on practical ways for people to remain sober, one day at a time.

On the surface, these programs appear to be centered around the subject of addiction. Indeed, these programs are designed to help people initiate and maintain sobriety. On a deeper level, however, these programs are centered around emotional, social, and spiritual growth. On a practical level, the Twelve-Step programs encourage identification with other addicts, promote peer confrontation of emotional dishonesty, model healthy behavior, and enable patients to participate in an established network of clean and sober people.[14]

Resistance to participation in the Twelve-Step process is often based on misunderstandings, especially incorrect assumptions about the supposed religious nature of the programs.[15] Such resistance may be a deeper sign of resistance to treatment in general. However, some programs encourage participation in meaningful alternatives for patients who refuse to participate in Twelve-Step programs.

There are different types of Twelve-Step meetings. Some meetings are "open" meetings, meaning that they are open to everyone. "Closed" meetings are limited to people who have a desire to stop drinking or using other drugs. Family members and people who are simply curious are always welcome at open meetings.

Family therapy. The addiction of one family member has a great effect on the other family members, and it affects the overall dynamics of the family. Similarly, the overall dynamics of a family can influence the onset and progression of a family member's addiction. Thus, family therapy is a critical aspect of addiction treatment, and should be one of the criteria used to select a treatment program.

Some families may want to send the addicted person off to treatment somewhere and not be personally involved with "their problem." In reality, addiction is a "family disease," because the addiction of one family member distorts the dynamics of the entire family. Thus, the most effective treatment of the addicted person includes treatment of the entire family.

When one family member is addicted, other family members adjust in some way, such as with silence, anger, disappointment, rage, workaholism, or fear. Shame is a common response and is often suffered in silence. Family therapy is designed to break this silence in a loving, constructive, healthy fashion. The goals of family therapy in an addiction treatment setting are to increase awareness of addiction, to enhance communication among family members, and to teach family members how to support the addicted family member's recovery.

Family programs often provide 1) patient education about the interplay between the family and addiction; 2) family education about the interplay between the family and addiction; 3) family education about addiction, drugs of abuse, treatment, and recovery; 4) family therapy sessions; and 5) participation in the Twelve-Step self-help groups for families of people with substance use disorders, which are called Al-Anon and Nar-Anon.

Family therapy often takes the form of multiple-family therapy sessions that involve three patients plus their families in a number of sessions over one or more days. After the therapy, there may be sessions for the family members to reflect on and discuss the therapy among themselves.

Family participation in Al-Anon and Nar-Anon is vital for the health of the entire family, and it is a practical way to support the addicted family member. These groups help family members address and resolve those problems that relate to the addicted family member's addiction. These groups also provide family members with practical guidance on how to stop unhealthy reactions to a family member's addiction and on how to enhance their own emotional and social health.

Relapse prevention. Patients should be taught relapse prevention throughout treatment, by means of lectures, videos, group sessions, written assignments, and drug refusal practice sessions. Relapse prevention involves an increased awareness of personal symptoms and signs that led to drug use in the past. This awareness may involve identifying and acknowledging certain people, places, situations, times, and emotions that increase the risk for relapse. For example, some people have a tendency to drink when they are sad; others have cravings for cocaine when they get paid on Friday afternoons.

Relapse prevention involves altering behavior so that high-risk situations are avoided. It also involves learning new response skills when these situations are unavoidably encountered. For example, patients can learn to go to an AA meeting when they feel sad or to go to a Cocaine Anonymous meeting on Friday afternoons.

Some people relapse because they want to see whether they are "strong" enough to be around drugs without using them. Relapse prevention teaches people to develop automatic responses, such as avoiding or immediately leaving high-risk situations.

Relapse prevention also teaches patients to become increasingly aware of specific thoughts and emotions that may lead to relapse. For instance, someone who normally attends AA meetings may begin to think of excuses for not attending. Although the thoughts may sound rational to the individual ("I'm just too tired to go"), they may represent one small step on the way to relapse. Thus, patients are taught to become more aware of how their thoughts and emotions could promote relapse. Because peers can often detect subtle changes in each other, patients also are taught to pay attention to the feedback they receive from others.

Relapse prevention groups provide a specific opportunity for patients to talk about their fears of relapsing. Without these supervised and safe opportunities, patients may silently cling to these fears, causing stress and anxiety and possibly promoting relapse.

Recreation, leisure, and stress reduction.   Some programs have comprehensive resources in these areas. Ideally, a program should have a certified recreation therapist who has specific training in teaching recreation skills, leisure activities, and stress reduction. Recreation skill enhancement involves recreational activities at the program, as well as teaching the value of such activities as an important aspect of recovery. Patients can participate in exercise routines, various sports activities, assorted arts and crafts endeavors, and therapeutic games.

Recreational activities are designed teach patients that stress and anxiety reduction do not have to involve drugs. These activities also help patients to learn social skills such as leadership, cooperation, healthy competition, and teamwork. Many of these activities—such as participatory games—teach valuable social skills such as learning to trust and to be trustworthy. Vigorous physical exercise helps patients to feel good about themselves, decreases anxiety and depression, increases appetite, and often helps patients sleep better.

Patients can learn how to learn to enjoy simple activities such as quiet walks, books, friendly conversation, and simple, drug-free entertainment. Patients are also taught various drug-free ways of reducing stress and anxiety, such as exercise, running, visualization techniques, communication skill exercises, progressive muscle relaxation, deep-breathing techniques, and sports. Patients may be asked to explore the ways in which they currently handle stress and to develop new, healthy responses to stress.

Special treatment groups. Depending on the treatment program, the available resources, and what the treatment program emphasizes, a number of groups and services may address specific treatment issues. These groups may take the form of educational classes, informal group sessions, or group therapy. In some situations, a number of topic-specific education and therapy groups may be combined to form a "track," or specialty emphasis within the program.

For instance, many programs have specialized tracks on cocaine addiction. A cocaine track is often a series of educational and therapeutic sessions that deal with cocaine-specific issues: psychopharmacology, neurotransmitters, psychiatric and medical complications, drug refusal skills, and relapse prevention.

Some programs have specialized tracks for impaired health care professionals, people who have recently relapsed, or people who have a dual diagnosis of a substance use disorder and a psychiatric disorder. In addition to specialized tracks, some programs are entirely designed for a specific group of patients. For instance, some treatment programs are specifically designed for gay men and lesbians, people from specific ethnic and cultural backgrounds, or people in religious orders.

Programs may have special-topic groups: for example, groups that help women discuss addiction-related problems that are specifically associated with being female. Many programs have groups that discuss men's issues, anger, violence, incest, codependence, pain management, grief, vocational skills, and the use of medication during recovery.

Continuing Care and Aftercare

After treatment in inpatient and intensive outpatient treatment settings, patients progress to a less intensive phase of treatment, often called continuing care or aftercare. This is a critical phase of treatment, because patients invariably live at home, return to work, and live more fully in their old environment. As a result, patients are more likely to encounter old drug-using friends and other high-risk situations.

Transition to the community. Ideally, participation in continuing care means that most of the treatment plan objectives have been met and that the unmet treatment goals can be met by a lower level of care. In reality, it may also mean that insurance coverage for more intensive treatment has expired, whether or not the treatment goals were met. Thus, some patients will be better prepared than others to enter continuing care.

Continuing care is a transition from the relative safety of treatment to the community. Many patients have intense fears about returning back to the "real world" of home, work, friends, and activities. Many patients have great fears about relapsing. Thus, patients are often exposed to continuing-care groups while they are in a higher level of care. This allows them to become familiar with their peers who have already made the transition to continuing care.

Continuing care often consists of one or two sessions of group therapy per week, depending on the needs of the individual patient and the available program resources. Many treatment programs allow ongoing participation, whereas others set a limit of 6 months to 1 year. In practice, and when requested, treatment programs tend to be flexible about the length of participation.

This phase is an opportunity to use in the real world the practical guidance and skills for living acquired during more intense treatment. Thus, the continuing-care groups often center around struggles with drug hunger at work, at home, or with other friends. Because patients are likely living at home, continuing care is an opportunity to discuss relationship difficulties, financial problems, dilemmas at work, and sexual issues.

Self-help groups. A dominant part of continuing care is continued participation in Twelve-Step self-help groups. During this treatment phase, vigorous participation in Twelve-Step programs is often symbolized by obtaining a Twelve-Step program sponsor. Getting a sponsor is an integral part of the Twelve-Step process (see Chapter 7).

Continuing-care group members will encourage participation in the self-help groups. They will likely confront peers who stop participating or who fail to get a sponsor. Dwindling participation in these activities is directly related to an increased likelihood for relapse.

Early in the continuing-care phase, patients often attend self-help groups each day. Indeed, patients are often advised to attend "ninety meetings in ninety days." Although this may seem excessive, it often represents a mere fraction of the time patients previously had spent involved with substance use, including finding the drug, using the drug, and recovering from the effects of drug use. Typically, patients attend meetings on a daily basis for a few months and then stick to three or four meetings per week for a year or more.

Liaison and advocacy. Because continuing care involves a therapist who has weekly (or more frequent) contact with patients, the therapist can be an objective observer of the patient's adjustment to sobriety. For instance, the therapist documents attendance at continuing-care sessions and the patient's level of participation. In addition, the therapist can document the resolution of previously unmet therapeutic goals.

As a result, the continuing-care therapist can be an effective liaison between the patient and the employer. For instance, people at the patient's workplace or union may require verbal and written communication with the treatment program. They will want to know how the patient is progressing in treatment and to be alerted of any significant problems. Similarly, people with legal problems may have a probation officer or judge who requests ongoing reports and evaluations regarding the patient's progress.

Often, the continuing-care therapist is asked to make recommendations about the patient returning to work or about other issues. Assuming that the patient is progressing well, the continuing-care therapist can play the role of patient advocate.

Monitoring and testing. An important role of continuing care is to monitor the quality of recovery and to test patients regularly for the use of psychoactive drugs. Drug testing is one way to prevent and identify early relapse and to intervene before an early relapse has the opportunity to progress. It should not be punitive.

In the context of continuing care and monitoring, two types of relapses have been described: recovery relapse and destructive relapse.[16] *Recovery relapse* is brief, and the patient takes responsibility both for the relapse and for full participation in resolving the problem. *Destructive relapse* is clandestine, and the patient is uncooperative regarding recovery goals and activities.

Even when the patient has not used drugs, resistance to drug testing may represent an overall resistance to treatment and recovery. It is generally considered a "red flag" that something is wrong, including but not limited to actual drug use. Resistance to drug testing may be an early sign of relapsive thinking.

In addition to preventing and identifying drug use, body fluid monitoring also provides the patients and others with proof of abstinence. Accumulating a series of negative drug tests often is a source of pride while patients begin to internalize deeper reasons for continued sobriety.

Continuum of Care

Addiction treatment programs vary widely in terms of the services that they offer, their settings, and how comprehensive their treatment is. Addiction treatment ranges from individual psychotherapy to comprehensive, multilevel treatment programs run by professionals from multiple disciplines who take a biopsychosocial approach.

Patients who have more severe addiction problems and thus

need more intense treatment require comprehensive addiction treatment services. Table 6–2 summarizes the elements of a comprehensive treatment program. All of these components do not need to be under one roof. Rather, families working in cooperation with health care professionals from different programs can organize a comprehensive treatment package for their addicted family member.

Some of the Benefits of Treatment and Self-Help

Several studies have documented the importance of treatment, continuing care, and participation in the Twelve-Step programs. In one study individuals were assigned to inpatient treatment (which included AA participation) or to AA participation only, or they could

Table 6–2. Components of a comprehensive treatment program

■ **Evaluations and assessments**	■ **Medical and psychiatric management**
Addiction screening	Detoxification
Diagnostic evaluation	Treat medical crises
Intake assessment	Manage psychiatric crises
Medical assessment	Treat other medical problems
Nursing assessment	Treat other psychiatric problems
Psychiatric assessment	
Psychological assessment	■ **Psychosocial rehabilitation**
Nutritional assessment	Group-oriented treatment
Family assessment	activities
Social assessment	Frequent group therapy
Recreation and leisure	Multiple educational activities
Stress assessment	Vigorous involvement in a
Legal assessment	Twelve-Step program
Vocational assessment	Family therapy and education
■ **Treatment planning**	Recreation and leisure activities
Develop treatment plans for	Ongoing stress reduction
treatment needs as identified	training
in the above assessments	Relapse prevention training
	Individual therapy when needed
	Frequent random drug screens
	Special-issues treatment groups
	Continuing care and monitoring

choose one of those two options. This study noted that people assigned to inpatient treatment fared best and had higher rates of abstinence.[17] Another study noted that individuals who attend AA after treatment are more likely to be sober than people not attending AA.[18] Studies have noted that individuals who attend AA and participate in aftercare are more likely to be sober than people who do not do so.[18,19] In one study, about 70% of those patients who attended AA regularly but did not go to aftercare remained sober; a comparable percentage of patients who attended at least 4 months of aftercare remained sober even when they did not attend AA. However, up to 90% of those who both attended AA on a weekly basis and went to aftercare for the entire year maintained their abstinence.[20] In this study, some of the benefits of treatment included dramatic decreases in job problems and absenteeism, dramatic declines in moving traffic violations and other arrests, and a significant reduction in motor vehicle accidents. In addition, treatment is associated with significant decreases in the use of expensive medical hospital services after treatment. Similarly, one study noted that among recovering people in Narcotics Anonymous, psychiatric symptoms decreased significantly after cessation of drug use, even below the level present before initiation of drug use.[21]

■ Summary

Addiction can affect every area of people's lives: physical, cognitive, psychological, emotional, social, and spiritual. Therefore, addiction treatment should address these biopsychosocial issues. Because addicted patients' problems vary in type and severity, addiction treatment is offered at different levels of care.

Outpatient treatment generally consists of fewer than 9 hours of treatment per week, often in the form of group therapy. Intensive outpatient treatment generally includes services that require patients to participate from 9 to over 60 hours per week. Partial hospitalization is a form of intensive outpatient treatment that typically involves treatment 8 hours daily for 5 or more days per week. Residential treatment describes several types of programs such as short-term halfway houses, social model detoxification programs, and long-term therapeutic communities. One type of treatment combines partial hospitalization with a residential setting: patients live in a special residence with other patients and attend treatment during the day. Inpatient hospitalization includes 24-hour medical and nursing care and enhanced psychiatric supervision. This level of care is extremely important for those patients who need medical detoxification or who have additional medical and psychiatric problems.

There are several phases of addiction treatment. Of particular importance are evaluations and assessments, treatment planning, psychosocial rehabilitation, and continuing care. In a comprehensive addiction treatment setting, a multidisciplinary treatment team evaluates patients regarding the biopsychosocial aspects of addiction. These evaluations include medical, nursing, psychiatric, and nutritional assessments. Similarly, therapists conduct family, social, recreation and leisure, and stress assessments. Some programs may also include legal and vocational assessments as necessary. Based on these assessments, the treatment professionals make specific treatment recommendations for each patient.

Based on the formal assessments and the specific needs of the patient, patients participate in psychosocial rehabilitation that includes group therapy, education, Twelve-Step self-help programs, family therapy, stress and leisure education and activities, and relapse prevention exercises and education. Many programs have specialized educational activities and group therapy on specialized subjects and themes, such as cocaine, relapse, spirituality, and women's issues.

Treatment generally begins at a high level of intensity, such as inpatient or perhaps intensive outpatient treatment. After participating in the initial intense phase, patients participate in continuing care, which is a less intense phase of treatment and provides a transition from the safe, protected, highly structured treatment environment back to living at home. During the continuing-care phase, patients are expected to participate actively in Twelve-Step self-help groups as well as continuing-care groups. The continuing-care therapist can provide liaison and advocacy assistance to patients, monitor recovery progress, and randomly test for drug use.

■ References

1. Milhorn HT Jr: Chemical Dependence: Diagnosis, Treatment, and Prevention. New York, Springer-Verlag, 1990
2. The National Association of Private Psychiatric Hospitals and the American Association for Partial Hospitalization: Definition of partial hospitalization. The Psychiatric Hospital 21(2):89–90, 1990
3. American Society for Addiction Medicine: ASAM Patient Placement Criteria for the Treatment of Psychoactive Substance Use Disorders. Washington, DC, American Society for Addiction Medicine, 1991
4. Barr MA: Evaluation and triage, in Handbook of Hospital Based Substance Abuse Treatment. Edited by Lerner WD, Barr MA. New York, Pergamon, 1990, pp 7–17
5. Lerner WD, Barr MA: The substance abuser as a high risk surgical patient. Problems in General Surgery 3:329–345, 1984
6. Selzer ML: The Michigan Alcoholism Screening Test: the quest for a new diagnostic instrument. American Journal of Psychiatry 127:1653–1658, 1971
7. Horn JL, Skinner HA, Wanberg K, et al: Alcohol Dependence Scale (ADS). Toronto, Canada, Addiction Research Foundation of Ontario, 1982
8. Horn JL, Wanberg KW, Foaster FM: The Alcohol Use Inventory. Denver, CO, Center for Alcohol Abuse Research and Evaluation, 1974
9. McLellan AT, Luborsky L, Woody GE, et al: An improved diagnostic evaluation instrument for substance abuse patients: the Addiction Severity Index. Journal of Nervous and Mental Disease 168:26–33, 1980
10. Graham JR: The MMPI: A Practical Guide, 2nd Edition. New York, Oxford University Press, 1987
11. Crist DA, Milby JB: Psychometric and neuropsychological assessment, in Handbook of Hospital Based Substance Abuse Treatment. Edited by Lerner WD, Barr MA. New York, Pergamon, 1990, pp 18–33
12. Lipman AG: Nutritional deficiencies: which to blame on alcohol abuse. Modern Medicine 61:77–78, 1980
13. Lieber CS: Alcohol and nutrition: an overview. Alcohol, Health & Research World 13:197–203, 1989
14. Muhleman D: 12-Step study groups in drug abuse treatment programs. Journal of Psychoactive Drugs 19:291–298, 1987
15. Buxton ME, Smith DE, Seymour RB: Spirituality and other points of resistance to the 12-Step recovery process. Journal of Psychoactive Drugs 19:275–286, 1987

16. Buxton M: Monitoring, reentry, and relapse prevention for chemically dependent health care professionals. Journal of Psychoactive Drugs 22:447–450, 1990

17. Walsh DC, Hingson RW, Merrigan DM, et al: A randomized trial of treatment options for alcohol-abusing workers. New England Journal of Medicine 325(11):775–782, 1991

18. Hoffman NG, Harrison PA: CATOR Report: Treatment Outcome—Adult Inpatients Two Years Later. St. Paul, MN, Ramsey Clinic, 1988

19. Hoffman NG, Harrison PA: CATOR Report: Perspective on Admission and Outcome. St. Paul, MN, Ramsey Clinic, 1988

20. Hoffman NG, Miller NS: Treatment outcomes for abstinence-based programs. Psychiatric Annals 22(8):402–408, 1992

21. O'Connor JE, Berry JW, Morrison A, et al: Retrospective reports of psychiatric symptoms before, during, and after use in a recovering population. Journal of Psychoactive Drugs 24:65–68, 1992

Chapter 7

The Recovery Process

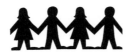

Recovery is the process which allows people to lead comfortable and responsible lives without the use of psychoactive drugs. Recovery is a personal program of living, based on changes in behavior and attitude and is best approached one day at a time. Recovery can begin once the destructive denial system is weakened, and distorted perceptions become replaced with accurate insights about oneself and others. Involvement in the Twelve-Step programs encourages self-growth, emotional health, and social interdependence. Relapse is a reversal of the recovery process. It begins when behavior and attitude begin to return to old, irresponsible patterns, and a return to distorted self-perceptions. This can occur long before people actually return to psychoactive drug use.

Donna Jackson, M.F.C.C.
Marriage, Family, and Child Counselor
Private Practice
Costa Mesa, California

■ What Is Recovery?

Recovering from a bout with the flu is an experience that most people have had. Some people experience a rapid onset or burst of symptoms, whereas others become ill gradually. After the worst of the symptoms have faded, people restabilize slowly. During this recovery period of restabilization, people are returning to normal but aren't quite themselves yet. Gradually, the symptoms and signs of the illness fade, and people are completely back to normal. After the experience, they may make certain life-style changes, such as increasing exercise, improving diet, getting appropriate rest, and avoiding excess.

Obviously, recovery from addiction is much more complicated than recovering from the flu. However, both are best understood as processes, not as events or single points in time.

The process of recovery from addiction can be described in terms of its various qualities: early-stage or late-stage recovery; good or poor; complete or incomplete; mature or immature; internalized or externalized motivation for change; strong or weak; and stable or precarious. In other words, recovery is indeed a process. It can differ from one person to the next, and it can mean different things at different times for the same person.

Various terms are used to describe aspects of recovery, such as "clean and sober," "abstinence," "sobriety," and of course, "recovery." These are not interchangeable terms. The term *abstinence* simply means being drug free. The main task of abstinence is learning to live without drugs. Abstinence does not describe quality of life or a life-style. It simply describes the absence of psychoactive drug use. As will be seen, abstinence from psychoactive drugs is not recovery from addiction but is necessary for the recovery process to begin. It is not uncommon for addicted people to have brief episodes of abstinence during long periods of addiction.

Abstinence alone does not imply that the addiction has been treated. For instance, some people are alcohol free and drug free for many years, but continue to have an extremely dysfunctional life-style with several areas of impairment. In fact, they are commonly called "dry drunks" because they appear to be dysfunctional like addicts, but are drug free.

Sobriety describes abstinence from psychoactive drugs in the context of a life-style that is focused on staying drug free. In other words, sobriety is not merely stopping the consumption of drugs (abstinence), but also includes creating a life-style centered around being drug free.

The task of sobriety is learning to cope with life without drugs. Sobriety describes an active decision to be free of psychoactive, mood-altering drugs and, in addition, to have a healthy life. People who describe themselves as "clean and sober" are referring both to their abstinence from psychoactive drugs and to their attempt to live a healthy life.

Abstinence and sobriety become the basis for recovery.[1] *Recovery* is a process in which the physical, psychological, emotional, and social damage caused by addiction is being healed.[2] Recovery involves abstinence and sobriety, resolving various biopsychosocial crises, and experiencing emotional, psychological, social, and even spiritual growth. Recovery is a process of healing and growth that goes far beyond mere abstinence from psychoactive drugs. Recovery involves learning to live comfortably, productively, and meaningfully while remaining abstinent and sober.

■ The Process of Recovery

Recovery implies that there is something to recover from. Thus, recovery from addiction involves reversing the impairments caused by addiction. If addiction is a biopsychosocial disease, and if addiction treatment is likewise biopsychosocial, then recovery must be biopsychosocial, too.

For example, addiction can cause impairment in people's physical, cognitive, emotional, psychological, social, and spiritual lives. Addiction causes more severe impairment in some of these areas than in others. Thus, the recovery process often involves the selective reversal of certain areas of impairment.

When does recovery begin? Although it may sound strange, some aspects of recovery may begin during active addiction. People who occasionally use and abuse drugs may not think about their drug use very much until adverse consequences occur. In contrast, people who are addicted generally experience an overwhelming compulsion for drug use and engage in powerful struggles over the control of their drug use. By definition, addiction involves losing these struggles for control of the drug use: addicted people use drugs more than intended or for longer than intended, or they lose control of their behavior during episodes of drug use.[3]

As addiction progresses, the loss of control becomes greater and the consequences become more severe. As a result, addicted people may psychologically redefine their personal identities from people who believe they can control their alcohol and drug use to addicted users who are not capable of such control.[4] This shift in personal identity may not represent a complete change in identity (and it may not be thoroughly conscious), but it may emerge at certain times, such as during crises.

Thus, during the active addiction, a small but important step is taken toward recovery: a glimmer of awareness that personal control over drug use is lacking. As the crises clear, people may reject this idea and repeatedly test their ability to control drug consumption. This helps to explain why many addicted people have alternating periods of abstinence and drug use.

The recovery process begins with crisis management and progresses to biopsychosocial problem resolution and personality change. Recovery starts with abstinence and sobriety and progresses to comfortable and productive living without psychoactive drugs. The process and progression of recovery can be divided into various developmental phases.[5]

Phase One: Biopsychosocial Restabilization

The recovery process begins in earnest during the treatment process. Beginning with the medical management of physical and psychiatric crises, patients begin a process of physical, psychological, and social restabilization.

Biopsychosocial crisis management. The initial phases of treatment can be described as "putting out fires." Physicians may need to

160

address detoxification concerns, manage medical problems that result from drug use, and treat medical problems unrelated to addiction. Similarly, psychiatrists may manage various psychiatric crises that result from recent drug use or that emerge during the withdrawal period. Once these medical crises are resolved, patients can begin to resolve other problems.

Various emotional and psychological crises may emerge during this initial phase. For some patients one of the initial aspects of the recovery process involves psychosocial crisis management. These crises may be internal, emotional crises or external crises such as family, job, and legal problems.

For example, patients may begin to realize how much harm they have caused their families and may have periods of intense guilt, low self-esteem, and feelings of worthlessness. They may become suddenly aware of the disasters that have been caused by their addiction and experience massive self-doubt and misgivings about their abilities in many areas of their lives.

In other words, people may become overwhelmed when they finally become aware of the full extent and consequences of their addiction. Thus, at this point, the task of recovery is to become aware of the consequences of addiction while not being overwhelmed by this knowledge.

Through group therapy, educational activities, and participation in the Twelve-Step programs, addicted people become aware that the destruction in their lives caused by addiction is similar to that in the lives of other people. As they identify with other addicted individuals, they become aware that other people have had similar experiences and that recovery is possible. In other words, a little hope goes a long way.

In addition to internal crises, psychosocial crisis management often involves the stabilization of external crises at home or work or crises involving financial or legal affairs. At this stage, addicted people may not find sophisticated solutions to long-standing problems, but they will be encouraged to make an effort to stop the crisis from exploding. This "first aid" may involve simply acknowledging the problem. For instance, they may not be able to solve a complicated financial problem immediately, but by speaking to the appropriate person and setting up appointments to discuss the problem, they may be able to demote the crisis to a manageable problem.

Biopsychosocial normalization. Many people in treatment have recently ended extensive periods of poor nutrition, lack of appropriate sleep, and absence of exercise. Thus, one of the first tasks of biopsychosocial normalization is to restore and encourage healthy eating habits. Some patients whose nutritional needs have been severely disrupted receive aggressive nutritional management. The nutritional needs of most patients will be met by having three healthy meals per day. Patients will likely be encouraged to discontinue using sugar and caffeine.

Similarly, patients are encouraged to manage their time in such a way that they receive a full night's sleep every night. Regular aerobic exercise can be an excellent way to decrease anxiety and depression and to promote a healthy appetite and normal sleep.[6]

After the resolution of psychosocial crises that may emerge during the initial treatment phases, patients can begin a period of "coming back to normal." Of course, some people have used psychoactive drugs for extremely long periods, and it may have been 10 or 20 years since they have been "normal." Also, people who began to use psychoactive drugs during adolescence may never have experienced extended periods without drugs. They may never have been "normal."

Psychosocial normalization is a phase of recovery during which addicted people attempt to use new solutions to solve problems. During active addiction, they use various solutions such as emotional distance, avoidance, denial, lying, and, of course, drugs to solve problems.

In contrast, during the early phases of recovery, recovering people may try new solutions they learned in treatment and in self-help groups. In fact, they may become eager to try new approaches to old problems. For this reason, self-help groups, drug-free recreational activities, and social activities with other people in recovery often become intense arenas for self-growth and therapeutic exercises.

During episodes of abstinence in an overall period of addiction, drug hunger is often endured in silence, expressed as an explosion of anger, or temporarily satisfied by drug use. In recovery, drug hunger may be handled by acknowledging it to oneself, talking about it with others, and employing stress reduction techniques. The same is true for other problems.

During this phase, recovering people may return to previous health habits or start new ones. For instance, they may begin an exercise program, make an effort to eat a balanced diet, and get a proper night's sleep most nights. They may begin to value emotionally healthy social relationships, use stress reduction techniques, and begin to feel and look better.

They may have episodes of depression, anxiety, frustration, and anger, perhaps related to prolonged withdrawal syndromes. But these episodes may be overshadowed by periods of relative normalcy.

Phase Two: Posttreatment Restructuring

After the more intense treatment phases, patients may begin to reorganize and restructure themselves. As they continue to face the reality of their loss of control over drugs and continue to acknowledge the severity of their addiction, their self-identity may change. They may increasingly identify themselves as people who are maturing emotionally, psychologically, and socially. They may distance themselves from their "old self" and focus on their new, healthier identity.

During active addiction, the addicted life-style of obtaining drugs, using drugs, and recovering from the effects of drugs becomes the framework and structure for living. During the intense phase of treatment, the rules of the treatment program become the structure. Later, during continuing-care phases of treatment, the self-help, Twelve-Step process becomes the predominant structure and framework.

People participating in the Twelve-Step self-help programs encounter a well-defined set of expectations. Participation in the Twelve-Step programs involves embracing a philosophy of a drug-free life-style with an emphasis on emotional, social, and spiritual health and growth, as well as personal honesty, interpersonal openness, and willingness to change.[7]

Importantly, people in the Twelve-Step programs provide one another with positive feedback for active participation and attempts at emotional, social, and spiritual growth. In other words, the

Twelve-Step programs provide peer support for growth, whereas drug-using acquaintances may provide peer pressure for using drugs. For many people, the healthy peer support that they receive in the Twelve-Step programs is the first time that they have received positive feedback for healthy activities.

Accordingly, one of the motivating factors for recovery during this period of restructuring is the sought-after approval of others. In fact, this positive feedback from others is central to the development of self-esteem.

Another motivating factor during this recovery phase is the need to comply with various authorities. Many addicted people enter treatment because of work problems, school problems, legal problems, or professional license issues. As a result, many people in early recovery are motivated by the need to comply with agreements they may have with their employer, school, parents, union, or licensing board. For example, they may make vigorous efforts to have a good recovery because they don't want to lose their job. This is another example of external motivation for recovery.

Phase Three: Mature Recovery

Initially, people depend on positive feedback from others as a guide for their behavior. In other words, during an early phase of recovery, people often rely on external guidelines for their behavior. Mature recovery describes a process during which people begin to internalize certain values and guidelines.

While participating in education, group therapy, and the Twelve-Step process, people are exposed to values that are likely different from the values they had during active addiction. For example, basic values such as honesty, openness, trust, and sharing are core features of the Twelve-Step recovery process.

For many people, internalizing these values is the beginning of a mature recovery process. During earlier phases of recovery, complying with the value system of others or of the self-help groups may be sufficient to sustain periods of recovery. Compliance with authority can be a motivating force to initiate recovery, but it may not be enough to sustain these efforts.

An admittedly clichéd phrase heard frequently in the Twelve-Step programs is "Bring the body and the mind will follow." This statement succinctly captures the essence of gradually replacing externally motivated lip-service participation in recovery with internally driven recovery.

As people begin to adopt certain values for themselves, they are in some sense restructuring their own personality. Priorities and personal philosophies may become reorganized, and people may change from destructive, self-centered, and compulsive loners to people who enjoy helping one another.

Indeed, mature recovery is generally characterized by a more balanced life-style. During active addiction, life is often associated with extremes, excess, competition, and rigidity. In contrast, mature recovery is associated with balance, moderation, cooperation, and flexibility.

Mature recovery is a time when people make serious attempts to restore balance in their social and family relationships. The friendships with other people in recovery may become particularly important. There may be sober attempts to heal old family wounds or talks about forgiveness and cooperation.

Above all, mature recovery involves a genuinely sobriety-centered life-style. During active addiction, obtaining drugs, using drugs, and recovering from the effects of drugs are the focus of living. During early recovery, people may attempt to accommodate desired aspects of sobriety into their prior life-style. For instance, people in early recovery may want to stay drug free and attend Alcoholics Anonymous (AA), but they may also want to spend time with drug-using friends or to continue to go to favorite bars.

In contrast, mature recovery involves the creation of a new life-style that is centered squarely on recovery from addiction. Once recovery becomes the focus, all significant decisions are made in terms of compatibility with recovery.

Phase Four: Late Recovery Period

During the earlier phases of recovery—restabilization, restructuring, and mature recovery—many people may become extremely enthusiastic about recovery-oriented activities. They may talk about recovery during nearly every conversation; they may attend Twelve-Step meetings every day or attend more than one per day. They may seem obsessed with recovery and engage in few activities that are not directly related to recovery.

During mature and late recovery periods, this seeming obsession may diminish. There may be a new balance between recovery-oriented activities and normal, healthy hobbies, activities, and events. Although the central focus of life may be a sober life-style, this new life-style may be expressed in a greater variety of experiences that are compatible with recovery.

The late recovery period, which may begin a year or two after treatment, is the time for resolving long-standing psychological issues through psychotherapy.[8] During this phase of recovery, people can resolve distorted attitudes or beliefs that were developed during childhood.

Earlier periods of recovery are concerned with behavioral changes and establishing healthy values, philosophies, and traits. Late recovery is a time for personality growth, such as resolution of self-esteem and intimacy problems. When a healthy personality is in place, long-standing emotional and psychological problems may be addressed without the severe risk of relapse.

Table 7–1 outlines the phases of recovery process and highlights the primary tasks within each phase.

■ Elements of Recovery

It is critical to understand that recovery from addiction is a process, not an event. Rather than being a "cure," recovery is an ongoing strategy, best understood as a life-style. Recovery can be good or poor; mature or immature; internalized or externalized; strong or weak; stable or precarious.

The recovery process can differ from one person to the next, and it can mean different things at different times for the same person. It is a ongoing, changing process. Even the goals of recovery change. The initial goals of recovery are crisis management and a subsequent increase in overall biopsychosocial health. Ultimately, the recovery

Table 7–1. Phases of recovery

Phase	Biopsychosocial crisis management	Biopsychosocial normalization
1. Biopsychosocial restabilization	Medical detoxification Psychiatric crisis management Critical medical treatment Emotional crisis management Psychological crisis management Family crisis management Social crisis management	Begins to eat healthy diet Begins to sleep normally Exercises and takes part in physical activities Learns communication skills Learns problem-solving techniques Talks about drug hunger Learns stress reduction techniques
2. Posttreatment restructuring	Changing self-identity Adaptation to external recovery rules	External motivation for recovery Feedback increases self-esteem
3. Mature recovery	Internal motivation for recovery Increasingly balanced life-style	Personality restructuring Increasingly sobriety-centered life-style
4. Late recovery period	Balanced, sobriety-oriented life-style Resolution of psychological conflicts	Personality growth

process is concerned with psychological and emotional growth and personality changes.

In some ways, recovery can be understood as a series of stepping-stones across a lake. To cross the lake, people will have to use all or most of these stepping-stones. In some ways, it takes a certain amount of faith and practice to learn how to rely on these stepping-stones. People can and do fall off, but they can get back on and continue the process.

However, some people never fully trust the process and see the stepping-stones more as hurdles. They may not make a good-faith attempt to cross, or they may give up during the attempt.

There are three underlying tasks of recovery. First, addicted people must recognize that they have a debilitating, life-threatening disease. The second task involves complete abstinence from all psychoactive drugs. Finally, addicted people must recognize their need for a program that provides them with support and assistance to stay sober one day at a time[5] and improves the quality of their life.

The following are fundamental elements of the recovery process. To the people who are earnestly pursuing recovery, they are stepping-stones to a vibrant and healthy drug-free life. To the people who are reluctant to engage in the recovery process, they represent areas of frustration and problems. Active participation in the recovery process can be assessed by evaluating participation in these elements of recovery.

Avoiding All Psychoactive Drugs

Recovery means abstinence from all psychoactive drugs, not just the primary drug of choice. Addicted people often have fantasies of controlling their addiction. Someone addicted to alcohol may wish to continue taking an occasional diazepam (Valium) tablet during periods of high stress, whereas someone addicted to cocaine may want to continue drinking, perhaps to enable sleep.

These people may insist that their addiction was to their primary drug of choice. In fact, their use of the secondary drug of choice may trigger relapse to the primary drug, as well as addiction to the secondary drug of choice.

Importantly, use of any psychoactive drug will cause distortions in thinking and effectively alter perception and feelings. Poor decisions may be made while using any psychoactive drug, including a return to use of the primary drug of choice, with the distorted belief that addiction will not occur.

Defusing Triggers for Drug Hunger

Drug use becomes associated with certain people, places, activities, behaviors, and feelings that act as cues and reminders of drug use. Consider someone who has frequently used cocaine and alcohol with certain friends at parties, bars, and clubs and who has regularly bought cocaine on payday Friday afternoons. For this person, parties, bars, clubs, and even Friday paydays can become triggers.

When people experience these cues and reminders, they have a strong desire to use drugs. Thus, the cues and reminders are called *triggers* because they trigger episodes of drug hunger. During active addiction, people are likely to seek out and use drugs after experiencing drug hunger.

Some triggers are related to external places or behaviors, whereas other triggers are internal, related to emotional states. Thus, some triggers are avoidable and others have to be defused.[9]

Identifying and avoiding external triggers.   External triggers include people, places, things, and activities that have become associated with drug use. For example, the drug hunger triggers for people addicted to cocaine and alcohol may be cocaine dealers, neighborhoods in which they bought the cocaine, certain types of music they listened to while high, and bars and nightclubs.

During recovery, experiencing external triggers leads to drug hunger. The drug hunger gnaws at people in recovery, making them agitated, nervous, irritable, and depressed. When they try to ignore these feelings, the feelings can become overpowering and lead to relapse.

Recovering people may not be aware that they have developed these external triggers. However, they can learn to identify these triggers and their reactions to the triggers. Importantly, they can learn

169

to avoid the triggers, by not going to certain neighborhoods or seeing certain people and by avoiding activities that were associated with drug use for them.

It is equally important for recovering people not to ignore the feelings they experience when near a trigger. It is vital that they speak with others about their triggers.

Self-help groups, group therapy, and counseling sessions are particularly good places for recovering people to talk about these experiences and to receive support and tips for avoiding them.

Identifying and defusing internal triggers. People can develop triggers that are associated with emotional states. Some people use drugs when feeling lonely, sad, and depressed. Other people may use drugs when feeling anxious, irritated, and nervous. Others may use drugs during times of sexual insecurity or to heighten or reduce certain feelings.

As a result, people may develop associations between emotional states and using drugs. These emotional states may become powerful triggers for causing drug hunger. At times these emotional states can be avoided. For instance, a diet high in sugar and caffeine may cause anxiety, agitation, and depression in some people. Avoiding these foods may decrease these feelings.

However, certain emotional states cannot be avoided. The death of a family member should cause sadness and depression. Some emotional states can be prepared for, such as the "holiday blues." When they cannot be avoided, internal triggers can be interrupted by engaging in healthy activity. For instance, people who experience emotional triggers during the holidays can plan to participate in healthy recreational or therapeutic activities.

Eliminating All Drug Paraphernalia

Early in recovery, people face the decision to throw away their drug paraphernalia. This may include wine and shot glasses for some alcoholic people, pipes for crack users, needles for intravenous-drug users, and rolling papers and bongs for marijuana users. These objects are powerful triggers for drug hunger.

Recovering people may have a hard time parting with these objects and rationalize keeping all or some of them. Family members can be supportive by encouraging them to talk about how it feels to get rid of these objects. It is a common and healthy reaction to feel sad and even grieve for drug paraphernalia.

Balanced Twelve-Step Group Participation

There are many different styles of participation in the Twelve-Step groups. Some people attend these meetings eagerly and participate vigorously. Some people are less than enthusiastic, attend irregularly, and participate minimally.

During early phases of recovery, some people attend Twelve-Step meetings every day or more than once per day. Depending on the individual's circumstances, that may be a good or a bad sign. Daily attendance is recommended and encouraged for the first few months of recovery. After a number of months, many people establish a balance between nonrecovery activities and recovery groups. For these people, Twelve-Step group attendance two to three times per week may be ideal.

On the other hand, some people attempt to meet all of their social, emotional, psychological, and spiritual needs through long periods of daily Twelve-Step group participation. This type of participation may be a sign that patients are avoiding problems in one area of life by focusing intensely on another. Although increased participation in self-help and therapeutic groups may naturally occur during times of high stress and problems, most people learn to balance these meetings with healthy nonrecovery activities.

In addition, some people are reluctant to attend the Twelve-Step groups. Discomfort with active participation in the self-help group process may be a sign of discomfort with recovery and a sign of impending relapse. Indeed, relapse is frequently preceded by a decrease in recovery activities such as Twelve-Step meeting attendance.

Creating a Sober Social Network

Some recovering people want to keep their drug-using friends while participating in the recovery process. These friends are often strong triggers for drug hunger. Also, these friends may purposefully or accidentally encourage drug use. The recovering person's goal of sobriety is generally at odds with friends' goal of drug-oriented recreation.

The creation of a new social network of sober people provides tremendous support for maintaining a drug-free life-style. Because people have the same goals, the new social network also is a tool for relapse prevention.

Avoiding Hasty Relationships

Drugs generally medicate feelings and emotions. After detoxification, normal feelings and emotions return. These include emotions and feelings associated with sex, intimacy, joy, and passion.

These feelings may have been dormant during the drug-using years. Because of poor memory of these emotions, some people experience them as extremely powerful and state that they are "in love." It is not uncommon for two people who meet during early recovery to have a steamy relationship that is high in passion and idealism and low in maturity and soundness.

In general, platonic relationships are encouraged during early recovery. Some recovering people have never experienced healthy nonsexual relationships with members of the opposite sex or with people who share their sexual preference. For these people, recovery becomes a time to experience healthy relationships based on trust, emotional honesty, and openness, not on sex or power.

Working the Twelve Steps

The Twelve-Step programs are more than meetings. In fact, the core of the programs are the Twelve Steps themselves. The Twelve Steps are suggestions for living a healthy life. They are recommendations for emotional, psychological, social, and spiritual growth.

In addition to the regular Twelve-Step self-help group meetings, there are also "Step Meetings," wherein participants explore these suggestions for living. Through these and other meetings, people can "work the steps," progressing from one level to the next. The process, which often takes many months or years, is growth oriented.

Steps One, Two, and Three describe, respectively, recognition of the disease, becoming aware that effective help is available, and making a decision to comply with that treatment. Steps Four and Five illustrate that personal insight is needed for full recovery. Steps Six and Seven describe a willingness to change what is found to be wrong. Steps Eight and Nine identify the responsibility for personal actions. Steps Ten and Eleven remind the patient that addictive disorders tend to be chronic and that an ongoing recovery effort is the best way to avoid relapse. Step Twelve represents altruism and service to others, a core feature of the Twelve-Step programs.

Twelve-Step Group Sponsor

It is generally considered essential for people in recovery to obtain a Twelve-Step group sponsor. The relationship between sponsor and "sponsee" has been described as the heart of the recovery process.[10] A Twelve-Step group sponsor is typically someone who has been in recovery for a number of years, who is not struggling with major problems associated with addiction, and who is an active and regular participant in the Twelve-Step process.

Sponsors help newcomers by explaining the self-help process and encourage active participation in recovery efforts. Importantly, they become a regular contact for the newcomer, and they can be a source of advice, encouragement, and inspiration. Sponsors can also play an important role in helping newcomers avoid relapse by confronting them about seemingly poor decisions that threaten to jeopardize sobriety. As recovery becomes more mature, sponsors may emphasize ways to work through the Twelve Steps and to make behavioral and psychological changes.[11]

The sponsor becomes a reliable person in whom to confide about struggles, mistakes, hopes, and successes. Twelve-Step group participants decide whether or not they want a sponsor. Although many people have good recovery programs without a sponsor, reluctance to obtain a sponsor may be a sign of reluctance to fully participate in recovery.

HALT!

The recovery process involves creating a healthy balance in all areas of life. For this reason, a popular acronym in recovery is HALT: "Don't get too hungry, angry, lonely, or tired." People in recovery begin to realize the importance of eating, sleeping, and resting to get recharged. Likewise, it is unhealthy to remain in a state of extreme emotion or to isolate oneself for extended periods of time. In brief, excesses are destructive.

Table 7–2. Characteristics of a healthy recovery

- Accepting addiction as a treatable disease
- Acknowledging the loss of control over drug use
- Abstaining from all psychoactive drugs
- Eliminating all drug paraphernalia
- Participating in all phases of treatment
- Participation of entire family in treatment process
- Family involvement in Al-Anon and Nar-Anon
- Early recovery: 90 Twelve-Step group meetings in 90 days
- Regular Twelve-Step group attendance and participation
- Obtaining a Twelve-Step sponsor during early recovery
- Working the Twelve Steps
- Creating a healthy and sober social network
- Avoiding new intimate relationships during early recovery
- Avoiding and defusing triggers for drug hunger
- Avoiding self-medication of emotional and social problems
- Seeking professional help for serious psychosocial problems
- Developing healthy leisure and recreational life
- Tendency toward trust, openness, and honesty
- Tendency to talk about personal feelings
- Concern for thoughts and feelings of others

■ Characteristics of Recovery

Recovery invariably involves significant changes in the way people think and what they believe. Recovering people may begin to perceive themselves, others, and their world differently. A number of characteristics are associated with these changes.[12,13]

Admission

One of the first steps in recovery is recognizing and acknowledging the existence of one's addiction. People often grudgingly admit their addiction, while secretly believing otherwise. It is for this reason that Twelve-Step group participants introduce themselves as follows: "Hi, my name is John, and I am an addict [or alcoholic]." By meeting others who admit their addiction, people may become more aware of their own addiction and less reluctant to believe it.

Recovery includes admitting that the addiction has become an overpowering part of the addicted person's life. This admission is stated in Step One of the Twelve Steps of Alcoholics Anonymous: "We admitted we were powerless over alcohol—that our lives had become unmanageable."

Thus, addiction is understood as something that becomes more powerful than willpower. Recovering people learn that the addiction somehow took over their lives and that recovery is a way to regain their lives.

Admitting or acknowledging the fact that one is addicted is a powerful psychological action that people often struggle against strongly. For instance, people in treatment might believe that they were hospitalized because another family member was mad at them or for reasons unrelated to addiction.

Acceptance

One of the characteristics of a vigorous recovery effort is acceptance of personal responsibility for the recovery process. Many people are powerfully aware of the severity and dangerousness of their addiction, realizing the risks they took and the harm they caused. These people may be more aware of the steps that they will have to take to have a meaningful and productive life without drugs. They begin to realize that recovery is not gloom and doom, but it is work and represents personal change.

Acceptance also means accepting the addiction for what it is. In other words, nothing can change the past, but active participation in recovery can change the present and thus the future.

Surrender

During active addiction, people often develop extremely rigid life-styles and attitudes. For instance, whereas everyone around the addicted person can plainly see the destructive path of addiction, that person may rigidly deny the existence of any problems. Because addicted people need a defensive shield to protect them from the comments of others, they may not take advice from others in any area of life. They become rigid.

During the recovery process, people are asked to drop their defensive shields and learn to listen to the feedback from others. They are asked to try new approaches to problem solving and replace their rigidity with flexibility.

Surrender does not mean giving up hope and quitting. It implies discarding old dysfunctional attitudes and behaviors and replacing them with new, healthy ones. Surrender also means to stop fighting the program, stop fighting the recovery process, and stop fighting oneself. Surrender means to stop fighting people who are trying to help. It means to let go of the need to have absolute control over everything and to yield to the recovery process.

Fellowship

A fundamental part of recovery is fellowship. Isolation from others encourages emotional isolation, distortions of reality, and relapse. Fellowship, or healthy relationships with others united in a common goal, is a key ingredient of sobriety.

The common experience of addiction, the common struggles associated with recovery, and the common goal of sobriety are powerful bonds. These bonds can transcend personalities and politics.

They become the basis of giving and receiving hope, encouragement, and support.

Restitution

The Twelve-Step programs teach the value of restitution to people who were harmed, except when doing so would cause harm. The nature of addiction is harm to self and to others. Addicted people often hurt others emotionally, physically, and financially and are often unaware of the severity and scope of damage they have caused until well into recovery.

At an appropriate time in recovery, people often make restitution to those they have harmed and hurt. By doing so, recovering people further their own healing process and reduce the emotional burden of having hurt others.

Service

During active addiction, people tend to focus entirely on their own needs and on trying to satisfy their addiction. During recovery, people learn the value of service to others. Of course, some people become more concerned with the problems of others than with themselves. But healthy service to others is an integral component of the Twelve-Step process and recovery.

Helping others in the self-help setting includes becoming a sponsor, lending a hand, or simply listening to the problems of others. It does not necessarily mean knowing how to solve other people's problems. Rather, it means being willing to help others when appropriate.

By learning to help others, recovering people learn to stop focusing on their own problems and to recognize the needs of others. Service is a way for people to help themselves by helping others.

One Day at a Time

The addiction process generally takes months and often years to develop and progress. Similarly, the recovery process takes time to develop, progress, and mature. There is a naive temptation to say, "I will never use drugs again, for the rest of my life." In practice, people can better handle planning one day at a time. A day is far more manageable than a lifetime.

Also, the focus on a single day helps people to "start over" after mistakes. For instance, people who relapse often feel depressed and inconsolable after the incidents. However, by learning from the past and focusing on staying sober one day at a time, they can shift the emphasis from failures to successful attempts at sobriety.

Most importantly, people in recovery often need to stop dwelling unnecessarily on past mistakes and to discontinue having unproductive anxieties about the future. Rather, people in recovery, like all people, can simply do the best that they can do today.

Belief in a Higher Power

Recovery includes but is not limited to the reversal of impairments caused by addiction. It also involves growth beyond the initial point of addiction and the addition of new experiences.[14] This growth and these new experiences include initiation and maintenance of a spiritual life. Indeed, in a study examining the recovery process of individuals, the development of spirituality was critical for personal change and alteration of addicted people's attitudes toward and interpretation of themselves and others.[4]

The first step of AA states that "We admitted we were powerless over alcohol—that our lives had become unmanageable." The second step of AA is "Came to believe that a Power greater than ourselves could restore us to sanity." These two steps work hand-in-hand. The first step is an admission that alcoholic persons have lost control over alcohol use and that the addiction has had a powerful and negative effect on their lives. This admission is an acknowledgment that the drug use is indeed a problem and that help is needed to solve the problem. The second step is an acknowledgment that the problem can be solved, that help from the outside is necessary to solve it, and that there is some Power greater than oneself. The Twelve-Step programs call this outside help a "Power," "Higher Power," or "God," but leave it to each individual to define what he or she means by these terms.

At its most simple level, recovering people come to realize that the ways in which they have attempted to arrest the addiction have failed. The second step is an admission that in order to succeed in recovery, they will need to rely on resources outside of themselves. Addiction promotes a self-centered life-style blinded to the concerns, needs, and pains of others. The development of spirituality is a shift away from this self-centered view of the world to a view that places the individual within the context of a larger universe. Essentially, it is an emergence of a self in relation to others.[4]

As a result, people may define their Higher Power as the group process, the Twelve-Step programs, their recovering peer support system, nature, treatment professionals, or more traditional concepts of God. Frequently, the Higher Power is interpreted by people as simply the faith and hope that there is a solution to the addiction. The Twelve-Step programs are not religious and do not promote a specific concept of God or Higher Power. But these programs are specifically designed to foster the development of spirituality and a belief in a Higher Power.

In some ways, belief in a Higher Power is the opposite of desperately clinging to delusional beliefs of personal control over drug use. Belief in a Higher Power makes it possible to relinquish this control and to surrender to the recovery process.

■ Recovery and Relapse

Various medical and psychiatric disorders are called chronic disorders because they persist for long periods of time; in fact, some are permanent. For instance, diabetes is often a lifelong disease. There is no "cure" for diabetes, but there is effective treatment and there are practical ways of managing the disease.

Like diabetes, addiction is described as chronic or permanent;[15] there is no "cure" that will permanently eradicate the condition. However, addiction treatment (and recovery activities) can arrest the addiction.

Some people get confused about the difference between the disease of addiction and symptoms of the addiction. The common cold is a good model for describing the difference between a disease and symptoms of that disease.

What people call "colds" are actually short-term illnesses caused by various viruses. The illness may cause the symptoms of stuffy nose, sore throat, cough, and chest discomfort. When people take over-the-counter cold medications, they are merely treating the symptoms of the virus-caused illness. They are not treating the illness itself.

Thus, people can take medications that will reduce or eliminate the symptoms of the cold without curing the cold itself. Despite the lack of symptoms, the cold can continue, progress, or run its course and stop.

The symptoms of the addictive disease include compulsive use of mood-altering drugs, loss of control over use of these drugs, continued use of these drugs despite adverse consequences, and distortions in thinking such as denial. In other words, compulsive drug use and distortions in thinking are symptoms, signs, and evidence of the underlying addictive disease.

People who are no longer using drugs may appear to be free of the addiction. But being symptom free does not mean that the person is free of the addictive disease. Rather, the disease can be compared with a hibernating bear, waiting to be roused. For example, when people resume drug use after a prolonged period of time, the severity of the drug use is generally at the same level as it was when they last used. In other words, when people relapse, they don't generally "start over" slowly. Rather, they resume about where they left off.

In fact, when some people relapse after a prolonged period of abstinence, the drug use is more severe than it was when they last used. This phenomenon is so common that addicted people describe it as "relapsing harder and faster than before" and "the disease progresses even when not using." In other words, the underlying addictive disease remains, and perhaps become more severe, even though the person is not using psychoactive drugs.[12]

Why is the difference between addictive disease and addiction symptoms important? In part because people who have been abstinent for some time may believe that they have been "cured" and are no longer addicted. People who believe this may entertain fantasies of controlled drug use. They may believe that they can return to experimental, situational, or social drug use without experiencing compulsion, loss of control, and continued use despite adverse consequences. They may be more likely to turn again to drugs to solve emotional, psychological, and social problems, rather than use other coping skills. They may be more likely to expose themselves to high-risk situations that may trigger drug hunger and relapse.[16]

The Road to Relapse

Relapse is not simply the act of using drugs after a period of abstinence. Rather, relapse is a process, much as addiction and recovery

Table 7–3. Characteristics of a poor recovery

- Reluctance to accept addiction as a disease
- Fantasies of controlled, social drug use
- Continued use of secondary drugs of choice
- Irregular attendance at treatment meetings
- Irregular attendance at Twelve-Step group meetings
- Continued social relations with drug-using friends
- Unsupportive, dysfunctional family
- Tendency toward secrecy and isolation
- Tendency toward distrust and dishonesty
- Conscious lying
- Unreasonable resentments
- Compulsive attempts to impose sobriety on others
- Ambitious beginnings but poor follow-through
- Irritation and annoyance with friends
- Easily angered and annoyed
- Overconfidence about recovery
- Poor eating habits
- Poor sleeping habits
- Prolonged, severe periods of stress
- Severe guilt over past behavior

are processes. Relapse is also progressive, meaning that without treatment or intervention, it will get worse rather than better. The relapse process may be described in three broad phases: relapse thinking, lapse, and full relapse.

Relapsive thinking. During active addiction, people have distorted thoughts, feelings, and beliefs. During the treatment and recovery process, thinking and feeling become normalized and undistorted. The relapse process begins when thoughts, feelings, and behaviors become distorted again.

Before the actual return to drug use, the relapse process often includes reactivation of denial as a prominent defense mechanism, a tendency toward isolation, examples of impaired judgment and decision making, and poor coping with periods of elevated stress.[17]

During this phase of relapse, people may entertain fantasies of controlled drug use. They may also question whether they are truly addicted. They may "find themselves" in high-risk situations such as with drug-using friends or at bars. These delusions and distortions pave the way for a "slip" or a "lapse."

Slips. Sometimes called a lapse, a slip describes an episode of drug use during an overall period of recovery. The slip does not suddenly emerge out of nowhere. As mentioned above, the slip is preceded by a return to distorted, relapsive thinking. Often, addicted people "give themselves permission" to experiment "just this once" or to test their ability to control the drug use.

Although a slip is dangerous, it is less severe than a full relapse. A slip is short in duration and may occur only once or a very few times. It may involve a mere taste of alcohol or a short-term binge. The patient takes responsibility for the episode of drug use and for participating fully in a rapid resolution of the problem.[18]

Full relapse. Ranging from a brief period of use to ongoing addiction, full-blown relapse is often clandestine and is accompanied by a full complement of severe distortions in thinking and feeling. During a full relapse, the patient is more likely to be uncooperative regarding the resumption of treatment and recovery activities.

During the relapse process, addicted people often experience a general loss of control over drug use. This loss of control is influenced by biological, psychological, and situational factors.[19] Psychological factors include the strength of the denial system, the level of emotional stress, and the strength of the individual's self-image. Biological factors include drug craving, medical and psychiatric disorders, and general issues such as sleep, nutrition, and fatigue. Situational issues include the strength of the social support for sobriety versus the social support for drug use and the overall intensity of stress.

In general, relapse can best be understood as a progressive process and as a transition between sobriety and active addiction.[20] Importantly, the relapse process can be interrupted, and it is far easier to interrupt during the early stages than during the actual return to drug use.

What Causes Relapse?

Only recently have researchers begun to study the causes of relapse. It is reasonable to assume that relapse can be triggered by various medical and psychiatric problems. Relapse may be more likely when patients receive poor or inadequate treatment or when their recovery program is insufficient or weak.

It has been suggested that the relapse mechanisms for various addictions include neurochemical, behavioral, and cognitive components.[21,22] Certainly, it appears that drug hunger and craving are important components of relapse.[23]

In addition, there are various psychosocial factors that may prompt relapse, including negative emotional states, stressful circumstances, interpersonal conflict, and, to a lesser degree, social pressure, drug availability, cues associated with drug use, and positive mood states.[20,24,25]

Negative emotional states. Negative emotional states include circumstances in which recovering people experience a negative or disagreeable mood, emotion, or feeling preceding or during the relapse process. These may include episodes of anxiety, depression, frustration, anger, and boredom.

Interpersonal conflicts. Interpersonal conflicts, which may be ongoing or recent, can occur within the context of a marriage, friendship, family, or occupation. These conflicts may take the form of arguments and confrontations.

Social pressure. In these situations one or more people pressure the recovering person to behave in a way inconsistent with recovery and sobriety. The pressure may be direct and straightforward, such as trying to talk someone into using a drug. The pressure may be indirect or even imagined, such as not wanting to be the only one without a drink at a party.

It is believed that the longer the period of recovery, the shorter the relapse, if relapse occurs.[26] It takes time to adapt fully and comfortably to a life of sobriety and recovery. During this time, a return to distorted thinking, slips, and even relapses may occur. Although relapse is not inevitable, families should have specific plans to deal with relapses should they occur.

Relapse is not failure. Although many people respond to a relapse with feelings of hopelessness and despair, relapse not only can be interrupted but also can be used to strengthen recovery. In particular, a relapse is an opportunity to help people identify the areas of their recovery that are weak and to strengthen them. For some people, a relapse dramatizes the fact that their hopes of returning to controlled drug use are delusional.

After going through a relapse, people often begin using learned but underused relapse prevention skills. Relapse can help people to more closely identify their drug hunger triggers and to strengthen their responses to those triggers.

Family Response to Relapse

Relapse is a well-recognized characteristic of addiction. People who participate in a recovery program can relapse, especially if their recovery program is incomplete or half-hearted; relapse can also occur during crises in other areas of life.

The relapse is itself a crisis and should be treated as an emergency. Ignoring the relapse or hoping that it will fade is a poor reaction. Immediate action should be taken.

It is important to interrupt the relapse as quickly as possible to reduce the damage to the recovery process. The family can participate in relapse crisis management by encouraging the following activities.[27]

Sponsor involvement. Ideally, recovering people call their sponsor before using drugs. However, after relapse, they should be strongly encouraged to contact their sponsors immediately. This simple action can help to bring the relapsed person back to the recovery process.

Attendance at a Twelve-Step meeting. Relapsing people should be strongly encouraged to attend a Twelve-Step self-help meeting immediately. They should once again be encouraged to attend 90 meetings in 90 days in order to jump-start the recovery process. Immediate attendance at Twelve-Step meetings can help to begin resolving the problem that may have initiated the relapse.

Pick up a white chip. At a Twelve-Step meeting such as AA, the white chip represents the desire to become abstinent and to begin the recovery process. Relapsing people should be strongly encouraged to begin again with Step One of the Twelve Steps.

Contact support group friends. During a relapse crisis, people need a lot of support. Support group members and Twelve-Step group members can provide nonjudgmental support for return to the recovery process. They may not be undergoing the emotional turmoil experienced by close family members, and they can help the individual make the transition back to the family.

Contact treatment providers. Depending on personal and community resources and on the nature of the relapse, additional treatment may be recommended. This treatment may involve personal physicians, psychiatrists, an individual or group therapist, or an addiction treatment program.

Complete family participation. Relapse is not the time either for ignoring the crisis or for furious tirades. Rather, it is a time for crisis management, problem solving, and open discussion of responses to the crisis. The lines of communication should remain open.

■ Summary

Abstinence describes being drug free or learning to live without drugs. Sobriety describes a state of abstinence within the context of a drug-free life-style and learning to cope with life without using drugs. Recovery describes a process during which the physical, psychological, emotional, and social damage caused by addiction is in the process of being healed. Recovery requires both abstinence and sobriety but also involves personal growth, living comfortably, and being productive. Recovery is a life-style and a multistaged process.

Because addiction causes deterioration in people's physical, cognitive, emotional, psychological, social, and spiritual lives, recovery involves healing the damage in all these areas. The first phase of recovery involves biopsychosocial restabilization. During this phase, there may be biopsychosocial crisis management, including medical detoxification, psychiatric management, other medical treatment, and management of emotional and family crises. After crisis management, a period of biopsychosocial normalization can help to bring disrupted processes back to normal. This phase may include a return to normal eating, sleeping, and physical exercise. It also includes restoration of normal emotional, psychological, and social processes. Posttreatment restructuring is concerned with changes in self-identity and personal growth. The Twelve-Step programs provide the structure needed for this externally motivated phase. Later, mature recovery represents an internally motivated phase of growth during which people begin to balance their recovery activities with other nonrecovery but healthy activities. Finally, the late recovery phase is a time for personality growth; it is also an appropriate time for treating long-standing psychological and emotional problems without jeopardizing recovery.

Several activities and behaviors characterize a comprehensive recovery program. Participation in these activities generally indicates good recovery, whereas nonparticipation characterizes poor recovery efforts. These activities include the avoidance of all psychoactive drugs and the identification and defusing of triggers for drug hunger. People in recovery should dispose of all drug paraphernalia because they are potent drug hunger triggers. Effective recovery involves the creation of a new sober social network while avoiding hasty intimate relationships during early recovery. Working the Twelve Steps, participating in the Twelve-Step group meetings, and obtaining a Twelve-Step sponsor are all critical issues for recovery.

In addition, healthy recovery is often evidenced by certain personal characteristics: admission, acceptance, surrender, fellowship, restitution, service to others, a belief in a Higher Power, and living one day at a time.

Like addiction and recovery, relapse is a process with multiple phases. It often begins with relapsive thinking, which is a return of distorted thinking and a reactivation of denial as the primary defense mechanism. Following relapsive thinking, a slip or lapse may occur, which is a short-duration episode of drug use after which people take responsibility for their actions and work to resolve the problem that may have initiated the lapse. A full-blown relapse involves an episode of binge drug use or a return to ongoing drug use. It is often clandestine and is generally accompanied by strong denial and a lack of cooperation about getting additional help.

Relapse is triggered by multiple factors, including medical, psychiatric, social, and family crises; negative emotional states; interpersonal conflicts; and social pressure. Relapse is a characteristic of addiction, and family members should have a specific plan ready to cope with it. Should relapse occur, a plan of attack should include immediate involvement of the addicted individual's sponsor and encouragement to immediately attend a Twelve-Step group meeting, where the relapsed person can pick up a white chip. Relapsing individuals should be encouraged to contact their clean and sober support group members immediately and to contact the treatment provider. Above all, a relapse should not be ignored. It should be treated as a crisis and an emergency that can be resolved and integrated into a healthy recovery.

8

■ References

1. Alcoholics Anonymous World Services: Living Sober. New York, Alcoholics Anonymous World Services, 1975
2. Milhorn HT Jr: Chemical Dependence: Diagnosis, Treatment, and Prevention. New York, Springer-Verlag, 1990
3. Landry M: Addiction diagnostic update: DSM-III-R psychoactive substance use disorders. Journal of Psychoactive Drugs 19:379–381, 1987
4. Brown S: Treating the Alcoholic—A Developmental Model of Recovery. New York, Wiley, 1985
5. Gorski TL, Miller M: Staying Sober: A Guide for Relapse Prevention. Independence, MO, Independence Press, 1986
6. Johnsgard KW: The Exercise Prescription for Depression and Anxiety. New York, Plenum, 1989
7. Alcoholics Anonymous World Services: Twelve Steps and Twelve Traditions. New York, Alcoholics Anonymous World Services, 1988
8. Gorski TT: Relapse prevention planning. Alcohol Health and Research World 2(1):6–63, 1986
9. The Koba Institute: Living in Balance Counselor Manual. Washington, DC, The Koba Institute, 1991
10. Bales RF: The therapeutic role of Alcoholics Anonymous as seen by a sociologist, in Society, Culture, and Drinking Patterns. Edited by Pittman DJ, Snyder CR. New York, Wiley, 1962
11. Alibrandi LA: The folk psychotherapy of Alcoholics Anonymous, in Practical Approaches to Alcoholism Psychotherapy. Edited by Zimburg S, Wallace J, Blume SB. New York, Plenum, 1978
12. Johnson VE: I'll Quit Tomorrow, A Practical Guide to Alcoholism Treatment, Revised Edition. San Francisco, CA, Harper & Row, 1980
13. Walker R: The Seven Points of Alcoholics Anonymous. Seattle, WA, Glen Abbey Books, 1989
14. Wiseman JP: Sober comportment: patterns and perspectives on alcohol addiction. Journal of Studies on Alcohol 42:106–126, 1981
15. Johnson VE: Intervention: How to Help Someone Who Doesn't Want Help. Minneapolis, MN, Johnson Institute Books, 1986
16. Marlatt GA: Cognitive factors in the relapse process, in Relapse Prevention: Maintenance Strategies in Addictive Behavior Change. Edited by Marlatt GA, Gordon JR. New York, Guilford, 1985
17. Gorski TT: The Relapse Dynamic. Hazel Crest, IL, Alcohol Systems Associates, 1982

18. Buxton M: Monitoring, reentry, and relapse prevention for chemically dependent health care professionals. Journal of Psychoactive Drugs 22:447–450, 1990
19. Gorski TT: Dynamics of relapse. EAP Digest 10:40–45, 1990
20. Sandberg GG, Marlatt GA: Relapse prevention, in Clinical Manual of Chemical Dependence. Edited by Ciraulo DA, Shader RI. Washington, DC, American Psychiatric Press, 1991, pp 377–399
21. Hunt WA, Barnett LS, Branch LG: Relapse rates in addiction programs. Journal of Clinical Psychology 27:455–456, 1971
22. Marlatt GA, Gordon JR: Determinants of relapse: implications of the maintenance of behavior change, in Behavioral Medicine: Changing Health Lifestyles. Edited by Davidson PO, Davidson SM. New York, Brunner/Mazel, 1980, pp 410–452
23. National Institute on Alcohol Abuse and Alcoholism: Relapse and craving. Alcohol Alert 6:1–4, 1989
24. Cummings C, Gordon JR, Marlatt GA: Relapse: strategies of prevention and prediction, in The Addictive Behaviors. Edited by Miller WR. Oxford, England, Pergamon, 1980
25. Tucker JA, Vuchinich RE, Gladsjo JA: Environmental influences on relapse in substance use disorders. The International Journal of the Addictions 25(7A & 8A):1017–1050, 1991
26. Goodwin DW: Is Alcoholism Hereditary? 2nd Edition. New York, Ballantine Books, 1988
27. Talbott GD: Elements of the impaired physician's program. Journal of the Medical Association of Georgia 73:749–751, 1984

Chapter 8

Defense Mechanisms: Living With Trauma

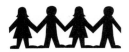

Defense mechanisms are an invariable consequence of the disease of addiction. These processes allow people to distance themselves from their own feelings, thoughts, and behaviors. By rationalizing, justifying, and minimizing, people are temporarily protected from the awareness of their own feelings, thoughts, and behaviors. The most common defense mechanism in addiction is denial. Denial protects addicts from the reality that they are addicted even though (or perhaps because) their lives are out of control. Defense mechanisms are commonly seen in the families of addicts. They allow family members to believe that the family is healthy and not in need of change. These mechanisms provide temporary shelter from the harsh realities of addiction. To understand addiction, one must understand defense mechanisms.

Eileen B. Kulp, A.C.S.W., L.C.S.W.
Director, Adult Chemical Dependency Treatment Programs
HCA Peninsula Hospital
Hampton, Virginia

■ Introduction

Nothing strikes fear in families living with addiction as much as the thought of the addiction going on without end—nothing, except perhaps the thought of confronting the addicted person. Family members often say, "The time is not right. Maybe things will get better. Later, not now."

For some people, merely thinking about confronting an addicted family member is enough to make hearts beat faster and palms get sweaty. They may decide that life is better with a quietly intoxicated shadow of a person they once knew, rather than arousing the violent alcoholic rage that ignites with a single conversation. Fear keeps these people silenced. They may say, "Don't bother your father; he needs his sleep."

For others, the idea of confronting the addicted family member seems completely out of the question. Their hope for a time when their family member would no longer be controlled by unseen compulsions has long faded into bitter pessimism. They may say, "Nothing will help," or "It's not that bad, really."

Some people have made numerous attempts to talk with, reason with, yell at, threaten, and cajole the addicted person out of his or her addiction. They may have elicited promises from or made promises to the addicted person. Anything to stop the madness. Nothing worked. They say, "I have already tried. It didn't work. I give up."

Throughout this book, addiction is described as a chronic and progressive biopsychosocial disease. It's not an attitude problem. It's not a lack of willpower. Addicted people are not stupid or bad. People do not choose to become addicted, in the same way that people do not choose to become delusional, depressed, or diabetic.

Rather, addiction is a disease, an abnormal medical condition with characteristic symptoms and signs that worsen when left untreated. This disease is influenced by, and in turn influences, behavior, thinking, feeling, perception, and physical processes. Impairment in these areas is not going to be reversed by forced promises, threats, or punishment. (Remember, one of the characteristics of addiction is the continued use of psychoactive drugs despite adverse consequences.)

Importantly, addicted people have severe and disturbing distortions in thinking and perception. Most prominent is the defensive mechanism of denial, which creates a powerful protective shield. Accordingly, rational persuasion, threats, and punishment are often futile to "get through" to the addicted person and are generally useless to stop the addiction.

Thus, to arrest the process of addiction temporarily and to lay the groundwork for biopsychosocial treatment, a special type of confrontation has been designed. This type of professionally led confrontation, called an *intervention,* is specifically designed to weaken the denial and defense system. With a weakened denial system, addicted people are able to get a glimpse of what others can easily see: that they are in trouble and that they need professional help for this problem.

■ Defense Mechanisms

The word *denial* as used in everyday language describes the conscious act of taking exception to a statement. In other words, the commonsense meaning of denial describes a conscious disagreement with a specific statement or belief. For instance, when asked, someone may deny having made a certain statement or perhaps deny participation in certain activities. However, the phenomenon of denial as a defense mechanism is quite different from the everyday meaning.

Consider the following true example. Both feet of a hospitalized white woman have gangrene. Anyone looking at her feet will immediately recognize that something is wrong. The flesh on her normally pinkish feet is dead, black, shriveled, rotting, and stinking. Physicians recommend that she consent to amputations to save her life. She refuses treatment, because when she looks at her feet, she sees nothing wrong.[1]

This woman does not simply have a opinion different from that of her physicians. It is not a matter of her lacking the medical expertise to realize that she has a serious problem. Nor is she disputing the significance of her physicians' medical findings.

Rather, this woman lacks the ability to perceive those medical findings. She just doesn't see the gangrene. Her perception is distorted, making her unable to recognize facts that are obvious to others. Because she cannot see the problem, she can deny the medical significance of the problem. Thus, she can refuse recommended treatment. She is experiencing an obvious distortion in perception.[2] This distortion in perception is a defense mechanism called denial.

What are defense mechanisms? *Defense mechanisms* are patterns and styles of behavior, thinking, and feeling that spring into action in response to perceptions of psychological danger. These responses are generally involuntary and are designed to conceal or reduce the psychological conflicts that cause anxiety.

But what is anxiety? In some ways, anxiety is a lot like pain. Pain is a warning sign that something is wrong. It signals the individual that there is a problem that needs attention. Pain motivates the individual to seek help for the problem. Pain protects people from ignoring injury.

In a psychodynamic sense, anxiety is a warning sign that something is wrong. It is a signal to the individual that there is a problem that needs attention. Ideally, anxiety motivates the individual to seek help for the problem, such as resolving some type of inner conflict.

For most people, much of the time, inner conflicts and anxiety can be handled by rational measures. For instance, when people accidentally hurt others, they feel guilty or embarrassed, or feel a sense of hurt themselves. They recognize the damage they have caused and take corrective measures to resolve the immediate problem and to avoid it in the future.

What kind of conflicts do addicted people experience? Perhaps the most basic conflict involves the loss of control over drug use and the continued drug use despite adverse consequences. There is a split between conscious intentions and behavior. The logical center of the brain (the cerebral cortex) is unable to control the intense cravings for psychoactive drugs that originate in the more primitive limbic system.[3] The limbic system is the part of the brain associated with feelings, emotions, and motivation. The limbic system also includes the body's pleasure center, where many psychoactive drugs exert their euphoric effect.

Further, addicted people often develop a sense of guilt because of their use of drugs, their inability to control the drug use, and the harm they cause themselves and others. In the drug abuser, this guilt may stop or curb further use. However, in the addicted person, whose powerful drug hunger is governed by the brain's limbic system, defense mechanisms such as denial serve to separate the cognitive and logical system from the emotional and feeling system. These defense mechanisms help to sustain the addiction.[4,5]

When people are overwhelmed by severe or constant crises and conflicts, they may be unable to handle and resolve them by rational measures. When that happens, largely unconscious and irrational defense mechanisms such as denial spring into action.

These irrational and unconscious defense mechanisms help to decrease or eliminate the anxiety caused by the conflicts and crises. They do so by pushing painful ideas out of conscious awareness and by giving people a distorted view of reality instead of a way to deal directly with the problem. As a result, there is an undesirable schism between objective reality and the individual's perception of reality.[6]

In the earlier example, if the woman acknowledged that her feet were gangrenous, she might reach the conclusion that amputations would be necessary. That awareness would cause great anxiety. Her inability to perceive her actual medical status results in her not experiencing psychological conflicts or anxiety.

Defense mechanisms can also be understood as enduring styles and patterns of coping with conflict. During severe crises, psychologically healthy people may unconsciously resort to irrational mechanisms. For example, immediately before an important business meeting, a businessman learns of the death of a close friend. He may initially doubt the truthfulness of the report and experience little or no internal reaction during the meeting. However, after the business meeting, he may suddenly "realize" that the report was probably true, become very sad and angry, and begin to mourn for his friend's death.

In this example, the businessman unconsciously shielded himself from the harsh reality of his friend's death just long enough to conduct an important business meeting. In effect, he temporarily denied the reality of his friend's death by initially disbelieving the report. At that point, his perceptions were distorted. After the meeting, he was able to perceive the reality of the death and became appropriately sad.

This type of psychological defense is normal and healthy. Everyone needs to be psychologically protected occasionally.

In these circumstances, psychological defense mechanisms are healthy and helpful. However, when these styles and patterns of coping become inflexible and rigid and don't allow the individual to perceive objective reality for extended periods of time, the defense mechanisms become unhealthy and dangerous.

Denial

As mentioned before, denial is an unconscious, irrational defense mechanism in which the individual fails to perceive and acknowledge an important objective truth that is obvious and apparent to others. It is a protection of the self from unpleasant reality by an unconscious refusal to perceive it.[7]

In terms of addiction, people may deny that their drug use is a problem; those who realize that a problem exists may deny that they need help to solve the problem. Others may deny that there are any solutions to the problem.

Example

John is the son of an alcoholic. His father and uncle were both alcoholics. They both died of cirrhosis of the liver. John has been informed that the likelihood of his becoming an alcoholic is substantial if he begins to drink alcohol. Even after reading literature from the National Council on Alcoholism and Other Drug Dependencies, John believes that his father and uncle were weak willed and simply didn't understand how to control their alcohol use. Even after repeated episodes of losing control of his alcohol intake and his alcohol-induced behavior, several blackouts, and driving-under-the-influence tickets, John believes that he can still learn to control his drinking if he tries hard enough.

196

Minimization

Similar to denial, minimization is the unconscious defense mechanism that allows some but not all of the objective reality to sink into conscious awareness. In other words, minimization is the awareness of only a part of the overall problem and thus a distortion of reality.

In relation to addiction, minimization can be seen in three classic ways. First, some people may unconsciously underreport the amount of their drug use. Second, people may have limited awareness that their drug use is a problem, but minimize the actual severity of the addiction. Also, people may believe that their drug use has caused limited adverse consequences, whereas in fact their drug use has caused severe adverse consequences to themselves and others.

Example

Julie describes herself as a social marijuana user. She has been smoking marijuana for the past 10 years. Although she began by smoking once or twice over an entire weekend, today she smokes marijuana nearly every night before bedtime, four to five times per day on weekends, and before most social occasions. When asked, "How much marijuana do you smoke?," she responds, "Not much." When asked more specifically how much marijuana she consumes per week, she states that she smokes "a little" during some weekends. Julie is not consciously lying. Rather, she unconsciously perceives her marijuana use to be the same as it was 10 years ago.

Rationalization

The unconscious defense mechanism of rationalization describes the use of socially acceptable but untrue explanations for inappropriate behavior.[8] The untrue explanations are self-serving and personally reassuring and are used to conceal or disguise unworthy motives for behavior. The individual believes these explanations, whereas others generally do not or should not.

Addicted people often use rationalizations to initiate drug use, to continue using drugs despite adverse consequences, to explain away drug-related problems, and to avoid going to treatment.

Example

Sam is an employee at a company that has an employee assistance program (EAP). Sam's EAP representative and supervisor have recommended that Sam enter a 90-day treatment program for his addiction, and they provide a written guarantee that they will hold his job for him. During the intervention process, Sam initially refused to enter treatment voluntarily, stating that he will lose his job.

Intellectualization

As an unconscious defense mechanism, intellectualization doesn't have much to do with being smart or intellectual. Rather, it refers to a tendency to avoid painful feelings by an enduring focus on thinking rather than feeling. In other words, some people cope with conflict and crises by focusing on thinking and logic, while ignoring their feelings.[9]

For example, when asked how they feel about their parents, people who have been physically and emotionally injured by their parents often say, "Well, they did the best they could. They didn't know what they were doing." In this example, it is not important whether the parents did their best or knew better. The important issue is the ability of the now-adult battered children to recognize their own feelings about such incidents. By coming to the defense of their parents, these people are unconsciously avoiding the experience of their own feelings.

Even when asked to do so, some addicted people are unable to describe how they feel. They appear out of touch with their feelings and unaware of the feelings of others. They tend to perceive their environment through nonemotional eyes. For instance, they may focus on rules, laws, and technicalities rather than on how a certain situation might make them feel. They may even state that how they feel is unimportant.

Example

Joanne's mother recently died. At the funeral, many family members and friends appear sad. Many are crying. Joanne appears calm.

A close friend asks Joanne how she feels at that moment. Joanne ignores her own feelings and states, "Mom had a good life and a painless death." The following year, when a few family members gather together to honor the memory of her mother, they watch a videotape of her. Everyone except Joanne is moved emotionally by the video. Every except Joanne cries for a few moments. Joanne is asked how she feels at that moment. She replies, "That was a long time ago, it doesn't affect me now."

Projection

Projection is an unconscious mechanism by which people falsely attribute their own unacknowledged feelings, beliefs, thoughts, impulses, and motives to others. In other words, they project their own beliefs, feelings, and troubles onto other people. As a result, people may accuse another of having certain motives or feelings that are really their own motives or feelings.[10] Addicted people often blame others for their own behavior or for the consequences of their own behavior.

Example

George has been using cocaine for about a year. He uses cocaine in binge episodes about twice per month. When he binges, he generally spends more money than he intends, money needed for the family budget, which causes severe arguments with his wife. During an argument with his wife, he tells her, "There wouldn't be any problem if it weren't for you. Get off my back and maybe we won't have these problems."

Repression

Repression describes a defense mechanism in which the individual is unable to remember specific, often traumatic experiences or disturbing thoughts, feelings, or wishes. In many ways, repression resembles an alcoholic blackout, except that repression is psychologically induced, not drug induced. As a defense mechanism, repression reduces conflict and anxiety by not letting painful, embarrassing, shameful memories into consciousness.

Repression can be a healthy and normal defense mechanism. Children who observe the hideous murder of their parents may repress the incident or be unable to remember details. Without repression, people might become overwhelmed with painful memories.

Addicted people may repress episodes of their own behavior. In particular, they may not remember their behavior that was embarrassing, shameful, and painful. This repression can be devastating because this is exactly the type of behavior they should remember, and thus correct. Increasing episodes of drug-related traumatic behavior may cause more frequent episodes of repression, widening and deepening the gap between an addicted person's awareness and the truth.

Example

Jody works at an auto parts store. She and her husband Tom attended a Christmas party sponsored by the store. Both Jody and Tom had used cocaine before attending the party. While Jody was at the party, her inhibitions were loosened, and she made a sexual advance to her boss in front of Tom and her boss's wife. This incident prompted a public argument between Jody and Tom, who left the party. After Jody wakes up the next morning, she briefly feels a sense of dread and horror, sensing that something is wrong. But having no memory of any specific problem, she begins to plan her day as if nothing is wrong. She is confronted by her husband, who is still angry, but she believes that he is making up a story about her.

Physical Isolation

As both an unconscious and a conscious defense mechanism, people can avoid relationships and situations that may threaten them psychologically. Solitude can be a healthy and enjoyable experience. However, some people engage in excessive isolation as a way to escape conflicts and to avoid the possibility of being confronted about changing certain behavior and ideas.

During active addiction, people may lessen their involvement in activities that they previously found enjoyable. They may discontinue attending social, recreational, and family events to avoid encountering obstacles to continued drug use. During early recovery and after hearing a talk about a deeply personal issue, some people tend to want to be alone rather than to process the information with others.

Example

Doris has been in recovery from her benzodiazepine addiction for about a month. She finds herself becoming increasingly uncomfortable around people, especially after group therapy. Although she still attends the group therapy, she immediately leaves the building after the session, whereas everyone else lingers for a few minutes and often socializes over coffee. She tells people, "I need to think, and I think better alone."

Blackouts and Euphoric Recall

Unconscious defense mechanisms such as denial, minimization, and projection are nearly universal and obvious features of addiction, but they are not unique to addicted people. Rather, these defense mechanisms are commonly encountered in various medical and psychiatric settings.

There are a few processes unique to addiction that are not defense mechanisms per se, but that serve to sustain the addiction process. These include blackouts and euphoric recall. In particular, blackouts and euphoric recall help to sustain addicted people's distorted perception of reality and create additional work for the defense mechanisms.[11]

Blackouts. Blackouts are drug-induced episodes of memory loss called amnesia. As described in Chapter 3, blackouts are periods of activity about which the individual has no or limited memory. People experiencing blackouts continue to function, make decisions, go to school and work, and interact with others. Others are unaware that anything is wrong. A blackout is not the same as passing out, which is losing consciousness. Rather, a blackout is a drug-induced impairment of memory, lasting for moments, hours, or days.

201

The awareness that one has no memory of periods of time can be extremely traumatic and frightening. People wonder: "What did I do? Where did I go? With whom was I with? What did I say? Did I become angry? Did I hurt someone? Did I lose my job? Did I wreck the car? How did I get home? Did I have sex with anyone?"

This psychological trauma is worsened by repeated blackouts. The trauma is worsened further by the reports of others who can describe details of what occurred during the blackouts. Over time, defense mechanisms help addicted people deal with this trauma by helping them pretend that blackouts aren't really happening or that blackouts are a normal part of life.

After receiving reports from someone else about their embarrassing behavior during blackouts, people may deny these reports and remain convinced that their behavior was socially acceptable. They may also believe that other people are creating lies and conspiracies about them, so strong is their desire not to believe reports of their own behavior during a blackout.

After repeated blackouts, addicted people may develop rigid defense mechanisms such as denial, minimizing, or projection to reduce the powerful psychological conflicts. These serve to strengthen the overall defense mechanism system.

Euphoric recall.   Like blackouts, euphoric recall is also a drug-induced impairment of memory. Whereas blackouts describe the inability to remember, euphoric recall describes a distortion in remembering and subsequent distortions in perception. More specifically, euphoric recall is the perception that one's memory of a drug-intoxicated episode is factual and accurate.[12]

During drug-intoxicated episodes, perceptions of the surroundings are distorted. Intoxication causes misperceptions, mistakes, poor judgments, and misunderstandings, although people are not always aware of these perceptual distortions and impairments.

Unless a blackout has occurred, people can remember events that took place during their intoxication. They may believe that their memory of events is accurate. However, because their perception during the intoxication was distorted, their memory will also be distorted.

For example, while intoxicated, a man tells a woman a sexual joke. Because he is intoxicated, he does not accurately perceive that she is irritated and annoyed at his joke. The next day, when he is informed by a colleague that the woman to whom he told the joke is still irritated and angry, he denies her ever being angry. He incorrectly recalls that she liked the joke.

A second aspect of euphoric recall has to do with the memory of events being distorted by the memory of feelings. People use psychoactive drugs because the drugs change their mood and feelings. Because this is a strongly sought-after effect, people often have vivid memories of how good they felt, or how euphoric they were, during specific episodes of intoxication. In fact, they may remember how they felt more than what they or others did or said.

For example, a normally anxious and socially quiet person may attend a party and use certain drugs. While at the party, she experiences a tremendous relaxing of inhibitions, a reduction in anxiety, and an increased ability to socialize. The next day, she remembers having a good time because she remembers feeling good. However, she does not remember spilling drinks, talking too loudly, and slurring her words.

Table 8–1 lists common defense mechanisms seen in addiction.

Table 8–1. Common unconscious defense mechanisms in addiction

Mechanism	Consequence
Denial	Failure to perceive reality or severity of addiction
Minimization	Partial awareness of reality or severity of addiction
Rationalization	Socially acceptable but false explanations for addiction and behavior
Intellectualization	Avoidance of feelings by focusing on thinking and logic
Projection	Blaming another for one's thoughts and behaviors and for the consequences of one's actions
Physical isolation	Avoiding interpersonal conflict by avoiding other people

■ The Addicted Family

Living with addiction and with addicted people who have rigid defense mechanisms can be confusing, troubling, and frightening. Their absolute denial of painfully obvious addiction may seem unbelievable. Their minimizing of the most severe consequences of their addiction is inconceivable. Their projection of blame for the consequences of their own behavior onto someone else is preposterous. Their repeated episodes of repression, blackouts, and euphoric recall can make other family members doubt their own perceptions and sanity.

Living with active addiction is traumatic. In many families, living with addiction is like living in a constant state of emergency, always prepared for the unpredictable.

Families respond to addiction in a variety of ways, ranging from healthy confrontation and intervention to unhealthy adaptation to the addiction. Unfortunately, many families learn to live with the addiction and make the family system adapt to it. Making a family adapt to addiction causes the family to become unhealthy.

In fact, as a way of adapting to addiction, family members often begin to use the same defense mechanisms as the addicted person. Thus, family members begin to deny, minimize, rationalize, isolate, and repress the trauma caused by someone else's addiction. They may deny the existence of the addiction in their midst, deny the adverse consequences suffered by the family, and deny that they have experienced any consequences.

Those families who have adapted to addiction in their midst can be described as addicted families. Addicted families may have one family member who is actively addicted, or they may have several. The coping strategies that addicted families use often cause further destruction in the family.

One of the most common coping strategies for addicted families is denial.[13] In various ways, family members may develop unconscious ways of denying the overpowering fact of addiction in their family. These families generally adapt to the addiction by experiencing shame, anxiety, and fear.[14]

If the addicted family were to be thought of as an individual, the individual would be described as sick and needing help. Like addicted people, the addicted family has a progressive sickness. The dysfunction begins with subtle changes, and it may not end until the family is severely unhealthy and dysfunctional. The sickness begins with very simple reactions to the addicted person, such as protecting, controlling, and blaming.

Enabling the Addicted Person

Assume that Joe was a heavy cigarette smoker and was hospitalized recently for a heart attack and a coronary bypass. Joe nearly died as a complication of smoking. He was put on a healthy diet and advised that continued smoking will result in further heart complications. Despite these instructions, Joe is openly smoking and refuses to remain on the diet.

The only healthy response to this potentially fatal disorder is confrontation and intervention. If Joe continues to smoke, it will threaten his life. He has a progressive and potentially fatal disease.

In contrast, people would enable Joe's heart condition to continue if they 1) ignore his behavior; 2) buy cigarettes for him; 3) make excuses for his behavior; 4) smoke around him; 5) avoid being around him because he smokes; 6) lie to his doctor and state that he is not smoking; 7) attempt to control his cigarette use by controlling and limiting his access to just a few cigarettes per day; 8) rationalize that Joe has lived a long life and he should do what he wants; 9) give up, saying "I just don't want to fight anymore"; and 10) feel "It's my fault that he smokes. If it weren't for me, he wouldn't smoke. I should be more understanding."

Addiction is a progressive and potentially fatal medical disorder. The only healthy response to a family member's addiction is confrontation and intervention, leading to treatment and the arrest of this medical disorder. Any other response allows the progressive and potentially fatal addiction to continue and worsen.

The term *enabling* refers to the behavior of a family member or friend that allows someone's addiction to continue or progress. In other words, enabling describes the actions of one person that promote the continued addiction of another. In this context, enabling is the opposite of confrontational intervention. People can be described as "enabling one another." Enabling can be a conscious or an unconscious behavior, and it can be done actively or by omission.

Conscious enabling describes the actions of an individual who knowingly and purposefully supports the drug use of another. For instance, two people who drink together enable one another. Conscious enabling also describes the creation of an atmosphere that is permissive for drug use. For example, a mother who believes that it is safer for her adolescent to buy marijuana from her rather than buy it on the street enables her child.

Unconscious enabling describes the behavior of an individual who unknowingly and unwittingly allows the drug use of another to continue uninterrupted. Consider the parents of an honor role student who refuse to believe the school nurse who calls to say their daughter became intoxicated during lunch. A wide variety of unconscious defense mechanisms may be at play here, such as denial, minimizing, rationalization, and projection.

Active enabling involves direct action and behavior that help to sustain the drug use of another. Examples include buying drugs for someone or calling in sick for someone who is experiencing a hangover.

Enabling by omission describes the indirect encouragement of drug use by failing to take some action. For instance, the spouse of an alcoholic person may fail to mention his drinking during couples counseling for sexual problems.

Institutional enabling describes the philosophy and perhaps rules of an organization or group that help to sustain drug abuse. Businesses that serve alcohol on the premises during lunch or during business meetings and groups that meet at bars to watch football games encourage the use of alcohol.

Effects of enabling. By reducing barriers to drug use, enabling creates an environment that advocates the continued use of drugs. Reduction of these barriers helps to strengthen the distortions in perception and delusions experienced by addicted people. Strengthening these distortions in perception increases the gap between what is real and what the addicted person perceives as real. As a result, the addicted person's ability to perceive the severity of the addiction objectively is worsened.

In addition, enabling affects the enabler. Enablers are generally unaware that they increase the severity of the addiction and thus increase the trauma with which they live. Enablers also experience distortions in perception and lose touch with their own feelings and emotions. As enabling becomes more entrenched and severe, enablers often become more concerned with the addicted person's feelings than with their own.

Types of Enabling Behavior

As with defense mechanisms, a variety of behaviors consciously or unconsciously support the drug use of another.[15]

Taking over responsibilities involves attempts to assume the personal responsibilities of someone else who cannot meet these duties because of drug-caused impairment.

Rationalizing and accepting entail the rationalization of obviously distorted thinking, behavior, and perception. They also include accepting the rationalizations and the excuses given by the addicted person.

Cooperation and collaboration include any involvement in the obtaining and using of drugs, as well as treating the individual's withdrawal from drug use.

Protecting and shielding. During the earlier stages of addiction, family members—consciously and unconsciously—do not want to believe that the addiction exists. However, they may see the addicted behavior themselves, observe the consequences of the addiction, and hear about addiction-related behavior from others.

In such a situation, seeing is not believing. Family members can see obvious examples of addiction and unconsciously deny what they have seen. They may minimize, rationalize, and repress specific observations, experiences, and feelings.

Thus, family members engage in three types of protecting as an unconscious defense mechanism. First, they protect themselves from the internal conflict of seeing evidence of addiction but not wanting

207

to believe it. Second, family members protect the addicted person from being identified as addicted. Also, family members protect the addicted person from the consequences of the addiction.

Example

Thirteen-year-old Bruce has been smoking marijuana for 2 years now, has replaced most of his lifelong friends with drug-using acquaintances, experiences memory and concentration problems, and will be expelled if he gets into another fight at school. He has been arrested for driving without a license and for driving while under the influence of marijuana. His father is an untreated alcoholic.

Bruce's father is emotionally distant but reacts with rage whenever Bruce gets into trouble. Bruce's father says, "He's no good. He'll never change." Bruce's mother refuses to believe that her son has a drug problem. She blames the school and the parents of Bruce's new acquaintances for "the way Bruce is treated."

In this example, the father creates a wall between himself and his son by being emotionally distant. He creates further distance by reacting with rage when Bruce gets into trouble. Unconsciously, Bruce's father knows that as long as the spotlight is on Bruce, his own alcoholism will be ignored.

Meanwhile, Bruce's mother cannot resolve the conflict of seeing the consequences of Bruce's addiction versus believing that it is not true. She unconsciously resolves this conflict by denying that Bruce is addicted and projecting blame onto other people.

Control and guilt. The use of protection and shielding during the early stages of a family member's addiction protects other family members from the harsh reality of the addiction and shields the addicted person from being identified. During this time, family members often believe that nothing is wrong.

However, this protection allows the addiction to continue and progress. As the addiction becomes increasingly severe—and the addicted person's defense mechanisms become more pathological—family members often believe that somehow they are responsible for the addiction. They may believe, "If I tried harder he wouldn't need to drink." They may think, "Maybe I've been too demanding. I'll try to be more supportive." "It's my fault."

Indeed, the underlying message that family members often receive from the addicted person is "If it wasn't for you, I would not have this problem." Family members may believe this delusion, accept responsibility for the drug use, and make attempts to rectify the situation. Because they believe they are responsible for the addiction, they feel they should try to stop it.

Importantly, the most destructive aspect of this delusion is that people's self-worth becomes linked to someone else's drug use.[11] People may believe that they can't feel good about themselves until they cure their family member's addiction. In other words, their own self-esteem is directly linked to their ability to control someone else's addiction.

Example

Patty has been married to Peter for 5 years. Peter has been drinking alcohol heavily for about 3 years and has recently experienced severe addiction-related consequences such as making extravagant purchases with family money budgeted for household expenses. After these purchases, Patty and Peter have violent arguments. Using projection, Peter frequently tells his wife that she is the reason he drinks alcohol. After a few years, Patty starts to believe it.

Believing that she is responsible for her husband's addiction, Patty begins a campaign to curb it. She takes over the family finances and buys only a limited amount of alcohol in the hopes that this will curb Peter's drinking. She declines invitations for social events at which alcohol is served. She stops participating in her various hobbies and activities so she can devote more time to her husband and try to be more attentive to his needs. Peter's addiction progresses unchecked.

Codependence

Family members who live with the trauma of addiction for extended periods of time can themselves experience severe psychological trauma. As described above, family members of addicted people often develop psychological coping strategies and enabling behaviors that initially protect the family member from psychological harm.

However, these coping strategies, defense mechanisms, and enabling behaviors can become rigid and inflexible and ultimately become more of a problem than a solution. As a result, family members of addicted people develop their own problems as a reaction to the constant trauma of addiction. This set of problems is called codependence.

The term codependence is derived from and replaced an earlier term called co-alcoholism. *Co-alcoholism* describes a recognizable pattern of behavior and attitudes characteristically found in members of alcoholic families.[16] Much as the terms addiction and chemical dependence describe addiction to alcohol and other psychoactive drugs, the term codependence describes the behaviors, attitudes, and psychological impairment caused by living with people who are addicted.

Codependence describes the psychological and behavioral reaction and adaptation by family members to the ongoing trauma of addiction in their family. There is some disagreement among experts about whether codependence is a personality disorder, the result of severe stress from another's addiction, or dysfunctional patterns of coping with addiction.[17]

Whatever the specific nature of codependence, it is a disorder with characteristic personality traits, coping styles, and behaviors.[16,18–22] There are five particularly characteristic elements of codependence: 1) currently or recently living with an actively addicted person, 2) an obsessional focus on the needs and behaviors of the addicted person, 3) a zealous tendency to please the addicted person and to deprive oneself, 4) identity confusion, and 5) dismally low self-esteem.[23]

Pleasing others and depriving oneself: focus on others.   The hallmark feature of codependence is the ongoing and excessive trait of pleasing other people while depriving oneself. Although in certain circumstances this behavior may be noble and generous, in the codependent person it is an inflexible, enduring pattern that causes suffering, dysfunction, and impairment.[24] In a healthy relationship, there is give and take between two people. In contrast, the codependent person unconsciously feels the intense need to please, serve, and satisfy the needs of others. Codependent people will nearly always defer to the wishes and whims of others, rather than state their own.

A central theme of codependence is fear of abandonment. Codependent people may unconsciously believe that if they state their wishes, they will be abandoned and rejected. They often have problems with low self-esteem and generally engage in people-pleasing behavior. As a result, they suppress their feelings of anger, rage, disappointment, and assertiveness.

To avoid abandonment and to please other people, codependent people deny their own needs and deprive themselves of pleasures. They will experience uncomfortable situations in order to make someone else feel more comfortable.

Codependent people spend most of their time and energy on issues that relate to the addicted person. In particular, they expend massive amounts of effort attempting to manage and control the addicted person, rather than satisfying their own needs. They often feel the compulsion to "fix" the addict. With continued excessive focusing on the addicted person's needs, codependent people may actually lose touch with their own needs, much less how to meet those needs.

Healthy adults organize their life around a core of personal integrity and self-esteem. In contrast, codependent people organize their lives around the values, standards, and needs of others.[25]

Identity confusion and self-esteem. Because codependent people ignore their own needs and place enormous weight on the needs of others, they literally confuse their own needs with the needs of others.

If the needs of the addicted person are unmet and if that individual is unhappy, the self-worth of the codependent person plummets. If the addicted person is unhappy, codependent people feel it is their "job" to make the individual happy. If the addicted person is happy, the self-worth of the codependent person rises. The self-worth and self-esteem of codependent people are not related to their own emotional health, but are related to the emotional health of the addicted person.

Because the self-worth of codependent people is directly related to another person, not being in a relationship can result in immeasurably low self-esteem. Psychiatrist Timmen Cermak quotes a patient: "I used to be half of something wonderful. Now I'm half of nothing, and half of nothing is nothing."[26] Because not being in a relationship is so devastating, codependent people often endure horribly unhealthy relationships, for example, with addicted people or batterers.

Other signs of codependence. Those who are in codependent relationships with addicted people may experience a variety of emotional, interpersonal, psychiatric, and even medical problems. These problems include the excessive use of denial and repression of emotions. Codependent people are often overresponsible caretakers and have compulsions and obsessions. They often have a distorted idea of trust and problems with intimacy, separation, and sex. They frequently experience inappropriate and excessive shame, guilt, and prolonged despair. Table 8–2 summarizes many of the symptoms and signs of codependence.

Beyond Defense Mechanisms

Remember that defense mechanisms are unconscious processes that are set into motion to protect the addicted person. Because of the overwhelming trauma of addiction on the addicted individual and the family members, these protective mechanisms can become rigid and inflexible. As they become rigid, severe, and constant traits, they stop protecting and start harming people.

As addiction progresses, and as unconscious defense mechanisms likewise progress, the ability of addicted people and their family members to communicate effectively with each other diminishes. At the same time, their ability to perceive reality becomes severely impaired. As time passes and these impairments progressively worsen, the health of the entire family diminishes. Tensions rise, frustrations are aggravated, and blame becomes more frequent.

As families focus on the dysfunctional behavior of the addicted person in their midst, it is easy to ignore their own needs. They may believe that "fixing" the addicted person is the first and final solution

Table 8–2. Symptoms and signs of codependence

Excessive use of denial
- Denial of what is seen
- Denial of what is felt
- Denial of what others tell them
- Belief that things will get better when they are getting worse
- Denial of their own needs
- Denial that they can't change someone else's behavior
- Denial of problems by becoming workaholic

Repression
- Excessive repression of feelings and emotions
- Excessive repression of opinions and beliefs
- Excessive repression of thoughts
- Excessive repression of own needs
- Repression of genuine personality
- Hiding behind a mask of rigidity
- Putting others' needs first and ignoring own needs

Low self-worth
- Excessive self-blame
- Excessive self-doubt
- Excessive shame
- Inappropriate feelings of guilt
- Fear of being abandoned and alone
- Frequently feeling like a victim
- Fear of making mistakes

Excessive caretaking
- Feels more comfortable giving than receiving
- Needs to be in charge and "fix" people
- Feels anxiety and guilt about other people's problems
- Is supersensitive and anticipates other people's needs
- Often feels used by others
- Overcommits and overextends self

Compulsions and obsessions
- Compulsion to keep family together
- Compulsion to keep addiction hidden from outsiders
- Compulsion to stay busy
- Compulsive behaviors: sexual, eating, spending
- Obsession about other people's problems
- Obsession about other people's behaviors

Distorted idea of trust
- Distrust of self
- Distrust of own feelings
- Distrust of others
- Distrust of God

to the problems in the family. In fact, getting help for that individual is merely part of the solution. The addicted person does not live in a vacuum, but exerts profound influence on the dynamics of the entire family system. Once the family dynamics begin to include enabling behaviors and codependence, simply interrupting the addiction will not be a complete solution to healing those dysfunctional dynamics.

For this reason family involvement is an integral component of addiction treatment. In some ways, the consequences of addiction can be understood as the "domino effect." As the domino of addiction falls, it causes other dominoes to fall. These other dominoes may represent normal, healthy family dynamics. Even if the addiction is interrupted, the other problems remain toppled. Thus, addiction treatment involves interrupting both the addiction and the dysfunctional and impaired family attitudes, defense mechanisms, beliefs, behaviors, and coping skills. In other words, comprehensive addiction treatment involves treating the addicted person and the entire family. Treatment becomes an opportunity for the family to identify, recognize, and reverse their unhealthy responses to addiction, as well as an opportunity for the addicted person to recover.

■ Summary

Defense mechanisms are generally involuntary patterns and styles of behavior, thinking, and feeling that spring into action to conceal or reduce the psychological conflicts that cause anxiety. For addicted

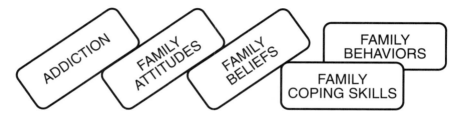

Figure 8–1. The domino effect of addiction on family function.

people, loss of control over drug use and continued drug use despite adverse consequences cause a split between conscious intentions and behavior. The logical center of the brain is unable to control the intense craving that originates in the brain's more primitive limbic system. Defense mechanisms such as denial serve to separate the cognitive and logical system from the emotional and feeling system. These defense mechanisms help to sustain the addiction.

These irrational and unconscious defense mechanisms push painful thoughts out of consciousness and cause a distorted view of reality. As a result, there is an undesirable schism between objective reality and perception of reality. Defense mechanisms can be understood as enduring styles and patterns of coping with conflict. Examples include denial, minimization, rationalization, intellectualization, projection, and regression.

Denial is an unconscious, self-protective refusal to perceive unpleasant reality. Minimization is the unconscious mechanism that allows some, but not all, of the objective reality to sink into conscious awareness. Rationalization describes the use of socially acceptable but untrue explanations for inappropriate behavior.

Intellectualization is a tendency to avoid painful feelings by an enduring focus on thinking rather than feeling. Projection is an unconscious mechanism by which people falsely attribute their own unacknowledged feelings, beliefs, thoughts, impulses, and motives to others. Repression describes a defense mechanism in which the individual is unable to remember specific, often traumatic experiences or disturbing thoughts, feelings, or wishes. Physical isolation is a way of escaping conflicts and avoiding the possibility of being confronted about changing certain behavior and ideas.

Like blackouts, euphoric recall is a drug-induced impairment of memory. Although blackouts describe the inability to remember, euphoric recall describes a distortion in remembering and subsequent distortions in perception. More specifically, euphoric recall is the perception that one's memory of a drug-intoxicated episode is factual and accurate.

Family members develop defense mechanisms to protect themselves psychologically from the trauma of addiction. Family members may develop unconscious ways of not admitting the overpowering fact of addiction in their family. Families can adapt to the addiction by experiencing shame, anxiety, and fear.

Enabling describes the actions of one person that promote the continued addiction of another. Enabling can be conscious, unconscious, active, by omission, and even institutional in nature. As enabling becomes more entrenched and severe, the enablers often become more concerned with the addicted person's feelings than with their own.

Codependence describes the psychological and behavioral reaction and adaptation by family members to the ongoing trauma of addiction in their family. Codependence is a disorder with characteristic personality traits, coping styles, and behaviors. There are five characteristic elements of codependence: 1) currently or recently living with an actively addicted person, 2) an obsessional focus on the needs and behaviors of the addicted person, 3) a zealous tendency to please the addicted person and deprive oneself, 4) identity confusion, and 5) dismally low self-esteem.

Because addiction causes severe dysfunction in both the addicted person and the family members, treatment goals should include the arrest of the addictive process, the cessation of family dysfunction, and improved psychosocial health for all members of the family.

■ References

1. State Department of Human Services v Mary C. Northern, 563 SW2d 197 (Tenn 1978)
2. Shelp EE, Perl M: Denial in clinical medicine: a reexamination of the concept and its significance. Archives of Internal Medicine 145:697–699, 1985
3. Milhorn HT Jr: Chemical Dependence, Diagnosis, Treatment, and Prevention. New York, Springer-Verlag, 1990
4. Van Cleave S, Byrd W, Revell K: If drugs are so bad, why do people keep using them? how denial and guilt perpetuate drug abuse, in Counseling for Substance Abuse and Addiction. Edited by Van Cleave S. Waco, TX, Word Books, 1987, pp 63–87

5. Milhorn HT Jr: Introduction to physiological control systems, in The Application of Control Theory to Physiological Systems. Philadelphia, PA, WB Saunders, 1966, pp 113–137

6. Coleman JC, Butcher JN, Carson RC: Abnormal Psychology and Modern Life, 2nd Edition. Glenview, IL, Scott, Foresman, 1984

7. Freud A: The Ego and the Mechanisms of Defense. New York, International Universities Press, 1966

8. Morrison MA, Smith QT: Psychiatric issues of adolescent chemical dependence. Pediatric Clinics of North America 34:461–480, 1987

9. American Psychiatric Association: Diagnostic and Statistical Manual of Mental Disorders, Third Edition, Revised. Washington, DC, American Psychiatric Association, 1987, pp 393–394

10. Hinsie LE, Campbell AJ: Psychiatric Dictionary. London, Oxford University Press, 1970

11. Johnson VE: Intervention: How to Help Someone Who Doesn't Want Help. Minneapolis, MN, Johnson Institute Books, 1986

12. Johnson VE: I'll Quit Tomorrow: A Practical Guide to Alcoholism Treatment, Revised Edition. San Francisco, CA, Harper & Row, 1980

13. Bean M: Denial and the psychological complications of alcoholism, in Dynamic Approaches to the Understanding and Treatment of Alcoholism. Edited by Bean M, Zinberg N. New York, Free Press, 1981, pp 55–96

14. Arentzen WP: Impact of alcohol misuse in family life. Alcoholism 2:345–351, 1978

15. Nelson CE: The styles of enabling behavior, in Treating Cocaine Dependency. Edited by Smith DE, Wesson DR. Center City, MN, Hazelden Foundation, 1988, pp 49–71

16. Cermak T: Diagnostic criteria for codependency. Journal of Psychoactive Drugs 18:15–20, 1986

17. Mendenhall W: Co-dependency definitions and dynamics. Alcoholism Treatment Quarterly 6:3–17, 1989

18. Mendenhall W: Co-dependency treatment. Alcoholism Treatment Quarterly 6:75–86, 1989

19. Potter-Efron RT, Potter-Efron PS: Outpatient codependency treatment. Alcoholism Treatment Quarterly 6:151–167, 1989

20. Mulry JT: Codependency: a family addiction. American Family Physician 35:215–219, 1987

21. Whitfield C: Co-alcoholism: recognizing a treatable illness. Family and Community Health 7:16–25, 1984

22. Coleman E, Colgan P: Boundary inadequacy in drug dependent families. Journal of Psychoactive Drugs 18:21–30, 1986

23. Cermak TL: Diagnosing and Treating Co-Dependence. Minneapolis, MN, Johnson Institute, 1986
24. Whitfield CL: Co-dependence: our most common addiction: some physical, mental, emotional and spiritual perspectives. Alcoholism Treatment Quarterly 6:19–36, 1989
25. Smalley S: Co-Dependency: An Intimacy Dilemma. New Brighton, MN, SBS Publications, 1984
26. Cermak TL: A Time to Heal: The Road to Recovery for Adult Children of Alcoholics. Los Angeles, CA, Jeremy P Tarcher, 1988

Chapter 9

The Intervention Process

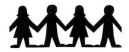

Addiction to alcohol and other drugs provokes the development of vigorous defense mechanisms, preventing addicts from being fully aware of the severity of damage that their behavior causes themselves and others. Because of this lack of insight, addicts are generally unaware of their own addiction and their need for help. Since spontaneous insight about addiction rarely happens, interventions allow the addicts to finally see their lives as others can. Since interventions include family education about addiction and involvement with Al-Anon and other self-help groups, they are vital for the growth and health of addicted families. Interventions can be the processes which result in treatment for the addict, but they can also be a new beginning of hope, healing, and growth for the entire family.

Nancy Miller, R.N.
Bay Area Advocates for the Impaired Nurse
Pregnant Addict Project, Kaiser Hospital
San Francisco, California

■ Why Intervene?

For most addicted people, the decision to begin addiction treatment is not the result of rational, thoughtful deliberations that conclude with a voluntary admission to treatment. Rather, most addicted people are coaxed into treatment because of legal, family, medical, and employment problems, or because they were court-ordered.[1] Impairment and dysfunction in these areas grow progressively severe, precipitating a crisis that results in admission to treatment. In addition, treatment can result from a special type of deliberately planned, organized, highly structured, and therapeutic crisis: an addiction intervention.

Although it may seem painfully obvious to some people, the question should be asked, "Why does there need to be an intervention?" The answer has to do with addicted people's formidable and unconscious defense mechanisms. Because defense mechanisms such as denial are effective in distorting addicted people's perception of reality, they cannot see the destruction of addiction in their own lives. But defense mechanisms have limitations and weak points, and interventions can break through these barriers.

■ What Is Addiction Intervention?

In some ways, a type of intervention occurs whenever people receive accurate and objective information about their drug use. For instance, when a family-practice physician informs patients that their use of alcohol may be making their sleep problems worse, that is an intervention. This type of intervention is best described as advice, and it may have an impact on people who are experimental users or perhaps abusers.

However, because of potent defense mechanisms, interventions such as medical advice may have minimal impact on addicted people, who are often bombarded with advice, complaints, arguments, and reminders of the consequences of their behavior. Their defense systems reject and repel these attempted interventions.

To have an impact, interventions should temporarily weaken the defense mechanisms, at least long enough for addicted people to accurately understand the consequences of their drug use and their need for professional help. The addiction intervention is needed to accomplish these goals.

An *addiction intervention* is a structured, organized, professionally led process in which the objective facts of addicted people's drug-related behavior and consequences are presented to them in such a way that their defense mechanisms cannot reject the information. Or more simply, an intervention is the presentation of reality to individuals out of touch with it—in such a way that they can accept it.[2]

Ideally, the intervention involves helping addicted people to recognize that their drug use is a major cause of the immediate and painful life problems, rather than the result of these problems. Also, interventions can help addicted people to realize that their impaired control over drug use is one aspect of an illness and that treatment is available and can lead to recovery and health.[3] The intervention marks the beginning of cessation of drug use: a transition between active use and treatment.

Intervention, Not Simply Confrontation

To be sure, an addiction intervention is not a pleasant experience. A well-designed, planned, professionally led intervention can nonetheless be an emotionally draining and difficult process for both family members and addicted people. However, this relatively brief experience cannot compare with the trauma of living with addiction.

Also, an intervention does involve directly confronting addicted people about their drug use. In fact, for many families, the intervention is the first time that family members have spoken directly to the addicted person about the drug use.

However, other family members have had innumerable confrontations with the addicted person in their family. These family members often describe their attempts at confronting addicted people as "talking to a brick wall." That's a relatively accurate way of characterizing a purely confrontational interaction. Such confrontations consist of two communication components: 1) the family member talking to the addicted person and 2) the addicted person deflecting the family member's message.

During an intervention, there are also two communication components: 1) the family member talking to the addicted person and 2) the addicted person listening to the family member. When the defense mechanisms are weakened, the addicted person can listen, understand, and perceive what the other family members are saying. Not perfectly, perhaps, but well enough to understand.

Characteristics of Addiction Interventions

Several characteristics differentiate addiction interventions from other confrontations with addicted people. The addiction intervention is confrontational yet also loving, nonjudgmental, humanistic, educational, professional, and organized, and it leads to treatment.

Loving and confrontational. The addiction intervention is confrontational, but it is done in the spirit of concern and love. Interventions are done because of a genuine concern for the addicted person's health. They are done because the people involved can no longer watch the addicted person's health deteriorate, and they are willing to become personally involved with supporting the individual's treatment and recovery.

Nonjudgmental. Interventions are nonjudgmental, and they are not forms of punishment. Rather, the goals of interventions include arresting the addiction and providing treatment for the disease. Interventions are nonjudgmental in that they are not designed to harass addicted people and make them feel bad. During the process, addicted people may indeed feel bad, but that is the result of their awakened consciousness of their own behavior; making them feel bad is not the goal of the intervention.

Humanistic. The intervention is an opportunity for family members to openly discuss their concerns about the addicted person's behavior, but it is not an opportunity to deprive addicted people of their dignity. The intervention is a process designed to weaken the individual's unconscious defense system without inflicting psychological harm.

Educational. Interventions are educational for both the addicted person and the family members. The intervention process should include educational sessions for family members that precede the intervention. The intervention is often the beginning of an educational process for the addicted person as well.

Professional. A botched, anger-filled, disaster of an intervention is worse than no intervention. Even a perfectly run intervention is never far from chaos. Counselors who are specifically trained in leading interventions are the most desirable people to organize and lead them. Health care professionals who are knowledgeable about addiction but not specifically trained in leading interventions can be well meaning but can cause problems. Families should seek intervention specialists.

Organized. Addiction interventions are not haphazard, loosely organized affairs. Rather, they are tightly organized processes with firmly established and agreed-on ground rules and with specific goals and consequences. Intervention specialists should insist that family .members obtain education about addiction, prepare for the addiction, practice the intervention, and attend Al-Anon or Nar-Anon.

Beginning of treatment. Interventions are the starting point for addiction treatment. In contrast, purely confrontational interactions with addicted people often lead to a worsening of family communications and further distortions of reality.

When to Intervene

Addiction interventions are appropriate at any point during an individual's addiction. However, because of fears, anxieties, ignorance, and their own defense mechanisms, family members often postpone interventions, hoping that things will "get better." As family members become aware that addiction is a progressive disorder, they realize that the longer they wait, the more severe the addiction becomes. Interventions made during earlier stages of the addiction encounter less powerful defense systems than are seen in late-stage addictions.

However, interventions should not be rushed. A critical aspect of the intervention process involves family education about addiction. No family should be rushed into an intervention before learning about the drugs of abuse, addiction, treatment, and recovery. Most importantly, family members should be given the opportunity to learn about the defense mechanisms of addicted people, because that is the fundamental reason why interventions are necessary. The addiction intervention is a useful therapeutic process that can be adapted to a number of situations.

An addiction assessment. Sometimes co-workers, friends, and family recognize that something is seriously wrong with a colleague, but aren't as certain about the cause. Similarly, many people refuse to enter a drug treatment program, stating that they are not addicted. In these cases, an intervention can be done with the goal of getting people into a setting for psychiatric and addiction assessments. Based on biopsychosocial assessments, treatment may be recommended. Through the intervention, people agree to undergo thorough assessment and to follow the treatment recommendations.

Initiation of treatment. Perhaps the most common use of intervention is to arrest the addiction and initiate treatment. These interventions may be initiated by families, employees, licensing agencies (such as nursing licensing boards), and member organizations (such as state medical societies).

Poor treatment participation. Interventions can be used during treatment. Consider the example of patients who attend treatment, but who do not fully participate and do not meet the treatment goals set out in their treatment plans. Their lack of participation and unmet treatment goals may make them good candidates for a higher level of more intensive treatment. An intervention may be necessary to prompt such changes.

Leaving against medical advice and relapse. Interventions may be necessary for patients who no longer agree to remain in treatment. Also, interventions may be necessary for patients who have left treatment against medical advice or for people who slip or relapse. The goals of such an intervention may be to have the patient reenter treatment or perhaps to reinstitute a full program of recovery.

Other medical problems. Interventions also can be adapted to suit other circumstances; for example, they can be used with patients in recovery who refuse to take prescribed medications. Also, interventions can be used to prompt patient compliance in other areas, such as with diabetic people who refuse to adhere to their physician's dietary and medical recommendations.

When Not to Have an Intervention

Because the primary goals of interventions involve helping addicted people to identify their drug use as problematic and to recognize the need for treatment, people who ask for help with their addiction may not need an intervention.

Sometimes addicted people "hit bottom" or otherwise become aware of the nature of their drug use and their need for help. During these times they may ask for help. This awareness is not evidence that treatment is unnecessary, but should prompt immediate assessment and addiction treatment. It is possible for this sudden awareness to fade just as easily as it appeared.

As should be obvious, people without substance use problems should not receive addiction interventions. The addiction intervention is not a "scare tactic," a game, or a type of punishment. Rather, it is an aspect of addiction treatment.

■ Intervention Preparation

A rushed and failed intervention, filled with angry accusations and threats, can result in a family that is more frightened, chaotic, and dysfunctional than before. A poorly organized intervention, like other crises, can prompt a drug use binge, divorce, violence, or suicide. However, families can take certain steps that increase the likelihood of having well-planned, organized, professional interventions.

Find an Intervention Specialist

Families are well advised to seek professional help before planning and initiating interventions.[4] *Intervention specialists* have training and experience specifically in organizing, preparing, and conducting addiction interventions. They can educate the family about the addiction process and the principles of intervention. An intervention specialist can also counsel family members about their anxiety over the intervention and will encourage participation in Al-Anon and Nar-Anon.

Depending on local resources, intervention specialists can be found through local, nonprofit addiction education and treatment programs, city- and county-funded agencies and treatment programs, and for-profit treatment programs. In fact, one of the advantages of fierce competition among addiction treatment programs is the availability of addiction-related services such as interventions, which are often free.

Many treatment programs offer free assessment and intervention services even if the family is unable to send the addicted person to these programs. In those cases, the treatment programs make recommendations for treatment based on the available resources. Family members with limited resources are encouraged to seek out this service. Many treatment programs offer free counseling to family members before the decision to intervene.

Employed people often have significant resources for interventions. For instance, it is increasingly popular for businesses to have an employee assistance program. Employee assistance programs use counselors and therapists who can work with the employees' supervisor to arrange appropriate time off for treatment. These counselors can often coax the employee into treatment without an intervention, but they can also organize or participate in an intervention.

Many unions have addiction- and intervention-related services. Some unions have representatives who organize interventions or who can participate in them. Often, union representatives make referrals to employee assistance programs. Some unions have peer intervention programs.[5] Many local membership groups such as city or county societies (for example, the San Francisco Medical Society) offer intervention services for group members.

Many state professional associations can provide help with interventions. These include various state medical, nursing, pharmacy, dental, bar, and social work associations (for example, the California Nurses Association). Many national professional membership organizations have local mechanisms to identify and intervene with addicted colleagues. These organizations include the American Academy of Physician Assistants, American Bar Association, American Dental Association, American Judicature Society, American Medical Association, American Nurses Association, American Osteopathic Association, American Psychiatric Association, American Psychological Association, American Veterinary Medical Association, and the National Association of Social Workers.

Team Building

Interventions are group efforts with a specific philosophical orientation and a definite goal of initiating treatment.

Motivation for participation. Participants in an addiction intervention should be motivated to participate because they are concerned for the health and well-being of the addicted person and want the addiction to be arrested. People who are motivated because of anger, hatred, revenge, and punishment should not participate. The motivation should be the initiation of addiction treatment.

Philosophical agreement. Participants in an addiction intervention often encounter fierce opposition from the addicted person, whose defense system will fuel vigorous resistance. Therefore, the participants must be tightly united in purpose and philosophy.

Dr. Vernon Johnson, often called the "father of interventions," describes five philosophical points of agreement.[2] Participants must understand 1) that addiction is a medical disease against which normal willpower is inadequate to control drug use; 2) that the effects of psychoactive drugs further reduce the strength of normal willpower; 3) that the addicted person has developed a defense system so effective that it causes pronounced self-delusion, including the inability to recognize the nature of the addiction; 4) that because of this defense system and distortion of reality, outsiders must present this information to the addict; and 5) that addiction is not simply a bad habit and that the intervention is an integral part of stopping the progression of addiction.

Participants who are not impaired themselves. People who have drug abuse and addiction problems themselves should not participate in an intervention. On the other hand, friends and family members of the addicted person who are currently participating in a recovery program are excellent candidates.

People in an unhealthy, enabling, or codependent relationship with the addicted person (or anyone else) are poor candidates for participation. Because of their own defense mechanisms, they might undermine the intervention. Similarly, people who believe that the intervention team members are overestimating the seriousness of the addiction are poor candidates.

People who have a primarily antagonistic relationship with the addicted person, people who do not support the team's treatment recommendations, and people who believe that the addicted person should be punished rather than treated should be excluded from the intervention.

Participants who are respected by the addicted person. It is critical that intervention participants be people who are respected and valued by the addicted person. Whether peers, subordinates, or superiors, the participants should be people whose opinions are valued and whose friendships are treasured by the addicted person. Ideally, they should be people to whom the addicted person has turned for advice, counsel, and friendship.

Family members. Naturally, family members are important participants in the intervention. Spouses and significant others are obvious participants. Less obvious are the children and parents of addicted adults. Children as young as 8, 9, and 10 years old may be appropriate participants, as long as they understand the process and can describe their feelings about the addicted person's behavior. Parents and children of addicted adults can be powerful participants and can help to bring the family secrets to light.

Friends. Depending on the stage of the addiction, the addicted person's friends may all have drug problems themselves or may include nonusers. An ideal participant would be a friend who knew the individual before the drug abuse and addiction and who noticed personality and behavioral changes after the onset of addiction.

Colleagues and supervisor. Depending on the circumstances, colleagues, co-workers, and supervisors may be appropriate participants. For instance, if the wife of a laborer received word from a co-worker that her husband was intoxicated on the job, that co-worker might be an appropriate participant. Similarly, the colleagues or partners of a physician or dentist who are aware of substance use problems would have an important role to play in intervention. Supervisors and employee assistance program personnel are particularly important, because they often approve time off for treatment and can deny continued employment if treatment is refused.

Pastor, clergy, or rabbi. Depending on the addicted person's religious involvement, clergy members can play a valuable role, especially if they have personal knowledge of the individual's addiction.

Organization member. Representatives of professional organizations to which the addicted person belongs can be an important asset to the intervention. For instance, representatives of national, state, or local membership organizations for nurses, physicians, and dentists will willingly participate—or indeed initiate the intervention. Often these representatives are themselves recovering from addiction. They are often part of "impaired professional committees" within their organizations. Members of the armed forces have access to addiction counselors and therapists.

Knowledge of the addiction. Intervention participants should have direct and personal knowledge of the addiction. This knowledge may include seeing evidence of drug use, identifying behavioral and psychological consequences of the addiction, and experiencing adverse consequences of the addiction. Some participants may have experienced adverse consequences or noticed significant behavioral or psychological problems without knowing the cause of those problems. Supervisors and co-workers may have noticed changes in work performance, and colleagues in professional organizations may have received complaints about the addicted person.

Intervention team size. Intervention specialists often have preferred ideal sizes for intervention teams. Therefore, intervention team sizes vary, but the team often consists of three to six people plus the intervention specialist. For example, a team might consist of a spouse, two children, a brother, a friend, a supervisor, and the intervention specialist. In situations where there are few available participants, families are encouraged to use whoever is available. Interventions should not be avoided because only a spouse and a friend are available.

Information Gathering

Once the intervention team has been selected, the members should engage in two types of information gathering: addiction education for themselves and lists of addiction consequences.

Addiction education. Participation in an addiction intervention should never be undertaken blindly. Rather, all participants should understand the addiction process, defense mechanisms, treatment, and recovery process. Written information—such as this book—is an excellent way to begin that educational process. Family members can attend lectures on addiction, participate in workshops on interventions, attend group sessions for people preparing interventions, watch educational videotapes, and read educational material about addiction and interventions.

Creating lists of addiction behavior. During the intervention, participants describe to the addicted person 1) examples of drug- and addiction-related incidents they observed, 2) consequences of the incidents, and 3) their concern for the health and well-being of the addicted person. Because these can be difficult things to say— and because the intervention experience is emotional—participants must make a written list of items. In fact, these lists will be read to the addicted person during the intervention.

The lists include specific circumstances and episodes of drug use and signs of addiction. These specific incidents may be evidence of drug use, compulsion to use drugs, loss of control over drug use, loss of control over drug-induced behavior, and evidence of continued drug use despite adverse consequences. When possible, participants should write down incidents that they observed directly or that affected them in some way. Each team member should prepare a list of five or more statements.

Videotapes. There are two particularly valuable uses of videotapes during an intervention. First, family members who are unable to attend the intervention can videotape their comments for playback during the process. This is an update of the technique of out-of-town family members writing their comments in the form of a letter to be read during the intervention.

Also, families may have examples of drug-related behavior on videotape. For instance, there may be a tape of the individual speaking in a slurred voice, walking in an uncoordinated way or falling, making drug-induced mistakes, wearing disheveled clothes, making lewd gestures in inappropriate settings, throwing up, and having sudden personality changes such as rapidly becoming violent. It would be difficult for someone to deny behavior that can be seen on tape.

Treatment resources. The family members should begin to research available treatment resources and to investigate what their insurance company will cover. Intervention specialists who work for specific treatment programs will encourage treatment within their programs. However, family members should be astute consumers and compare treatment programs.

Treatment programs can differ in terms of the number of services offered, the quality of services, and the price. At the same time, insurance companies will likely make certain demands, agreeing to pay for certain types of treatments and declining to pay for others. Thus, treatment program selection should be a balance of treatment need, treatment quality, and available financial resources.

Many intervention specialists recommend narrowing the treatment options down to a single choice. Others may recommend offering the addicted person a few choices. Either way, before the actual intervention, all arrangements should be made, including financial arrangements, time off from work, and securing available bed space in a treatment program.

Family member resources. The intervention tends to put the focus on addicted people and their addiction. However, family members undertaking an intervention have their own emotional needs and will experience stress during the process. During this time, family participation in recovery-oriented activity is crucial. For this reason, most treatment programs strongly encourage active involvement in Al-Anon, Nar-Anon, and Alateen.

Indeed, participation of family members in these self-help groups should begin before intervention planning and should continue throughout the addicted person's treatment and recovery. Importantly, family members new to these groups meet family members who went through the same processes some time ago. These "old-timers" can help the newcomers by explaining what to expect and how to avoid problems, and by giving support.

In addition to Al-Anon and Nar-Anon, treatment programs may offer courses, lectures, workshops, and also counseling for family members.

Intervention Planning and Rehearsal

Once the members of the intervention team have been selected, are becoming actively educated about addiction, and are taking steps to take care of their own emotional needs, the intervention can be planned.

Determining leverage. A critical aspect of making an intervention succeed involves determining the type of leverage that can be used to prompt voluntary treatment.[6] In other words, is there something so important to the addicted person that it could be used to prompt entry to a treatment program, if necessary?

Ideally, leverage need never be used. In many interventions, the impact of a group of family members and friends confronting the addicted person openly and honestly is enough to weaken the defense mechanism and enable the addicted person to accept the team recommendations for treatment. In other cases, the addicted person rejects the team recommendations for treatment.

To prepare for this possibility, the team should decide ahead of time what specific leverages can be used. The selection of leverage is extremely sensitive and serious. Although leverages might diplomatically be described as contingencies, they are in fact threats. In essence, a leverage is an action that will be taken if and only if the addicted person does not follow the intervention team's treatment recommendations.

Leverages vary depending on the addicted person's occupation, social circumstances, and degree of impairment. If the employer is involved in the intervention, job loss could be the leverage necessary to coax the addicted person into treatment. Also, people who have licenses in the health care field—such as physicians, nurses, and pharmacists—would rarely refuse to go to treatment if it meant losing their license.

Leverage may include severed social relationships, such as a wife using divorce as leverage to get her husband into treatment. Friends may be willing to risk their relationship with the addicted person to prompt treatment. Business partners may demand a resignation unless treatment is accepted.

Again, selecting leverage is serious business. It is important to note that 1) leverage should be used only as a last resort, 2) leverage should not be threatened unless it absolutely will be carried out, and 3) leverage should be agreed on and supported by the entire team.

Details and homework. During the information-gathering phase of the intervention preparation, the team will learn about the available community resources for treatment and explore personal resources, including insurance limitations. Based on this information, the appropriate team members should finally decide on one to three treatment programs that will be offered to the addicted person. The team should call and verify that beds are available. The team should decide the time and location of the intervention and who will drive the individual to treatment.

In preparation for the intervention, a specific decision must be made regarding how the addicted person will be brought into the intervention. For example, a member of the team may drive the individual to a prearranged site where the other members are waiting. The specialist can provide additional alternatives that may be appropriate for the individual and the team.

Addicted people may refuse or want to postpone treatment because of outstanding obligations and responsibilities. Thus, every attempt should be made to provide a way to meet those obligations that must be met. This is easiest when the individual works for an employer who can make the necessary adjustments to cover the work. In other situations, business partners can take over the work load. Plans should be made to take care of children, pets, bills, picking up the laundry, and outstanding errands. Appointments can be canceled or postponed until the future.

To postpone treatment, the addicted person may use the excuse of needing to go home and get some clothes. Having a packed suitcase removes one more obstacle to compliance. Table 9–1 is a checklist of details that should be addressed prior to an intervention.

Team member guidelines. Team members must be in complete agreement on several issues and must completely support one another. The slightest hint of disagreement among intervention team members can be used to create discord and division. All disagreements about treatment goals and leverage should be ironed out before the intervention.

The intervention needs a chairperson—ideally, the intervention specialist—to keep things running smoothly. The chairperson should not be personally or emotionally involved in the family's life, except for the intervention itself, so as to be more objective and less emotional about the process. Each member should agree to follow the lead of the chairperson during the intervention. The chairperson will "direct traffic" and interrupt the addicted person and team members who begin arguing. The lead of the specialist-chairperson should be followed without argument.

The team members must agree to make no concessions during the intervention. No member should back down because of pleas, threats, and emotional outbursts. Each team member should be prepared for threats of lawsuits and threats of lost friendship. The addicted person will be scared and may say and do anything to stop

Table 9–1.   Checklist for interventions

Intervention preparation
- Find a professional intervention specialist
- Participate in Al-Anon, Nar-Anon, and Alateen immediately
- Assemble an intervention team
- Learn about drugs of abuse, treatment, and recovery
- Review examples of addiction-related behavior
- Learn about local treatment resources
- Research insurance coverage of treatment
- Examine personal financial resources

Intervention planning
- Have statements written down and prepared
- Determine leverage to be used if treatment is refused
- Select treatment programs to offer
- Verify that treatment space is available
- Decide time and place of the intervention
- Decide how the individual will arrive at the intervention
- Decide how the individual will be driven to treatment
- Arrange time off from work for treatment
- Cancel appointments, handle obligations, do errands
- Review reasons for wanting to do the intervention
- Have "walk-through" rehearsal to learn the format
- Have "dress" rehearsal with someone playing the role of the addicted person
- Pack suitcase

the intervention. These defensive maneuvers should not make team members retract anything they have said or decisions they have made.

Also, team members must be prepared to follow through with leverage and be fully prepared to support other members who will initiate that leverage. Thus, if a wife states that she will leave her husband if he does not enter treatment, the other team members must be fully prepared to support the use of that leverage and have a specific plan ready to help her to accomplish that task, even to the point of planning how and when to remove her belongings. With guidance from the intervention specialist, the team should rehearse the intervention at least once, if not twice.[7]

"Walk-through" and "dress" rehearsals. Intervention team members should attend addiction education lectures and workshops together to facilitate discussion of learned material. The team should participate in one walk-through to understand the intervention format and a dress rehearsal to increase familiarity with the format.

Review of purpose. At the beginning of each rehearsal, the team members should review briefly the reasons for their coming together and the purpose of the eventual intervention. They should review briefly the evidence and progression of the addiction, why they feel an intervention is necessary, and what they are willing to do to coax the individual into treatment.

Review of format. The team should decide specifically where each intervention team member and the addicted person should sit. The team should decide the order of presentations: who will go first, who will go last.

Role-play. The specialist or a colleague can play the role of the addicted person because he or she can mimic the type of defenses that may be used by the addicted individual. To make the rehearsal authentic, the "addict" should interrupt, make snide comments about the process, and be slightly uncooperative. This provides an opportunity to practice appropriate responses.

Rehearsal and Intervention

During rehearsals and the intervention itself, the tone of the process should be one of serious concern. The addicted person will likely be scared and anxious, and these fears may be exhibited through signs of anger. In some ways, this level of anxiety can be productive, because the ultimate outcome involves presenting to the individual a way to decrease that anxiety: treatment.

Initial statement to the addicted person. The rehearsal, as well as the actual intervention, begins in earnest with an initial statement to the addicted person. This initial statement will set the tone of the process. The intervention specialist will read or make a statement of general purpose and a request to the individual. The statement will likely be similar to the following.

"John, this group, consisting of your family, friends, and employer, have gathered together because they care about you and because they want to help you. Because they care about you and because they want to help you, they have one simple request. They request that you listen to what they have to say. That's all. After they are finished, you will have an opportunity to reply. But for now, they ask you for one simple request, to listen to what they have to say to you without interruption. We know you may have some questions, and those questions will be answered shortly. Will you agree to listen to what this group has to say to you?"

Naturally, responses may vary. Some people will simply agree to listen. Many will agree, but will interrupt with questions. Many will be resistant to the process, but ultimately will agree to listen.

Team members' statements. Under the direction of the intervention specialist, the team members should read their statements aloud to the addicted person. The team members' statements should not be generalized comments ("You're hard to live with"), value judgments ("I think you drink too much"), or emotional opinions ("I don't deserve this").

Team members' statements should be descriptions of specific prior events that are directly related to drug use; these events should be described in as much detail as possible and in a way that shows concern for the welfare of the addicted individual.[8] The selected incidents should have produced adverse consequences such as damage, harm, or injury to the addicted person or to others, whether this harm was physical, social, or emotional. The incidents may also show evidence of the progression of drug use or the progression of adverse consequences. They may also show evidence of progressive deterioration of health, hygiene, and job performance. These statements document by date, time, and place those specific incidents when the individual demonstrated addictive behavior that affected himself or herself and others.[9]

Each team member should have a list of five or more statements. Each statement should contain four elements: 1) a positive declaration, 2) a specific incident of addiction, 3) the consequence of that incident, and 4) a statement of concern.

The *positive declaration* should be a general, positive statement about the individual. A few examples follow: "John, you have always been a great provider for me and the children." "John, I have always looked to you as a great friend." "John, you have always been a valued employee." "Daddy, I am proud to be your daughter."

The *specific incident of addiction* should be simple, specific, and detailed descriptions of addiction-related behaviors. They should not be generalized statements, nor should they be value judgments, accusations, or emotional opinions.

A few examples follow: "Last month, you attended the PTA meeting with alcohol on your breath, and spoke to Johnny's teacher with slurred speech." "John, I've known you for 10 years. But since you started using cocaine, you have been a different person. This past month you borrowed $300 dollars from me in order to pay the kid's hospital bill, but I found out you bought cocaine with it." "John you used to be one of the best workers that I know. But since you started using cocaine, your job performance has decreased, and you have been late for work and absent more than ever before. You have had a few small accidents at work, and I am concerned that you will become even less safe." "Daddy, you promised to bring me to the circus for my birthday. That day, you said that you had the flu, but you smelled like whiskey and yelled at mommy."

The *consequence of that incident* may be mentioned during the statement. The consequences can be included to make it clear to the individual that the addiction behavior did cause repercussions that affected other people.

A few examples follow: "After you spoke to Johnny's teacher with slurred speech and alcohol on your breath, my heart sank, and Johnny's teacher and I became embarrassed, scared, and worried." "After I realized you borrowed the money from me to use cocaine, I felt hurt and saddened." "Since your job performance has decreased and your safety record has deteriorated, I have had to hire someone else to take up the slack." "When you missed my birthday and yelled at mommy, I got real angry and scared."

Also, each statement should end in a *statement of concern*. For example, "I know that this isn't really you. I am concerned that the real you will get lost, if you don't get help for your addiction." "My friendship with you is important, but I am more concerned with your deteriorating health. I want to see you get better." "Your recent accidents are damaging the good safety record you otherwise have. I don't want to see you jeopardize your position at the company."

Prepare for interruptions. Obviously, listening to these types of statements will be difficult. Some people will express a profound sense of relief and show appreciation for the concern. They may actually say, "What took you so long," and immediately ask about treatment options. More commonly, they will react with defiance, threats, denial, excuses, promises, and bargaining.[6] These defense mechanisms often will occur as interruptions, outbursts, and crying.

When team members are interrupted during their statements, they should ignore the interruptions. Importantly, they should not engage in a heated discussion or argument over specifics. Rather, the team member should simply say, "Please hear me out. All I am asking you to do is to listen to what I have to say." If the interruptions become severe, the intervention specialist will try to enforce the promise to listen.

Offering treatment options. After the team members have presented their statements, the intervention specialist will briefly summarize the reason for the intervention. The specialist may make a statement similar to the following: "These friends of yours have gathered together because they love you, because they are concerned for you, and because they realize that you have a problem which is out of control. Because of their concern for you, they want you to get help for your problem. In fact, they are willing to help you get help for your problem. They have selected three programs that treat drug problems like you have. They need your help in selecting the program you would like to go to."

The addicted person's reactions. The reactions of addicted people to the statements and the treatment recommendations will vary depending on each individual's defense mechanisms and on how smoothly the intervention operates. If the intervention is successful in weakening the defense mechanisms, the individual may experience a grieving process that may include denial, anger, bargaining, depression, and acceptance.[6]

When addicted people accept the treatment recommendations, they may attempt to control the way in which the recommendations are carried out. For instance, there may be requests to go home and pack, to cancel appointments, to go to the office and finish up a few things, to run some errands, to make some calls, to write some letters, to do some research on the treatment programs, or to get the car out of the shop.

It is critical that the intervention team present a very strong, unified, and clear message: the time is now. The team members must inform the individual that the errands have been done, the appointments have been canceled, and the suitcase has been packed. The team members should make it very clear that the only thing to do now is to go to treatment. However, offering more than one treatment program gives the individual some choice in the matter, so that he or she does not feel that all his or her dignity has been stripped away.

Using the leverage. In the event that the individual refuses the treatment recommendations or insists on conditions that differ from the intervention team's goals, the use of leverage comes into play.

Often, the best leverage relates to professional and vocational issues. For example, the employer may make continued employment contingent on receiving treatment.

Depending on the circumstances, there may be only one significant leverage, or there may be more. Because leverages should be used only when it is absolutely necessary, they should be presented one at a time. Continued refusal can be met with additional leverage.

Although the intervention team clearly exerts strong pressure, the decision of the addicted person is ultimately voluntary. If the addicted person absolutely refuses to attend treatment, the leverage must be applied, and each team member must support those who actually apply it.

Refusal to attend treatment. If treatment is rejected, leverage must be applied immediately. On occasion, addicted people will "test" the commitment level of the intervention team by attempting to coax the members to reduce, modify, or eliminate the leverage, as well as to attempt to create division among the members. Thus, it is crucial that the team members keep their resolve, communicate openly with one another, and attend Al-Anon and Nar-Anon.

Refusal to attend treatment after an intervention does not mean that the intervention has completely failed. Rather, it means that this particular phase of the intervention process has not yet resulted in the desired effects. In fact, addicted people may decide to enter treatment when they discover that the intervention team will indeed apply the leverage as promised.

Example

John was intervened on by a team that included his wife, employer, and two best friends. John was informed that his failure to attend treatment would result in 1) potential job loss (employer), 2) separation and initiation of divorce proceedings (wife), and 3) discontinuation of friendships (friends). After the intervention, John refuses to attend treatment. He promises not to drink anymore, threatens to sue his employer if he loses his job, vaguely threatens his wife, and curses his friends.

The next day, John goes to work as if nothing is wrong. His employer tells him to meet with the employee assistance counselors. The employee assistance counselors remind John that the company's drug policy stipulates that he attend treatment for his addiction. He reiterates his refusal to attend treatment. They inform John that because his refusal to attend treatment violates the company's drug policy rules, he is now suspended. He is given a written notice that failure to obtain treatment within 21 days will result in loss of his job. He leaves angrily for home.

When he arrives home, John is surprised by the presence of three cars in his driveway. His wife, accompanied by John's friends who participated in the intervention, are packing Mary's clothes. She informs John that as promised, she will no longer live with him if he does not get treatment. She also informs John that she will meet with her attorney about initiating divorce proceedings if he refuses treatment within a certain time frame.

Shortly before the 21 days run out on his suspension, John calls the employee assistance program and asks the counselors what he needs to do to keep his job. He is reminded about the treatment options previously given him. Although he feels that he does not have a problem and that other people have conspired against him, John finally agrees to enter treatment.

In this example of John's initial refusal to participate in treatment, his ultimate treatment could have been jeopardized at a number of critical points. If any of the team members had backed down during the intervention and accepted John's "promise" to stop drinking, John would still be drinking. If John's business had not established a drug policy mandating treatment, he might have ended up at another job without being treated. If John and Mary's friends had not fully supported the decision for John to get treatment, John might have talked Mary out of leaving.

An intervention that does not immediately result in an admission to treatment may appear to be a complete failure. In practice, however, the effects of the intervention process are cumulative. If someone does not enter treatment after an intervention, the combination of consistently applied leverage plus a second intervention may have the desired results.

Benefits of Interventions and Self-Help for Family Members

The goal of intervention is not limited to getting the addicted person into treatment. Rather, there are impressive benefits for family members even if the individual does not go to treatment.[4] Indeed, the intervention can have a powerful effect on individual family members and on family dynamics irrespective of the outcome for the addicted person. This is especially true for family members who also participate in the self-help Twelve-Step programs of Al-Anon, Nar-Anon, and Alateen.

In addition to prompting the addicted individual to receive treatment, interventions increase family members' awareness of their power to make effective choices for themselves, whether the addicted person accepts treatment or not. The intervention teaches family members to practice new and constructive behaviors to solve their own problems. In fact, the intervention becomes an opportunity for family members to look at themselves and identify areas of dysfunction. It can become a first step in the family's recovery process.

Examples of benefits for family members often include 1) becoming aware of their rights as individuals and family members and being able to exercise these rights without feeling guilty or disloyal; 2) learning to set boundaries for themselves within the family; 3) learning to trust their own intuition for validation, rather than judging themselves by how others would react; 4) realizing that each member of the family system is equally valued and important; 5) learning how to communicate openly and honestly; and 6) feeling hopeful rather than hopeless.[10]

Breaking the silence.   One of the most critical benefits to family members is breaking the silence of addiction. The intervention is often the first time that family members have openly and honestly talked about the addiction in their family, how it affects them, and how they feel about it.[11] They often realize that their thoughts and feelings were not "secrets" but were shared by other family members. Thus, the intervention and attendance at Al-Anon and Nar-Anon allow family members an opportunity to talk about and process their experiences and to realize that they are not alone. They meet others who have had the same experiences. Participation in self-help activities fosters a healthy supportive network.

Education, understanding, and recognition. People who participate in interventions become more knowledgeable about drugs of abuse and addiction, and they become more aware of the symptoms and signs of abuse and addiction. They are capable of earlier identification and thus earlier intervention. This education, coupled with enhanced communication with other family members, makes it less likely that they will believe in the addiction-induced delusions and distorted perspectives of addicted people. They become less likely to believe that they are the cause of another person's addiction. They become more likely to believe in themselves and to trust their own feelings.

Change of family focus. Before the intervention, family members probably communicated with each other indirectly and poorly, promoting broad communication problems. Similarly, the focus may have been on denying, minimizing, and hiding from the addiction in their midst. Many families experience severe fear, guilt, and shame. They may feel overwhelmed and believe that they are unable to change their problems.

After an intervention—and especially with participation in Al-Anon and Nar-Anon—families learn how to communicate with each other more effectively, how to solve problems, and how to deal better with problems that they cannot solve. Thus, families often stop focusing on problems and start focusing on problem solving; they stop living in fear and begin living with empowered, mutual support. Participation in an intervention is a therapeutic and educational opportunity for family members, and it results in changes in attitude, outlook, and perspective.[12]

New family rules. To survive living with addiction, family members often follow three unwritten, unconscious rules: don't talk, don't feel, and don't trust.[13] For example, family members often avoid talking about important issues that are greatly affecting them and other members. Similarly, family members may learn to deny their own feelings and inappropriately care more about the feelings of others. Also, family members often stop trusting their own perceptions, feelings, and values.

After an intervention, the family may develop new, healthy rules that foster open and routine communication. They may begin new traditions such as family meetings or engage in family outings to increase solidarity. They may begin to inquire openly about other people's feelings, while taking care of their own needs. As a result, they may learn to trust one another again and learn to trust their own strengths, perceptions, and feelings.

Family health. As with other crises, the intervention is an opportunity for family members to come together and solve a problem as a family. For many families, the intervention is the first time in a long while that they have become organized with a unified goal. That process alone can help families to put aside differences and modify existing priorities.

Family participation in Al-Anon, Nar-Anon, and Alateen helps family members to learn a common language of recovery through the therapeutic experiences of admission, acceptance, and surrender.[14] This new language of recovery provides a forum for problem solving, personal growth, and family health. For family members, the emphasis of recovery becomes self-growth and support of the self-growth of others.

Self-help groups help family members learn to stop trying to control the behavior of other people and to stop feeling responsible for a family member's addiction. Through such participation, family members can experience a reversal of depression, problems with coping, substance abuse, and intimacy problems.[15] But family recovery is not limited to a reversal of problems. Rather, participation in these programs promotes spirituality, which often takes a back seat to the chronic crises of addiction in the family.[16]

Living With Addiction

Sometimes the addicted person refuses treatment despite the efforts of family members. It is imperative to recognize that family recovery can, and indeed should, occur despite active addiction in the family. Family recovery is not pursued for the sake of the addicted person; it is done for the health of the family. Nor does family recovery depend on the future sobriety of the addicted person.[2] Indeed, active addiction is a powerful reason for families to initiate and pursue active family recovery.

However, the pursuit of family recovery in the face of active addiction requires philosophical and emotional adjustments. These adjustments can be called toughlove. Toughlove is both a philosophy and a program. Toughlove was developed as a self-help program for the parents of severely acting-out teenagers.[17] As a program and a philosophy, Toughlove involves the use of self-help support groups, education, parental rights, and limitations. As a philosophy, toughlove involves the use of open acceptance, assigning responsibility, and allowing consequences.[18]

Responsibility and consequences. In the face of active addiction, family members frequently rescue addicted people from the consequences of their behavior. When family members deny, minimize, excuse, rationalize, or cover up the adverse consequences of addiction, they are assuming responsibility for the addicted individual's behavior. The toughlove approach demands that people be responsible for their own actions and that they experience the consequences of their own behavior.

■ Summary

An addiction intervention is a structured and organized, professionally led process in which the objective facts of addicted people's drug-related behavior and consequences are presented to them in such a way that their defense mechanisms cannot reject the information. An intervention is not merely an angry confrontation; it is a presentation of reality to individuals out of touch with it, done in such a way that they can accept it. Interventions are loving yet confrontational, nonjudgmental, humanistic, educational, professional, and organized. They are the starting point for addiction treatment.

Interventions can be used to prompt an addiction assessment; to initiate treatment; to respond to relapse, poor treatment participation, or leaving treatment against medical advice; and to encourage compliance with treatment in patients with severe medical problems.

One of the first steps in intervention preparation involves finding a professional intervention specialist. In addition, an intervention team should be assembled. Intervention team members should agree on the goal of the intervention: to coax the addicted person into treatment. They should not be impaired themselves, should be respected by the addicted person, and may include family members, friends, colleagues, supervisors, and clergy. Intervention team members should become educated about drugs of abuse, addiction, treatment, recovery, and relapse.

The intervention team creates lists of examples of addicted behavior that resulted in adverse consequences that they saw or experienced personally. These lists ultimately will be read to the addicted person during the intervention. The team learns about treatment resources and resources available to help the team members themselves. Importantly, the team determines appropriate leverage that can be applied if treatment is refused. In preparation for the intervention, appropriate team members should secure the time off from work, cancel appointments, and even pack a suitcase. Before the intervention, team members should review the reasons for doing the intervention and their reasons for participation. There should be a "walk-through" rehearsal and a "dress" rehearsal for the intervention, involving someone who role-plays the addicted person. After the team members read their statements, the individual is offered specific treatment options. The individual should be brought to treatment immediately after accepting the options. Refusal to participate in treatment should be met with immediate application of leverage as previously determined. Continued application of leverage may ultimately lead to treatment.

Family members gain multiple benefits by participating in interventions, whether or not the addicted individual enters treatment. Interventions are opportunities for family members to communicate openly and honestly with each other about the addiction. Family members become educated about the causes and effects of addiction, learn to realize that they are not responsible for the addiction, and learn to identify symptoms and signs of the disorder. Interventions and participation in Twelve-Step self-help groups such as Al-Anon, Nar-Anon, and Alateen foster a change in family focus: from an overwhelmed and scared family to an empowered, openly communicating, problem-solving unit. In general, interventions and participation of family members in self-help programs improve family health, personal growth, and spirituality. Family recovery does not depend on the ultimate recovery of the addicted person. Rather, family recovery is pursued for the sake of improving the health of the family.

■ References

1. Van Cleave S, Byrd SW, Revell K: What really works in treatment, in Counseling for Substance Abuse and Addiction. Edited by Van Cleave S. Waco, TX, Word Books, 1987, pp 133–143
2. Johnson VE: Intervention: How to Help Someone Who Doesn't Want Help. Minneapolis, MN, Johnson Institute Books, 1986
3. Blume SB: Psychotherapy in the treatment of alcoholism, in Psychiatry Update: The American Psychiatric Association Annual Review, Vol 3. Edited by Grinspoon L. Washington, DC, American Psychiatric Press, 1984, pp 338–346
4. Beamer B, Collins BR: Intervention as a therapeutic process for the families of alcoholics. Journal of Applied Social Sciences 7:187–202, 1983
5. Molloy DJ: Peer intervention: an exploratory study. Journal of Drug Issues 19:319–336, 1989
6. Crosby LR, Bissell LeC: To Care Enough: Intervention With Chemically Dependent Colleagues. Minneapolis, MN, Johnson Institute, 1989
7. Spickard A, Thompson BR: The family trap, in Dying for a Drink: What You Should Know About Alcoholism. Edited by Spickard A, Thompson BR. Waco, TX, Word Books, 1985, pp 68–75
8. Johnson VE: I'll Quit Tomorrow: A Practical Guide to Alcoholism Treatment, Revised Edition. San Francisco, CA, Harper & Row, 1980
9. Root LE: Treatment of the alcoholic family. Journal of Psychoactive Drugs 18:51–56, 1986

10. The Johnson Institute: How to Use Interventions in Your Professional Practice. Minneapolis, MN, Johnson Institute Books, 1987

11. Caldwell J: Preparing a family for intervention. Journal of Psychoactive Drugs 18:57–59, 1986

12. Trama J-A, Newman BM: A comparison of the impact of an alcohol education program with Al-Anon on knowledge and attitudes about alcoholism. Journal of Alcohol and Drug Education 34:1–16, 1988

13. Black C: It Will Never Happen to Me. Denver, CO, M.A.C. Publications, 1981

14. Ehrlich P, McGeehan M: Cocaine recovery support groups: the language of recovery, in Treating Cocaine Dependency. Edited by Smith DE, Wesson DR. Center City, MN, Hazelden Foundation, 1988, pp 73–90

15. Cutter CG, Cutter HS: Experience and change in Al-Anon family groups. Journal of Studies on Alcohol 48:29–32, 1987

16. Young E: Co-alcoholism as a disease: implications for psychotherapy (special issue: professional treatment and the 12-Step process). Journal of Psychoactive Drugs 19:257–268, 1987

17. York D, York P: Toughlove. New York, Bantam, 1985

18. Van Cleave S, Byrd W, Revell K: Addiction is a family affair, in Counseling for Substance Abuse and Addiction. Edited by Van Cleave S. Waco, TX, Word Books, 1987, pp 76–88

Table 10–1.   Screening questionnaire for parents of adolescents

Drug use

- Have you found drugs or drug paraphernalia around the house?
- Have you noticed that prescription drugs are missing?
- Have you noticed that alcohol is missing from the house?

Social changes

- Does your adolescent have a new group and type of friends?
- Do your child's friends come to the house for only a few minutes and then leave? Do they come late at night for only a few minutes?
- Does your adolescent seem to spend a considerable amount of time alone?

Behavior

- Does your adolescent seem less motivated and more lazy than before?
- Does your adolescent seem to have erratic behavior, more than before?
- Have the grades of your adolescent dropped considerably?
- Has your adolescent gotten into trouble at school or with the police?
- Does your adolescent seem to have considerable amounts of money that you cannot account for?
- Has your adolescent recently purchased expensive items beyond the reach of his or her allowance or job?
- Has your adolescent gotten into fights or accidents that involved alcohol or other drugs?

Note. A drug abuse screening questionnaire is a tool that can help to determine whether there is a likelihood that drug abuse exists. A positive screening test means that a formal evaluation should occur. Three or more "yes" answers may suggest a possible drug abuse problem.

Chapter 10

Adolescent Addiction

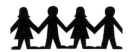

Of the challenges facing health care professionals, none are greater than the problems presented by the young person with a substance use disorder. Addicted youths often have troubling family histories of alcoholism and other addictions that create great dysfunction and entirely unwholesome family environments. They enter treatment today with multiple problems, including severe learning disabilities, personality and thought disorders, and problems arising out of childhood abuse, molestation, and incest. In order to understand and treat adolescent addiction, it is crucial to understand adolescence itself. This includes learning about the development tasks faced by adolescents. It involves knowledge of the triggers for adolescent problems. It requires an understanding of addiction in general, and how addiction affects younger people.

Paul Ehrlich, M.A.
Director
Institute of Addiction Studies
John F. Kennedy University
Orinda, California

This chapter was written by Mim Landry and Martha A. Morrison, M.D. Dr. Morrison is a specialist in adolescent psychiatry and addiction medicine. She is the Medical Director of the Talbott Recovery System in Atlanta, Georgia.

■ Adolescence

There was a time, perhaps, when adolescence was a period of carefree and untroubled living, a period of maturation unencumbered by significant danger. Expectations, rules, and guidelines were clear; parents were a protective shield from—not a source of—stress, conflict, and harm. Whether this time ever existed, or if it is just a fantasy of what could have been, it is certainly clear that childhood and adolescence today are complex and challenging experiences for both parents and youth. The image of the extended family that gathered together each Sunday for dinner, as idealized in Norman Rockwell's paintings, has been all but displaced by single-parent families, fast food, crack cocaine, and MTV.

Even in altogether healthy family environments where there are no drug abuse and addiction problems, adolescence can be a chaotic and tumultuous process. And indeed it is a process, a period of transition from childhood to adulthood. Adolescence can be a period of turmoil, conflict, and confusion. It may be only partially in jest that frenzied parents and health care professionals sometimes refer to adolescence itself as a psychiatric disorder, with time being the primary "cure."[1]

Certainly, adolescents are subject to tremendous pressures from within and without. Hormonal alterations promote emotional and behavioral changes, which may be severe enough to have the appearance of psychiatric problems.[2] During this time, adolescents often have severe struggles with autonomy and identity that may approach the level of emotional and social crises.[3] Peer pressure is particularly relentless during a time when adolescents' need for acceptance, praise, and approval is at its highest level.[4]

During this tumultuous process, adolescents face a number of developmental tasks.[5] The ability to resolve or accomplish these tasks has an impact on ultimate development, maturation, and styles of coping.[3,6–10]

Struggle for Independence

Adolescents' struggle to achieve independence begins with creating goals and assuming personal responsibility for meeting these goals.

This struggle for independence often includes a not-unhealthy period of testing the limits of parents, challenging authority, and contesting the values and attitudes of the family and family members.

Although this struggle is frustrating, through it adolescents can develop a sense of personal meaning and significance, a sense of personal direction in life, and a sense of identity and self-esteem. The inability to achieve a sense of independence can result in feelings of rejection and low self-esteem.

Meaning, Morals, and Values

One of the developmental tasks of adolescence is forming a sense of the meaning of life. Why am I here? What am I supposed to do? Why do bad things happen? It is important for adolescents to be encouraged to grapple with their own sense of morals and values.

Although adolescents may observe and challenge the values and morals of others, the developmental process includes the integration, internalization, and clarification of the meaning and importance of these values for themselves. An important element of this process is the development of a personal belief in and a sense of need for a spiritual dimension of life. Failure to find meaning and failure to develop personal morals and values generate a self-image of inferiority and lack of integrity.

Interpersonal Relationships and Intimacy

Much to the chagrin of many parents, adolescence is the time for observing, examining, and experiencing interpersonal relationships and various levels of intimacy. During adolescence, there is often intense exploration of relationships with friends, adults, and people to whom adolescents are sexually attracted. There is frequent experimentation with self-disclosure and intimacy.

Interpersonal interactions are vital for fulfilling adolescents' needs for acceptance, affiliation, and self-esteem. Adolescence is also a period of exploring personal sexuality issues and developing attitudes about sexual relationships.

These experiences may result in a tendency toward safety and trust or a need for protection and distrust. Poor resolution of interpersonal relationship and intimacy issues promotes a sense of insecurity and a lack of interpersonal connectedness.

Sense of Autonomy and Uniqueness

During adolescence, young people begin to discover and acknowledge who they are and develop a sense of autonomy and uniqueness. They increasingly become aware of the differences between themselves and their family members.

A sense of personal responsibility may surpass a previously external source of motivation. There is a heightened awareness of personal individuality and identity. Poor development of a sense of autonomy and uniqueness promotes a sense of hopelessness and a tendency toward depression.

As adolescents plow through this period of transition before adulthood, and as they struggle through these developmental tasks, their behaviors can be annoying, extreme, and even frightening. Because of these developmental tasks, behavior is often rooted in deeper and more primitive emotions, rather than rooted in logic. These struggles for independence, meaning, and values, explorations of interpersonal relationships and intimacy, and discovery of a sense of autonomy are emotionally potent experiences.

Especially if these developmental tasks are poorly met, these experiences may provoke powerful internal experiences that the adolescent may want to self-medicate with psychoactive drugs. In addition, a number of circumstances are common triggers for substance abuse, addiction, and other adolescent problems.

Triggers for Adolescent Problems

Some adolescents accomplish certain developmental tasks better than others. For some, however, these and other developmental tasks will be largely unmet. As a result, many adolescents experience identity crises and don't know who they are, what they are doing, where they are going, or why.

One expression of these identity crises is called "acting out," or behaviors that express various internal conflicts that adolescents are not able to acknowledge directly. These acting-out behaviors include substance use, sexual promiscuity, and criminal behavior. A common theme among these behaviors is a tendency toward impulsiveness, destructiveness, mistrustful behavior, and irresponsibility.

Psychoactive drug use is often perceived as one of the few pleasurable options that helps to self-medicate the turmoil, confusion, and identity crises. Initial exposure to mood-altering drugs may reduce anxiety and tension, increase self-esteem, and strengthen affiliation with peers. Initial drug use is often perceived as a solution to other, larger problems.

Parent-adolescent relationship. A number of factors contribute to or promote problems commonly seen in adolescents. Dysfunctional and impaired parent-adolescent relations are a frequent trigger for problems. Parent-child relations that are characterized by extremes are particularly noteworthy. Parental rejection, excessively strict parenting, excessively lenient and negligent parenting, inconsistent parenting, and parental overprotection may lead to severe difficulties in communication and relationships.

Adolescent peer relationships. As adolescents experiment with new behaviors and experiences, they adopt new sets of values held by their friends. Adopting new values and beliefs promotes conflict between the old system created by their parents and the new system supported by their peers. The new system is symbolized by their music, language, style of dress, role models, and goals. This conflict distances children from their parents and puts additional strain on communication efforts.

Chronic medical and psychiatric problems. During adolescence, various psychiatric and medical problems may emerge. For instance, anxiety disorders, mood disorders, personality disorders, and chronic medical problems may put considerable stress on both parent and child. Importantly, addiction—which may already be present in another family member—may emerge in adolescence.

Family crises. An unfortunately long litany of problems may beset families. Many problems are crises per se, whereas other problems are mishandled and elevated to the level of crisis and emergency. These include medical emergencies, parental separation or divorce, family death, parental job loss, and family relocation. During these crises, communication may become intense and volatile, followed by guilt and remorse over heated exchanges. Adolescents may inappropriately accept guilt over circumstances outside of their control, or they may sustain a level of anger at parents over circumstances outside of parents' control

■ Adolescent Addiction

Initial Exposure to Psychoactive Drugs

Adolescence can be a chaotic and stressful phase of life filled with potent peer pressure, passionate family conflicts, parental neglect, personal frustrations, formidable physiological changes, rapidly changing roles and expectations, and sustained periods of stress. Because of intense inner changes, periods of emotional turmoil, potent family dynamics, peer pressure, and drug availability, the use of psychoactive drugs to decrease stress and alter mood is increased during adolescence.[2] Thus, adolescents, like adults, use psychoactive drugs to decrease external stressors, as well as to medicate internal conflicts.

In addition to drug use for decreasing stress and escaping problems, adolescents engage in more drug experimentation than adults. Drugs are often used out of curiosity and to "have a good time." Adolescents frequently use mood-altering drugs because they believe drug use strengthens peer bonding and because they perceive it as an act of defiance, as well as a way to combat boredom.

The initial exposure to psychoactive drugs often occurs at a very early age. Table 10–2 shows the average age of initial drug use among people who have ever used psychoactive drugs. For instance, among the group ages 12–17 years, the average age of initial drug use is about 13.5 years. Consider that these figures are averages.

Large numbers of adolescents in treatment began their drug use as young as 9, 10, and 11 years of age.

Increasingly, exposure to psychoactive drug use occurs in the home, often with parental supervision. Adolescents' awareness that their parents use drugs and personally accept such behavior increases the risk that adolescents will initiate drug use.[11] Similarly, the risk of drug use is increased if older siblings living in the home are also users. The increased risk of drug use relates to having family models of drug use, family value systems that condone drug use, and family drug sources.[12]

Crossing the Line: Abuse to Addiction

It is critical to understand the distinction between adolescent drug abuse and addiction. As described in Chapter 1, abuse and addiction are separate diagnostic categories. Abuse describes the use of mood-altering drugs in such a way as to cause some level of dysfunction in the individual's life. In contrast, addiction (which may vary in severity) describes a process of compulsive use of drugs, loss of control over the drugs or over drug-induced behavior, and continued drug use despite adverse consequences.

During drug use and drug abuse, the behavior controls the drugs.

Table 10–2. Average age at time of initial drug use by age group

Drug(s)	Age group (years)				
	12–17	**18–25**	**26–34**	**35+**	**All ages**
Alcohol	12.8	15.5	16.2	18.5	17.2
Marijuana	13.4	15.6	16.6	23.2	18.7
Inhalants	12.4	15.7	16.9	19.5	16.6
Cocaine	14.6	18.1	20.8	26.5	21.7
Psychedelics	14.5	17.2	18.1	21.6	18.9
Heroin	13.7	14.1	18.5	26.1	21.7

Source. Adapted from the National Institute on Drug Abuse: *National Household Survey on Drug Abuse.* Washington, DC, U.S. Department of Health and Human Services, 1990.

Although it may be a poor idea, the decision to abuse drugs is made by cortical areas of the brain: those areas concerned with rationality and logic. In contrast, addiction is characterized by the drugs controlling the behavior. In particular, addiction is controlled by deeper, more primitive, lower centers of the brain.[13] The addicted person's compulsion to use the chemical arises from more primitive central nervous system instinctual centers, where imbalances in neurotransmitters occur.[4] In other words, for the addicted person, the choice to use or not use drugs no longer exists, and continued drug use precludes logical and rational thought processes.[14]

One way of describing this phenomenon is to say that people who abuse drugs can "cross the line" into addiction, but cannot cross back into controlled use.

Early-Stage Addiction

Psychoactive drug use during adolescence invariably interacts with the various developmental tasks necessary for normal maturation. Initially, adolescent drug use and the subsequent pleasurable alteration of mood may result in a false sense of independence, grandiosity, and invulnerability. Similarly, adolescents may report increased feelings of self-assurance, security, and belonging.

Based on these exaggerated or delusional perceptions, adolescents may develop the belief that the strength of their willpower will prevent future problems. The adolescent's developmental need for independence and growth may impede the ability to assess the dangers of drug abuse objectively.

Sustained and increased levels of drug use promote an arrest in emotional maturation. Adolescents will begin to use mood-altering drugs as abnormal coping mechanisms for normal emotional problems. They may appear to regress to a more immature state, using relatively primitive and immature defense mechanisms, especially denial and lying. Normal nondrug coping skills are inhibited, reflecting stunted developmental growth. As a result, adolescents in an early addiction phase begin to react in a more impulsive, immature, and irresponsible fashion. Table 10–3 summarizes many specific symptoms and signs of early addiction among adolescents.

Intermediate-Stage Addiction

As the process of addiction increases in severity, there is a corresponding increase in adverse consequences, an escalation in the severity of the adverse consequences, and an increase in observable

Table 10–3. Stages of adolescent addiction

Early addiction

- Experimental drug use
- Use is pleasurable, rewarding
- Many friends are nonusers
- Using as act of defiance
- First intoxication or hangover
- Increase in tolerance
- Decrease in attention span
- Some adverse consequences
- Some effect on maturation
- Episodes of impulsiveness
- Uses drugs when offered
- May feel invulnerable
- Use becomes more regular
- Using to escape boredom
- First blackout
- Using to relate to others
- Low frustration tolerance
- Some loss of control
- Inhibition of coping skills
- Episodes of irresponsibility

Intermediate addiction

- Use may be more frequent
- Using to feel good about self
- Using to reduce feelings
- Compulsion and drug hunger
- Most friends are drug users
- More time spent using drugs
- Loss of control over drugs
- Mood swings
- Impaired thinking
- Increased problems at home
- Denial and frank lying
- Isolation, hiding drugs
- Inconsistent behavior
- Promiscuity, negativity
- Family becomes aware
- Binges may be more severe
- Using to escape problems
- Using to strengthen bond with friends
- Using despite adverse consequences
- Begins to buy drugs
- More time spent finding drugs
- Poor control of drug-induced behavior
- Guilt and shame over loss of control
- Changes in appearance
- Increased problems at school
- Truancy, school performance drops
- Fighting, hostility, defensiveness
- Decreased extracurricular activities
- Possible legal problems
- Confrontation by parents

(continued)

Table 10–3. Stages of adolescent addiction *(continued)*

Advanced addiction

- Using to feed compulsion
- Loss of control over use
- Using to feel normal
- Episodes of withdrawal
- Episodes of overdose
- Failed attempts to control use
- Denial is prominent feature
- Uses in isolation
- Dishonesty becomes frequent
- Excuses become exhausted
- Despair and self-hatred
- Chronic depression
- Multiple fears and anxieties
- Acting-out behavior increases
- Most friends are drug users
- Friends and peers concerned
- Family conflicts about drugs
- Addiction progression is rapid
- Drug hunger drives behavior
- Continued use despite consequences
- Blackouts and memory impairment
- Drug-related physical injury
- Delusions of controlled use
- Obsession, preoccupation with use
- Blames others for problems
- Increase in risk-taking behavior
- Lies about amount of drug used
- Changes in appearance
- Resentments, hatred of others
- Poor self-esteem
- Frequent agitation
- Promiscuity and fighting increase
- Often has drug supply
- School and legal problems
- Drug-induced medical problems likely
- Severity of consequences increases

problems related to the addiction.

Addicted adolescents begin to experience problems related to obtaining drugs, using drugs, and drug withdrawal. These problems may emerge in many different areas of adolescents' lives: legal, social, familial, psychological, emotional, and physical. In particular, addiction-related problems are observed in school, at work, and at home.

Increased addiction severity further impairs developmental maturation. Addicted adolescents shift personal priorities, experience an attitude change, and increasingly use denial as a primary defense mechanism. The dominance of denial as a defense mechanism does not allow adolescents to view themselves or their relationship with drugs objectively. As a consequence, denial promotes a delusional belief in their control over mood-altering drugs. Table 10–3 lists numerous symptoms and signs of intermediate addiction among adolescents.

Advanced Addiction

As the addiction further increases in severity, addicted adolescents often find themselves surrounded by enablers: people who wittingly or unwittingly help to sustain the addiction. Parents and family members may unknowingly shield the addicted adolescent from authorities by assuming that drug-related problems are unrelated to drug use. Similarly, they may protect the addicted adolescent by ignoring, hiding, or making excuses for obvious adverse consequences of drug use. Drug-using peers may enable their friends' addiction by conscious lying and acts of omission.

During the advanced stages, progression of the addictive process can be rapid. Adverse consequences become compounded and are increasingly noticeable to objective observers. Addicted adolescents experience an increase in emotional pain, low self-esteem, and existential loneliness. They also experience a cycle of compulsive use; adverse physical, emotional, and social consequences; negative feelings about self; and further drug use to self-medicate these feelings. Unless intervention takes place, adolescent addiction will continue to progress to imprisonment, institutionalization, or premature death. Table 10–3 illustrates the stages of adolescent addiction.

Addiction Progression in Adolescents

Luckily, not all adolescents who experiment with psychoactive drugs become addicted. If they did, nearly every adolescent in the United States would become addicted. For instance, in the 1990 National High School Senior Survey on Drug Abuse, about 90% of the students had used alcohol at least once, about 50% had used "any illicit drug" at least once, and 40% had used marijuana at least once.[15]

The 1990 National High School Senior Survey on Drug Abuse also estimated alcohol binge drinking, defined as having five or more drinks in a row during the past 2 weeks. Binge alcohol drinking had been done by about 30% of the seniors, about 23% of the tenth-graders, and about 13% of the eighth-graders.

The percentage of adolescents in school who did become addicted can be estimated by looking at the percentages of high school seniors who used specific drugs on a daily basis over the past month. In the same national survey of high school seniors, 3.7% of the students used alcohol on a daily basis, 2.2% used marijuana on a daily basis, and 0.1% used cocaine on a daily basis over the past month. Of course, these figures are for high school students and do not include those students who were expelled, dropped out, were jailed, or died under drug-related circumstances.

As can be seen, more adolescents experiment with psychoactive drugs than become addicted. The progression from experimental use to addiction is influenced by a number of biopsychosocial risk factors, which are detailed in previous chapters. However, this information can be incorporated into a model that helps to describe the progression of addiction among adolescents.[16]

Consider the following formula:

$$\begin{array}{rl} & \text{predisposition} \\ + & \text{drug effect} \\ + & \text{enabling system} \\ \hline = & \text{addiction} \end{array}$$

The essential idea illustrated here is that addiction is a biopsychosocial process that is influenced by 1) factors relating to individual drug users, 2) factors relating to the drug being used, and 3) various social factors. The reality is that addiction is created and shaped by many different variables. This model helps to explain why some people become addicted and others do not.

Predisposition. In this context, predisposition describes genetic, constitutional, psychological, and sociocultural influences on the development and progression of addiction.[17] The *genetic* influences, as described in Chapter 13, suggest a genetically acquired higher risk for developing addiction after exposure to psychoactive drugs.[18] *Constitutional* influences include the various biological markers that suggest areas of biological differences between people who are addicted and those who are not.[19] *Psychological* influences for adolescents include failure to complete developmental tasks, emotional trauma, personality deficits, and traumatic events.[20] *Sociocultural* factors such as age, peers, status, social class, poverty, cultural issues, and other social factors contribute to the development of addiction.[21,22]

Drug effect. When people have a predisposition or a higher risk for developing addiction, but never use a psychoactive drug, they obviously won't become addicted. Thus, drug availability is necessary for becoming addicted. Drug availability may be influenced by finances, surroundings, or cultural issues. People are more likely to use drugs if the drugs are easily accessible.

As described in the chapters on the specific drugs of abuse, psychoactive drugs cause distortions in feelings, sensations, perceptions, thinking, and behavior. Some reduce pain, others reduce anxiety, and most produce some type of euphoria, which is positively reinforcing. In addition, most drugs have a withdrawal effect, which prompts people to use more of the drug to avoid the withdrawal. Also, the route of administration can dramatically alter the drug experience; for example, smoking cocaine produces a far more intense euphoria than snorting cocaine. Thus, the pharmacologic properties of drugs make some drugs more likely to be used repeatedly—and used in higher doses.

Enabling system. In general, the enabling system is a structure that enables the drug user to keep using drugs. In this context, the enabling system refers to both internal and external enabling factors.

Internal enabling factors refer to the powerful defense mechanisms that addicted people develop. The most prominent of these mechanisms is the denial system, which allows the addicted person to have the delusion that no problem exists, that any problems that do exist are not related to the addiction, and that any problems that might occur can be easily handled by the addicted person.

External enabling factors include the modeling of drug use by parents, peers, or society; the approval of drug use by parents, peers, or society; and the removal of adverse consequences that might deter use.[23]

In general, the enabling system creates an environment that is supportive of drug use and helps to reduce obstacles that are hostile to continued drug use. It creates a shield that protects the drug user from being confronted about the drug use.

The biopsychosocial model of addiction illustrated here describes addiction as influenced by predisposition factors, variables related to drug availability and pharmacology, and an enabling system. Each of these variables contributes to the development and progression of addiction.

Some adolescents are at very high risk of addiction before they ever try a drug because of a preexisting enabling system and predisposition factors. When exposed to drugs, they may experience an explosive addiction process: rapid, intense, and severe. Some adolescents who do not have these preexisting risk factors may also experience a rapid and severe addiction process if they begin their drug experimentation with smokable cocaine or amphetamine. In those cases, the intense effects associated with the route of administration make up for the lack of other high-risk variables.

In contrast, some adolescents may experiment with drugs for many months or even years before progressing to addiction (if they

Table 10–4. Factors associated with progression of adolescent addiction

Predisposition	Enabling system
Genetic	User's denial system
Constitutional	Delusions of controlled use
Psychological	Parent's denial system
Sociocultural	Peers' denial system
Drug effect	Peer pressure to use
Drug availability	Modeling of drug use
Drug type	
Potential for euphoria	
Potential for withdrawal	
Route of administration	

progress at all). This lack of progression may be because they have few or no predisposition risk factors, use a drug that creates only a mild euphoria, use a route of administration associated with less effects, and have no enabling system.

Habilitation, not Rehabilitation

For adolescents, rehabilitation efforts should be tailored to meet their developmental needs, which may be striking. As indicated in Chapter 6, rehabilitation describes the process of putting the treatment plan into action. Rehabilitation and recovery begin with biopsychosocial restabilization, including the management of medical and psychiatric crises, and biopsychosocial normalization. After that, adult patients begin the process of restructuring. However, before there can be restructuring, there needs to be something to restructure.

Adult rehabilitation and recovery depend on the existence of an adult personality and adult development. Although the personality may be unhealthy and there may be noticeable developmental deficits, adult patients can reinterpret certain values, relearn various experiences, and be retaught new coping skills. In this sense, rehabilitation means relearning.

In contrast, the personalities of adolescents are still in the process of growing. Addicted adolescents, in particular, have largely unmet developmental needs. These adolescents need to be habilitated (taught), not rehabilitated (retaught). In other words, the recovery process for adolescents involves initial learning (habilitation), not relearning (rehabilitation).[24]

Habilitation can be understood as provision of conditions that allow the adolescent to grow and mature emotionally, while acquiring nondrug coping skills. Both peers and healthy adults are necessary participants in this process, acting as role models for healthy behavior. Important in this process is the modeling of respect for the addicted adolescent, an important recovery task, as is the establishment of open communication. Open communication involves both sharing true feelings and ideas, which decreases misinterpretations, and confronting problems in a loving and caring fashion. In addition, open communication involves compassionate support and reassurance. These behaviors help to provide an environment of trust, honesty, and openness.

■ Summary

Adolescence is a process—a frequently tumultuous period of transition between childhood and adulthood. During this transition, adolescents face a number of developmental tasks. The ability to resolve or accomplish these tasks affects ultimate development, maturation, and styles of coping. The struggle for independence is a developmental task that often includes testing limits, challenging authority, and contesting the values and attitudes of the family. Achieving this goal of independence increases a sense of personal meaning, personal identity, and self-esteem. Another developmental task is forming a sense of the meaning of life. Developmental goals include the formation of personal values, morals, and personal meaning, including the development of a sense of spirituality. Adolescence is also a time for the exploration of relationships, friendships, self-disclosure, intimacy, and sexuality. These explorations are vital to meet the adolescents' needs for acceptance, affiliation, self-esteem, and interpersonal skills. Also, adolescents are faced with the task of discovering a sense of autonomy and uniqueness.

The inability to resolve some of these developmental tasks may result in identity crises, which are expressed through "acting-out" behaviors. These behaviors tend to be impulsive, destructive, and irresponsible. Often, psychoactive drugs initially are used to provide some respite from the turmoil, confusion, and frustration of these identity crises. A number of circumstances contribute to or promote the problems seen during adolescence. Parent-adolescent relationships, adolescent-peer relationships, chronic medical and psychiatric problems, and family crises all can be the source of tension, stress, and frustration—which may provide perceived justification for the adolescent to use psychoactive drugs for self-medication.

Initially, psychoactive drugs are often used to self-medicate frustration, tension, anxiety, depression, and social pressures. Also, adolescents experiment with drug use out of curiosity, for peer bonding, as an act of defiance, and out of boredom. Initial drug use

266

may occur in the home under the supervision of a parent or sibling. Initial drug use and abuse are governed by areas of the brain concerned with logic and rationality. During this phase, the behavior controls the drugs. As the adolescent "crosses the line" into addictive use, the drugs control the behavior. At this point, the drugs affect the more primitive areas of the brain, which in turn control the addictive behavior. Adolescents experience three progressive stages of addiction: early-stage, intermediate-stage, and advanced addiction. As the addiction progresses, developmental maturation is progressively impeded, the number of adverse consequences increase, and the negative consequences become progressively more severe.

Finally, adolescents require habilitation, not rehabilitation. Rehabilitation of adults involves relearning values and morals and restructuring their personalities. However, adolescents do not have fully developed personalities, and they have not yet fully developed personal values and morals. Thus, adolescents need habilitation, which is the initial learning of these values and morals, not a relearning process.

■ References

1. Smoller JW: The etiology and treatment of childhood. Journal of Polymorphous Perversity 2:3–7, 1985
2. Milliam R, Khuri E: Substance abuse: clinical problems and perspectives, in Adolescence and Substance Abuse. Edited by Lowinson J, Ruiz P. Baltimore, MD, Williams & Wilkins, 1981, pp 739–751
3. Betelheimn B: Surviving and Other Essays. New York, Knopf, 1979
4. Morrison MA, Smith T: Psychiatric issues of adolescent chemical dependence. Pediatric Clinics of North America 34:461–480, 1987
5. Morrison MA, Hayes HR, Knauf KJ: Progression of chemical dependence and recovery in adolescents. Psychiatric Annals 19:666–671, 1989
6. Schaefer D: Choices and Consequences. Minneapolis, MN, Johnson Institute Books, 1987
7. Freud A: Ego and the Mechanisms of Defense. New York, International Universities Press, 1967
8. Blos P: On Adolescence. New York, Free Press, 1962
9. Erickson EH: Identity, Youth and Crisis. New York, WW Norton, 1968

10. Svobodny LA: Biographical, self-concept and educational factors among chemically dependent adolescents. Adolescence 17:847–853, 1982

11. Baumrind D: Family antecedents of adolescent drug use: a developmental perspective, in Etiology of Drug Abuse: Implications for Prevention (National Institute on Drug Abuse Research Monograph No 56). Edited by Jones CL, Battjes RJ. Rockville, MD, National Institute on Drug Abuse, 1985, pp 13–44

12. Clayton RR, Lacey WB: Interpersonal influences of male drug use and drug use intentions. International Journal of the Addictions 17:655–666, 1982

13. Suojanen WW: Addiction and the minds of mind, in Management and the Brain: An Integrative Approach to Organization Behavior. Edited by Bersinger RC, Suojanen WW. Atlanta, Georgia State University, 1983, pp 77–92

14. Talbott GD: Substance abuse and the professional provider. Alabama Journal of Medical Science 21:150–155, 1984

15. National Institute on Drug Abuse: The 1990 National High School Senior Survey on Drug Abuse. Washington, DC, National Institute on Drug Abuse, 1991

16. Chatlos JC: Adolescent dual diagnosis: a 12-Step transformational model. Journal of Psychoactive Drugs 21:189–201, 1989

17. Donovan JM: An etiologic model of alcoholism. American Journal of Psychiatry 143:1–11, 1986

18. Goodwin DW: Hereditary and alcoholism. Annals of Behavioral Medicine 8:3–6, 1986

19. Schuckit MA, Gold EO: A simultaneous evaluation of multiple markers of ethanol/placebo challenges in sons of alcoholics and controls. Archives of General Psychiatry 45:211–216, 1988

20. Kernberg OF: Borderline Conditions and Pathological Narcissism. New York, Jason Aronson, 1975

21. Vaillant GE: The National History of Alcoholism. Cambridge, MA, Harvard University Press, 1983

22. Carroll JF: Treating multiple substance abuse clients, in Recent Developments in Alcoholism, Vol 4. Edited by Galanter M. New York, Plenum, 1986

23. Chatlos JC: Crack: What You Should Know About the Cocaine Epidemic. New York, Putnam, 1986

24. Morrison MA: Addiction in adolescents. Western Journal of Medicine 152:543–546, 1990

Chapter 11

Dual Diagnoses: Dual Disorders

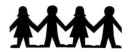

Until recently, my life has been a bizarre roller coaster ride. I guess that I shouldn't be surprised that I ended up with a problem with alcohol since my uncle died of liver damage and my father died in an alcohol-related accident. But I was surprised that even when not drinking, I still had serious problems. Every time that I got sober, it seems that I got crazier. After being arrested for disturbing the peace (while sober), I was examined by a psychiatrist who diagnosed my bipolar disorder. For a while, I used the medication on and off. When I was off the medication, I got really crazy, made people angry, and I drank to forget. Today, I am grateful for my sobriety, and thankful for having medication to keep me from getting manic. I have had to educate my friends in AA about my need for lithium. I think they understand.

Clarence T.
Washington, D.C.

■ Drug Use and Psychiatric Symptoms

Psychoactive, mood-altering drugs will—by definition—cause alterations of mood as well as changes in behavior, thinking, perception, and memory. These alterations may be mild or severe, brief or long lasting, desired or unwanted.

These drug-induced alterations in mood, thinking, and behavior can 1) cause psychiatric symptoms of varying intensity, 2) initiate or worsen existing psychiatric disorders, 3) mask existing psychiatric symptoms and disorders, and 4) cause withdrawal-related psychiatric symptoms.[1] In addition, psychiatric disorders can cause behavior that resembles the behavior associated with addiction.

Drugs Can Cause Psychiatric Symptoms

Psychoactive, mood-altering drugs are consumed specifically because they alter the central nervous system and thus alter mood, thinking, and behavior. Stimulants cause mental and behavioral stimulation, sedative-hypnotics cause sedation and sleep, and psychedelics alter sensory perception.

High-dose, long-term drug use causes the intensity of drug-induced symptoms to increase. Indeed, the symptoms may become severe enough to become psychiatric symptoms. Thus, intense use of stimulants can cause anxiety, agitation, and paranoia; intense use of sedative-hypnotics can cause depression; and intense use of psychedelics can cause symptoms similar to those of psychotic disorders.[2]

The symptoms caused by psychoactive drugs may appear identical to symptoms and signs of various psychiatric disorders. However, psychiatric disorders that are not drug related have a different course and often a different treatment.

In particular, drug-induced psychiatric symptoms are generally short-lived and temporary, whereas psychiatric disorders are often chronic and long lasting. For example, anxiety, depression, and thought disorders are often chronic problems that require prolonged and intensive treatment.

In contrast, symptoms of anxiety, depression, and disordered thinking caused by stimulants, depressants, and psychedelic drugs, respectively, generally fade as the drug effects fade. Treatment for such problems may range from supportive counseling to medical management, depending on the severity of the symptoms, the dosage of the drug ingested, and the psychiatric stability of the individual.

A recent study evaluated the presence of psychiatric symptoms among recovering people participating in Narcotics Anonymous. It was noted that psychiatric symptoms were significantly higher during periods of drug use. After cessation of drug use, psychiatric symptoms significantly decreased, even to a level below that reported as present before initiation of drug use.[3]

Withdrawal Can Cause Psychiatric Symptoms

Drug withdrawal can cause psychiatric symptoms in much the same way that drug use can. In general, drug withdrawal symptoms are the opposite of the effects of those drugs. For instance, withdrawal from stimulants is a period of depression, lethargy, and agitation. In contrast, withdrawal from depressants is a period of anxiety, tension, and agitation.[4]

Just as anxiety and depression can be symptoms of withdrawal, they can also be symptoms of psychiatric disorders such as panic disorder and major depression. For this reason, withdrawal from stimulants and depressants can mimic psychiatric disorders.

Thus, health care professionals should be immediately informed of the relationship between the current symptoms and recent drug use if the individual is brought to a medical setting during a withdrawal syndrome.

Drugs Can Provoke or Worsen Psychiatric Disorders

The use of psychoactive drugs can provoke or cause a psychiatric disorder to appear, as well as exacerbate an already existing psychiatric disorder.[5] For example, the use of cocaine can be the initial cause of an episode of panic, which may reappear even during times of abstinence from cocaine. In this example, the future use of caffeine may provoke further episodes of panic and anxiety.

Similarly, someone with previous episodes of depression may

reexperience depressive states during and after alcohol, opiate, and benzodiazepine use. Repeated use of depressants may cause the depression to resurface or to become more intense.

Importantly, if drug use prompts the appearance of a psychiatric problem, and if that problem becomes chronic, the psychiatric problem is now an independent psychiatric disorder that requires treatment. Thus, once a drug-initiated psychiatric problem develops a life of its own, the initiating drug experience becomes important mostly as it relates to the prevention of additional psychiatric episodes and to the avoidance of future substance use problems.

Also, drug use can provoke the reemergence of a preexisting but dormant psychiatric disorder, or it can worsen the intensity of an active psychiatric disorder. For instance, use of marijuana by an individual with a thought disorder such as paranoia may result in that person becoming vividly suspicious and paranoid.

Drugs Can Mask Psychiatric Symptoms

Psychiatric symptoms such as depression and anxiety are uncomfortable and cause personal distress. Some people who experience psychiatric disorders try to diminish their symptoms with psychoactive drugs.[6] Although addiction is not the result of people self-medicating their psychiatric symptoms, self-medication may sometimes be the reason for initial drug use.

For instance, some people may use alcohol to diminish the symptoms of anxiety and agitation. Someone else may be prescribed a sedative-hypnotic such as a benzodiazepine for the same purpose. The drug consumption of some of these people may progress to addiction.

For these people, drug use may mask psychiatric symptoms. As they stop using drugs, the psychiatric symptoms may reemerge. Indeed, these people may require treatment for both their substance use and their psychiatric disorders.

Psychiatric Disorders Can Mimic Addictive Behaviors

Addiction is not the only possible cause of erratic, impulsive, and dysfunctional behavior. In fact, various psychiatric, behavioral, and emotional problems can cause the same type of defense mechanisms (e.g., denial, projection, and minimization) and maladaptive behavior (e.g., anger, isolation, and lying). For this reason, psychiatric disorders may cause behavior that is similar to the behavior of addicted people.

For example, people with untreated bipolar disorder may experience disturbing episodes of mania and depression that are similar to some aspects of stimulant and depressant use. More importantly, the crises and psychosocial problems with family, friends, and employers caused by psychiatric disorders are similar to those caused by addiction.

■ Dual Disorders: Addiction Plus Psychiatric Disorders

As can be seen, the use of psychoactive, mood-altering drugs can cause alterations in mood, behavior, thinking, and perception that resemble, provoke, exacerbate, or mask psychiatric symptoms. This is important to understand because the same psychiatric symptoms in different people can have different causes.

Example

Dwight and Joe enter an addiction treatment program on the same day. They both have a 5-year history of alcohol addiction and about the same level of tolerance and intake. During the acute withdrawal, they both experienced significant anxiety, agitation, and insomnia, and both required medication to treat those symptoms successfully.

However, 1 month after detoxification, Dwight is beginning to feel "normal" again, whereas Joe still feels anxious and agitated and frequently has trouble sleeping. Although they both experienced anxiety related to alcohol withdrawal, Joe appears to be exhibiting symptoms of generalized anxiety disorder. Indeed, Joe can be described as having the dual disorders of addiction and a psychiatric disorder.

273

The Chicken or the Egg?

There are controversies in the addiction and psychiatric fields about the relationships between dual disorders. These controversies are often related to the best way to treat patients who have dual disorders.

For example, some experts believe that addiction is caused by psychiatric and emotional disorders. They argue that successful treatment of the underlying psychiatric disorder will prompt the addiction to fade.

Some experts believe that the best way to treat people with dual disorders is to treat the disorder that emerged first and to treat the more recently emerged problem later. Others believe that the disorder that is the most severe, intense, and debilitating should be treated first. In some ways, these debates reflect the different treatment approaches seen in addiction medicine, mental health, psychiatry, and primary-care medicine.

However, there is a growing awareness that the optimal way to understand and to treat patients with dual disorders is to conceptualize dual disorders as two separate and independent problems that each require treatment. Indeed, the term *dual disorders* can be used to describe a coexisting psychiatric disorder and a substance use disorder.

Examples of Dual Disorders

People with dual disorders have at least one substance use disorder involving abuse or addiction. In fact, more than one drug may be involved. For instance, someone may be diagnosed as having cocaine addiction and episodic alcohol abuse.

People with dual disorders have at least one psychiatric problem, such as depression, anxiety, psychosis, bipolar disorder, personality disorders, or attention-deficit disorder.

Although there is often some degree of interaction between the two disorders, neither necessarily relies on the other for its existence. Also, both disorders typically are influenced by biopsychosocial factors and in turn influence biopsychosocial factors. All of these factors need to be considered for effective treatment.

Treatment Approaches

Patients with dual disorders have special treatment needs that other patients do not have. Even among patients with dual disorders, there is great variability regarding treatment needs. There are also regional differences with regard to treatment resources.

The sequential approach. Sequential treatment for patients with dual disorders means receiving treatment for one disorder, followed by treatment for the other disorder. For some patients, this type of treatment may be appropriate and effective. For example, Bill is diagnosed as having alcohol addiction as well as phobias related to elevators and the subway. Because Bill does not have to ride the subway or elevators during treatment, he can fully participate in treatment of addiction, after which he can be treated for his phobic disorder.

Sequential treatment is inappropriate for other patients. For instance, in the earlier example, Joe was diagnosed as having alcohol addiction as well as generalized anxiety disorder. Because symptoms of his anxiety disorder emerged after detoxification, he would be unable to continue his participation in addiction treatment if his generalized anxiety disorder was not treated at the same time.

One of the risks of sequential treatment is that one health care provider may unwittingly sabotage the treatment of the other unless they work in harmony. This sabotage can easily happen because patients with dual disorders may be receiving treatment from two or more different treatment systems. However, sequential treatment can be appropriate and effective for some patients when there is close communication between providers and when those providers share the same treatment goals.

The parallel approach. The parallel treatment of dual disorders means that the addiction and the psychiatric problems are treated simultaneously but through different treatment providers. For instance, Eddie has been diagnosed as having cocaine addiction and bipolar disorder (manic-depressive disorder). For 2 months, Eddie participated in an intensive outpatient treatment program for his cocaine addiction. His counselors recommended that he see a private psychiatrist for the management of his bipolar disorder. His bipolar disorder is now successfully controlled with lithium, and he is in the continuing-care phase of addiction treatment.

As with sequential treatment, there is a substantial risk that one health care provider may sabotage the treatment efforts of the other unless there are intense coordination and cooperation and shared treatment goals.

The integrated approach. Some addiction, psychiatric, and mental health programs have developed special treatment units that are specifically designed for patients with dual disorders. These programs integrate elements of both psychiatric treatment and addiction treatment into a unified approach. Ideally, these programs have clinical staff who are well trained in treating psychiatric and substance use disorders.

The integrated treatment approach is especially valuable for patients who have severe, intense, and chronic dual disorders. For example, Jerry has a 10-year history of heroin addiction and alcohol abuse. He has occasionally experienced disturbing episodes that include hearing voices and seeing religious "visions."

Two years ago, Jerry received integrated treatment for his dual disorders. The clinical team helped him realize that when he stopped taking his prescribed medication, the voices and hallucinations would return. They also helped him realize that when he drank because of the anxiety associated with hearing voices, his impaired thinking and alcohol-induced drug craving prompted his relapse to heroin.

Reviewing these different treatment approaches, as well as reviewing different levels of care (see Chapter 6), is central to the placement of patients in the appropriate treatment program. For instance, patients with dual disorders often have more treatment complications, require more medical services, and make slower treatment and recovery progress than other patients. It is likely that the severity of the psychiatric disorder contributes more to treatment complications than does the specific type of psychiatric disorder.[7] For these reasons, patients with severe dual disorders require treatment involving a high level of care with an integrated treatment approach.

■ Treatment Concerns

The treatment of depression, bipolar disorder, schizophrenia, and many other psychiatric disorders often involves medications that may have a long-term effect on mood or thinking but that are not psychoactive, mood altering, or euphoric. Thus, the treatment goal for addiction (sobriety from psychoactive drugs) does not conflict with the medical management of these disorders.

In contrast, some of the medications used to treat anxiety and panic disorders include the benzodiazepines, which are psychoactive, mood-altering drugs. Although these drugs do not generally pose a risk of addiction for the average patient with anxiety, they can trigger compulsive addiction in high-risk patients, such as those who have a personal history of addiction.[8]

Accordingly, it is the treatment of anxiety disorders that poses the most significant treatment conflict. The use of benzodiazepines to reduce anxiety and promote sedation conflicts with the goal of addiction treatment: sobriety from mood-altering drugs.

Luckily, the benzodiazepines are not the only treatment for anxiety disorders. For people with anxiety disorders who are at high risk for addiction, nondrug treatments and nonpsychoactive drug treatments are used.[9] Nondrug treatments include therapy, stress reduction, relaxation techniques, meditation, biofeedback, acupuncture, hypnotherapy, self-help groups, support groups, exercise, and education. A number of nonpsychoactive drugs also help to decrease anxiety, such as buspirone (BuSpar), beta-blockers such as propranolol (Inderal), and various antidepressants.[10]

Recovery Conflicts

People who have dual disorders may encounter conflicts in group therapy, recovery groups, and self-help Twelve-Step groups. People participating in these groups become extremely adept at identifying evidence of drug use in others. Furthermore, they are encouraged to confront each other about apparent drug use and the evidence of relapsive thinking, which includes dishonesty and a lack of openness.

Although most Twelve-Step groups are not specifically designed for people with dual disorders, they are not incompatible with the treatment goals of people with these disorders. However, conflicts may emerge between the opinions of some self-help group members and the treatment goals, complicated somewhat by the style and recovery goals of the Twelve-Step groups.

Recovering people with dual disorders, like other people in the Twelve-Step programs, are continually encouraged to be honest and open. If patients with dual disorders who are appropriately prescribed medication mention their use of that medication, they may receive feedback about it and be encouraged to stop. Some recovering peers may not be sophisticated about specific medications, and they may not know whether the medication is psychoactive. Also, a few people may have personal biases against physicians and all medication.

Therefore, one recovery conflict centers around the dually disordered individual's struggle with openness and honesty versus nonprofessional advice about prescribing. In this situation, dually disordered people in recovery can receive counseling about how and where to appropriately discuss their medication during certain meetings.

Many settings are appropriate for these discussions, including certain Twelve-Step groups that are specifically designed for people with dual disorders ("Double Trouble meetings"). Other Twelve-Step groups are tolerant about this issue. People with dual disorders should not stop or change their medications without knowledgeable professional advice.

It should be mentioned that the tendency to confront recovering peers about use of psychoactive drugs, even when the drugs are prescribed, is overall a desirable situation. Addicted people without an appropriate diagnosis frequently seek out and obtain prescription medication. Although some addicted people consciously lie to obtain drugs from physicians, others may believe that their prescription drug use is legitimate and necessary, although it may be an example of drug-seeking behavior and drug hunger. Thus, peer confrontation is a valuable way to break through the delusional denial system and intervene before more significant addiction emerges.

Psychoactive Medications During Recovery

Psychoactive medications should only be prescribed for people at high risk for addiction when 1) the severity of their psychiatric problem is extreme and threatens their ability to function; 2) the physician and patient are working collaboratively and openly; 3) the medications are provided on a daily basis with very close supervision and contact; and 4) the psychoactive drugs are meeting an emergency need for a brief duration of time, during which period alternative treatments are initiated.[9]

Some examples include the temporary management of severe, debilitating panic attacks with benzodiazepines, during which time alternative nonpsychoactive medications and nondrug treatments are initiated. Similarly, recovering patients who undergo surgery require pain medication during the operation, and they may need pain medication after the operation.

Importantly, the decision to prescribe either psychoactive or nonpsychoactive medication should be made by a treatment professional who is specifically expert in treating people with dual disorders. This physician, working with a multidisciplinary team, should be the major facilitator in the patient's treatment and recovery program.

Ideally these treatment decisions are made based on open collaboration between the patient and the providers. This situation is substantially different from that of an individual who attempts to obtain psychoactive medication from a primary-care physician or psychiatrist who is not part of the treatment team.

Double Recovery

Although people diagnosed with addiction and a psychiatric disorder have two separate disorders, the disorders often interact with and influence each other. For instance, people with addiction plus an anxiety disorder often use depressants such as alcohol and benzodiazepines to self-medicate episodes of anxiety. Although their anxiety may be temporarily relieved, the use of depressants may trigger the return of active symptoms of addiction.

For the average addicted person, the recovery process describes the period of abstinence and sobriety from psychoactive drugs and reversal of drug-induced impairment. However, for people with a diagnosis of addiction and a psychiatric disorder, the recovery process includes the dual processes of recovery from addiction and recovery from the psychiatric disorder.

In other words, for people with dual disorders, the recovery process includes recovery from both problems. For these people, the goals of recovery include being free of psychiatric symptoms and not experiencing the compulsive use of psychoactive drugs.

Sometimes the emergence of psychiatric symptoms in a person recovering from dual disorders may be incorrectly interpreted as incomplete or half-hearted recovery efforts. Rather, psychiatric symptoms can interfere with patients' motivation and ability to participate in addiction recovery.

Double Relapse

In general, relapse often begins with relapsive thinking, which is a return of distorted thinking and a reactivation of denial as a primary defense mechanism. After this, people may experience a complete relapse to active addiction with compulsion and adverse consequences. Relapse is generally accompanied by strong denial and a lack of cooperation about getting additional help.

For people with dual disorders, relapse can refer to the psychiatric disorder, to the addiction, or to both disorders. In other words, people with dual disorders may reexperience deteriorating psychiatric health while remaining abstinent; they may experience an addiction relapse while remaining free of their psychiatric symptoms; or they may experience a relapse of the addiction and a return of the psychiatric disorder.

People with dual disorders have an additional area of concern in relation to relapse: the relapse of one disorder may trigger the relapse of the other.

Psychiatric relapse triggering addiction relapse. During a period of recovery from the dual disorders, the reemergence of a psychiatric disorder may trigger relapse of the drug addiction.

Patients with bipolar disorder are often successfully treated with lithium, a nonpsychoactive, non-mood-altering, noneuphorigenic drug. This medication is used to suppress the severe episodes of depression and mania, both of which are generally uncomfortable experiences.

People who have bipolar disorder often become resentful about having to take a medication. Many will stop taking the medication and experience profound mania or depression. Because these experiences are uncomfortable, people may medicate themselves with alcohol, marijuana, stimulants, or other drugs. Patients with dual disorders who self-medicate their bipolar disorder with psychoactive drugs may trigger a return of their drug addiction.

In a similar way, symptoms related to anxiety, depression, schizophrenia, delusions, sleep disorders, sexual disorders, and personality disorders may reemerge during recovery from addiction or perhaps surface for the first time. If people attempt to ignore these symptoms and not receive appropriate medical treatment, the symptoms are likely to escalate and progress.

These people may turn to the use of psychoactive drugs as a way to reduce the psychiatric symptoms—or perhaps to reduce the anxiety associated with the return of these symptoms. This psychoactive drug use may then trigger a return to active drug addiction.

Addiction relapse triggering a psychiatric disorder.   During a period of recovery from dual disorders, an addiction relapse may prompt the return of the psychiatric disorder.

Again, addiction relapse generally includes a period of relapsive thinking before actual drug use. Essentially, relapsive thinking is delusional. Addicted people believe in things that are essentially unbelievable, such as their ability to control the use of drugs or to control their behavior while under the influence of drugs. If left uninterrupted, this delusional thinking will likely lead to unsuccessful experiments with control over drug use and a subsequent return to active addiction.

Even if the individual is not yet using psychoactive drugs, delusional, relapsive thinking can trigger the reemergence of a psychiatric disorder. For instance, people who are experiencing relapsive and delusional thinking may falsely believe that they do not need to use their prescribed medications. They may falsely believe that their will-power can effectively manage their psychiatric disorder. As a result, they may discard their medications and reexperience the psychiatric problem. At this point, the relapsive thinking may lead to full relapse of both disorders.

In addition, recovering people who return to drug use experience various drug states that may trigger the return of a psychiatric disorder, or even initiate a new psychiatric disorder. For example, people with depression and alcohol addiction who return to active alcohol

Table 11–1. Relationships between drug problems and psychiatric problems

Relationship	Example
Drugs can cause psychiatric symptoms	Person drinks caffeine and feels anxious
Withdrawal can cause psychiatric symptoms	Person undergoing detoxification from alcohol feels anxious
Drugs can provoke or worsen psychiatric disorders	Depressed person feels more depressed while using benzodiazepines for insomnia
Drugs can mask psychiatric symptoms	Person diminishes panic associated with phobia by drinking
Psychiatric disorders can mimic addictive behaviors	Manic patient denies that problem exists and has severe social problems; manic symptoms mimic cocaine intoxication
Addiction can coexist with psychiatric disorders	Person with personality disorder is also addicted to marijuana
Psychiatric relapse can trigger addiction relapse	Alcoholic person with schizophrenia stops taking antipsychotic medications; drinks to diminish psychotic symptoms; relapses
Addiction relapse can trigger psychiatric disorder relapse	Recovering person with bipolar disorder and polydrug addiction uses stimulant; person feels good, stops using prescribed medication; addiction and bipolar disorder symptoms emerge

use may experience a temporary alcohol-related depression, which may then trigger the more serious reemergence of a depressive disorder. Similarly, people with depression and cocaine addiction may experience a depression related to cocaine withdrawal, which may then trigger the more serious reemergence of a depressive disorder.

Because the return of one disorder may activate the other disorder, relapse prevention for both disorders is critical.

■ Summary

Psychoactive, mood-altering drugs cause alterations in mood, behavior, thinking, perception, and memory. The relationships between drug use and psychiatric symptoms include the following: drugs can cause psychiatric symptoms; drugs can initiate or worsen existing psychiatric symptoms and disorders; drugs can mask psychiatric symptoms; withdrawal can cause psychiatric symptoms; and psychiatric disorders can cause behavior that resembles the behavior associated with addiction. Also, addiction can coexist with psychiatric disorders.

People with dual disorders have special treatment needs. The goal of addiction treatment is to learn to live a healthy and productive life without psychoactive drugs. The goal of psychiatric treatment includes eliminating or reducing psychiatric symptoms. There are different treatment approaches for people with dual disorders.

Sequential treatment involves first treating one disorder and then treating the other disorder. Parallel treatment describes simultaneous treatment of the addiction and the psychiatric disorder, but through different treatment programs or providers. Integrated treatment involves specialized treatment programs that provide simultaneous treatment for both disorders through the same program with the same staff. Integrated treatment is especially necessary for people with severe psychiatric and substance use problems.

For people with dual disorders, several potential treatment conflicts can occur. For instance, some of the medications used to treat anxiety and panic disorders are psychoactive and pose a threat to sobriety. Thus, for people with addiction and an anxiety disorder, nonpsychoactive and nondrug treatments should be used to treat anxiety.

Another potential conflict for people with dual disorders has to do with participation in the Twelve-Step groups. Participants in Twelve-Step meetings may not be knowledgeable about medications and may give inappropriate advice to others about stopping their medications. Thus, people with dual disorders should be prepared to educate their Twelve-Step peers, and they should be guided to participate in Twelve-Step meetings that are sensitive to people with dual disorders.

There are unusual situations in which recovering patients with dual disorders are appropriately prescribed psychoactive drugs. These are generally emergency situations, and the prescribing is done under very specific circumstances. These circumstances include close collaboration among all the providers and the patient, very close supervision of drug use, and prescription of these drugs only for very brief periods of time.

People with dual disorders have treatment and recovery goals that include sobriety and treatment of psychiatric problems. However, poor recovery from one disorder can lead to problems with the other. Generally, relapse begins with relapsive thinking, which is a return of distorted thinking and a reactivation of denial as a primary defense mechanism. As a result of this distorted thinking, patients may cease to take medication required for the management of psychiatric problems, or they may return to drug use. Relapse prevention involves learning the early warning signs of relapsive thinking, rather than waiting until late-stage symptoms emerge.

■ References

1. Landry MJ, Smith DE, McDuff D, et al: Anxiety and substance use disorders: a primer for primary care physicians. Journal of the American Board of Family Practice 4:47–53, 1991
2. Smith DE, Landry MJ: Psychoactive substance use disorders: drugs and alcohol, in Review of General Psychiatry, 3rd Edition. Edited by Goldman HH. Norwalk, CT, Appleton & Lange, 1992, pp 172–188

3. O'Connor LE, Berry JW, Morrison A, et al: Retrospective reports of psychiatric symptoms before, during, and after drug use in a recovering population. Journal of Psychoactive Drugs 24(1):65–68, 1992

4. American Psychiatric Association: Diagnostic and Statistical Manual of Mental Disorders, 3rd Edition, Revised. Washington, DC, American Psychiatric Association, 1987

5. Bukstein OG, Brent DA, Kaminer Y: Comorbidity of substance abuse and other psychiatric disorders in adolescents. American Journal of Psychiatry 146:1131–1141, 1989

6. Weiss RD, Mirin SM: Substance abuse as an attempt at self-medication. Psychiatric Medicine 3:357–367, 1987

7. Stoffelmayr BE, Benishek LA, Humphreys K, et al: Substance abuse prognosis with an additional psychiatric diagnosis: understanding the relationship. Journal of Psychoactive Drugs 21:145–152, 1989

8. Zweben JE, Smith DE: Considerations in using psychotropic medications with dual diagnosis patients in recovery. Journal of Psychoactive Drugs 21:221–228, 1989

9. Landry MJ, Smith DE, McDuff DR, et al: Anxiety and substance use disorders: the treatment of high-risk patients. Journal of the American Board of Family Practice 4:447–456, 1991

10. Landry MJ, Smith DE, Steinberg JR: Anxiety, depression and substance use disorders: diagnostic, treatment and prescribing practices. Journal of Psychoactive Drugs 23(4):397–416, 1991

Chapter 12

Treatment, Recovery, and Medication

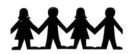

Psychoactive drugs, whether prescribed or not, are the triggers neces-sary for the expression of the disease of addiction. However, for some people, and in some situations, prescribed medications can be an ap-propriate, but generally limited, aspect of treatment. For example, med-ications are appropriately used for the treatment of the initial, acute withdrawal and to diminish cravings or symptoms of prolonged with-drawal. Medications such as Antabuse and naltrexone are used to block impulsive alcohol and opioid use. Also, medications are often required for those patients who have a dual diagnosis of addictive and psychiatric disorders. Recovery from addiction requires a comprehen-sive program of full recovery. Medications can be one aspect of that recovery program, but their use is generally time-limited. At present, there is no "drug treatment" that fully and specifically resolves or "cures" drug addiction.

John R. Steinberg, M.D.
Clinical Assistant Professor
University of Maryland School of Medicine
President, Maryland Society of Addiction Medicine
Baltimore, Maryland

■ Medication Confusion

The use of prescribed medications during various phases of addiction treatment is often bewildering for patients, family members, and even some health care professionals. On the one hand, the central philosophy of addiction treatment is learning to live a comfortable and responsible life without the use of psychoactive drugs. At the same time, physicians may prescribe medications—some of them psychoactive—as part of treatment.

Family members may become alarmed when they learn that their alcohol- and benzodiazepine-addicted relative was indeed prescribed benzodiazepines shortly after arriving at the treatment program. They may not realize that medical management of benzodiazepine withdrawal involves prescribing and then gradually tapering the dosage of benzodiazepines or related medications.

Some health care professionals may not understand the purpose of prescribing antidepressant drugs for patients experiencing stimulant withdrawal. It would be incorrect to assume that these patients have preexisting depressive disorders. In fact, antidepressant medications are routinely used to manage stimulant withdrawal and even some anxiety disorders.

Also, people can easily confuse one medication with another. For example, family members and people in recovery may not know the difference between Librium and lithium. And they may not understand why these differences can significantly affect recovery from addiction. Whereas Librium (chlordiazepoxide) is a psychoactive, rapidly mood-altering, benzodiazepine sedative-hypnotic and a significant threat to sobriety, lithium is a slow-acting, nonpsychoactive, noneuphorigenic medication that is used to treat the manic phase of bipolar (manic-depressive) disorder. Lithium is not a threat to sobriety.

A medication used during the detoxification phase may be completely inappropriate during the recovery process. Certainly, psychoactive, mood-altering drugs pose a grave threat to sobriety, whereas other medications such as naltrexone (Trexan) and disulfiram (Antabuse) may actually help to strengthen sobriety during difficult times.

The purpose of this chapter is to familiarize the reader with medications commonly used in various phases of the treatment of addiction. In addition, this chapter contains a brief review of medications frequently used for patients with dual disorders. There is a focus on identifying psychoactive, mood-altering medications that represent great risk for relapse. In addition, the chapter includes a description of the role of alpha- and beta-blocking agents and methadone.

However, this chapter is not a review of the mechanisms of action or efficacy of these drugs. Nor is it a critical review or analysis of the pharmacologic management of addiction-related syndromes or psychiatric disorders. To gain a comprehensive understanding of these medications, the reader is encouraged to review the references provided.

■ Medications Used to Manage Withdrawal[*]

People who have developed tolerance to and physical dependence on psychoactive drugs experience withdrawal syndromes when they stop or reduce their drug use. The severity of these withdrawal syndromes varies in relation to the specific drug used, the amount of drug used, the overall drug combinations, and the chronicity of drug use. As described in Part One of this book, many people experience two phases of withdrawal: acute and prolonged. Every person who has developed physical dependence on and tolerance to a drug experiences an acute withdrawal syndrome. A subgroup of addicted people go on to experience a significant prolonged withdrawal syndrome.

Acute withdrawal is the set of symptoms and signs that begin shortly after reducing or stopping drug use. They last up to 1 or 2

---

[*] For a critical review of approved and experimental medications used in addiction, see Wesson DR, Ling WL: "Medications in the Treatment of Addictive Disease." *Journal of Psychoactive Drugs* 23:365–370, 1991. For a comprehensive review of medications used in treating withdrawal syndromes, see Sees KL: "Pharmacological Adjuncts for the Treatment of Withdrawal Syndromes." *Journal of Psychoactive Drugs* 23:371–386, 1991.

weeks, depending on the drug and the severity of the withdrawal syndrome. The prolonged withdrawal syndrome may emerge days, weeks, or sometimes months after detoxification, and it may occur within the first year of being drug free.

Because withdrawal syndromes vary in severity, they also vary in seriousness and dangerousness. In general, the higher the daily drug dosage and the longer the period of drug use, the more severe and possibly more dangerous the withdrawal syndrome is. Depending on the drug of addiction, the withdrawal may include problems with insomnia, anxiety, depression, psychosis, seizure, gastrointestinal distress, muscle pain, and drug craving.

Most of these symptoms and signs can be treated with prescribed medications. The treatment of acute withdrawal is generally the same across treatment settings, whether they are inpatient hospital settings, outpatient clinics, or through primary-care physicians. Inpatient settings allow for closer supervision of symptoms and signs and stricter regulation of medication. Similarly, it is safer (and therefore preferable) for outpatient clinics to dispense medication on a daily basis rather than dispense detoxification medications in larger-than-daily dosages.

Irrespective of the medical setting, the medical management of withdrawal is a humane and ethical aspect of treatment. Patients need not suffer the effects of withdrawal when treatment is available. However, some treatment programs do not offer medical detoxification services. For instance, some social model detoxification facilities provide shelter, nutrition, counseling, and care with a minimum of medical attention. Although these resources are vital aspects of our health care system, people with severe tolerance and physical dependence should have access to medical detoxification.

Sedative-Hypnotic Withdrawal

Withdrawal from alcohol, the benzodiazepines, and the barbiturates may produce an acute withdrawal syndrome followed by a prolonged withdrawal syndrome. Acute sedative-hypnotic withdrawal generally consists of anxiety and apprehension, insomnia and nightmares, and emotional and behavioral stimulation, including agitation and irritability. In general, patients experience stimulation of the autonomic system, which stimulates the "fight or flight" syndrome, including elevated heart rate, blood pressure, and respiration rate. Tachycardia, muscle pain, weakness, nausea and vomiting, and a slight tremor of the hands and eyelids may occur. The possibility of seizures is high for patients undergoing withdrawal from short-acting barbiturates; it is less likely for patients undergoing withdrawal from alcohol and the benzodiazepines.[1]

The basic concept of medical management of sedative-hypnotic withdrawal is to avoid or minimize withdrawal symptoms by administering a cross-tolerant sedative-hypnotic and gradually tapering the dosage. First, physicians estimate the approximate total amount of sedative-hypnotic drug used each day. Then they administer that amount to the patient, enough to stop withdrawal symptoms or perhaps cause a brief and mild intoxication. Once it appears that they have approximately matched the amount of sedative-hypnotic administered to the patient's tolerance, they begin gradually to diminish or taper the drug dosage. In general, longer-acting drugs provide a smoother, more gradual withdrawal. For this reason, the longer-acting benzodiazepines such as chlordiazepoxide (Librium), diazepam (Valium), clorazepate (Tranxene), oxazepam (Serax), and lorazepam (Ativan), as well as the long-acting barbiturate phenobarbital, are commonly used.[2]

For example, withdrawal from the benzodiazepines may include 1) the graded dosage reduction of the benzodiazepine of addiction, 2) the substitution and graded dosage reduction of a long-acting benzodiazepine for the benzodiazepine of addiction, and 3) substitution and graded dosage reduction of the long-acting barbiturate phenobarbital.[3] The medical management of alcohol withdrawal generally includes the substitution and graded dosage reduction of a long-acting, cross-tolerant sedative-hypnotic such as a benzodiazepine or phenobarbital.[4,5]

Because sedative-hypnotics generally produce sedation and sleep and reduce anxiety, many patients do not experience significant anxiety and insomnia during the withdrawal phase. However, some patients experience episodes of anxiety and insomnia that require medical management. For the management of insomnia, physicians may prescribe the sedative-hypnotic chloral hydrate or the antihistamine tripelennamine.[6]

For the management of physical symptoms of anxiety, physicians may prescribe the beta-blockers propranolol (Inderal) or atenolol (Tenormin). Beta-blockers (beta-adrenergic blocking agents) are drugs that slow heart rate and regulate abnormal cardiac rhythms such as tachycardia. They can reduce the physical symptoms of anxiety such as palpitations, excessive sweating, sweaty palms, and muscle tremor.

A similar approach to reducing physical symptoms of anxiety involves the use of alpha-blockers (alpha-adrenergic agonists) such as clonidine (Catapres) and clonidine patches (Catapres-TTS) during withdrawal from alcohol, benzodiazepines, opiates, and nicotine.[7] Clonidine inhibits the firing of norepinephrine neurons in a part of the brain (locus coeruleus)[8] responsible for the "adrenergic storm" that promotes panic and other symptoms of anxiety.[9] Clonidine can be taken in capsule form or worn as a patch on the skin.

Some physicians prescribe the nonsedating antianxiety drug buspirone (BuSpar) as an adjunct in acute benzodiazepine withdrawal syndromes,[10] as an adjunct in acute alcohol withdrawal syndromes,[11] for treatment of prolonged withdrawal from sedative-hypnotics,[12] and as adjunctive treatment of alcohol craving.[13] There has been some research regarding the use of the opioid antagonist naltrexone (Trexan) for alcohol-dependent patients as an adjunct to treatment after alcohol detoxification. Research indicates that naltrexone appears to decrease alcohol craving and relapse rates and helps to stop the resumption of binge drinking typically seen in placebo-treated subjects.[14]

Alcohol is absorbed primarily from the small intestine, the site of absorption of many vitamins and other nutrients. Alcohol interferes with nutrient absorption and promotes increased excretion. Thus, even apparently well-nourished people with alcoholism are assumed to be possibly deficient in folic acid, thiamine, and niacin,[15] as well as in electrolytes and carbohydrates. As a result, physicians may administer vitamin, mineral, amino acid, electrolyte, and nutritional supplements in capsule form (e.g., Special Amino Acid and Vitamin Enteral [SAAVE])[16] or in liquid form (e.g., Oral Alcohol Treatment Solution [OATS] and Oral Electrolyte Supplement [OES]).[17]

Stimulant Withdrawal

The acute withdrawal from cocaine and the amphetamines generally lasts 1–2 weeks and can include agitation, insomnia, loss of appetite, and drug craving, followed by fatigue, exhaustion, depression, abnormally increased appetite, and excessive sleeping.[18] After the acute withdrawal phase, many people experience prolonged stimulant withdrawal syndromes that may last 1–18 weeks, consisting of dysphoria, loss of energy, lack of pleasure, depression, and intense drug craving.[19] After this phase, intense stimulant craving is replaced by episodic craving, which may be triggered by internal and external triggers.

Many patients experience intensely dysphoric symptoms accompanied by potent drug craving. This may lead the patient back to stimulant use, including high-risk behaviors to obtain more stimulants. Without medical management, an outpatient would likely relapse, and an inpatient would likely leave treatment against medical advice.[20] For some, the stimulant withdrawal symptom of depression may be severe and lead to suicide.[21]

Chronic use of stimulants causes depletion in the number of neurotransmitters, which in turn causes dysphoric symptoms, depression, agitation, and drug craving. The medical management of stimulant withdrawal often includes antidepressants, dopamine agonists, and neurotransmitter precursors, all of which help to increase neurotransmitter levels and hence to reduce withdrawal symptoms.[18,22]

Tricyclic antidepressants such as imipramine and desipramine cause an increase in the concentration of the neurotransmitters serotonin, dopamine, and norepinephrine in the synaptic gap of nerve cells. However, the tricyclic antidepressants may take 2–4 weeks to have clinical effects. Some physicians use drugs called dopamine agonists, such as bromocriptine and amantadine. These drugs help to increase the amount of the neurotransmitter dopamine in the nerve cells. Similarly, many physicians prescribe products such as Tropamine, which consist of amino acids that are precursors (or building blocks) of dopamine, serotonin, norepinephrine, and the enkephalins (opiate-like neurotransmitters).[23]

Opioid Withdrawal

Except in newborns, opioid withdrawal is an uncomfortable but not life-threatening experience. In general, symptoms of withdrawal from opioids are surprisingly similar to symptoms of influenza or the flu. During opioid withdrawal, people often experience symptoms and signs of muscle aches and pain; gastrointestinal distress including diarrhea, nausea, or vomiting; runny noses and eyes; insomnia; fever; sweating; piloerection ("goose bumps"); and yawning. People may experience tachycardia, anxiety, restlessness, and irritability.

Withdrawal symptoms from heroin or morphine may begin about 6–8 hours after the last dose. These symptoms peak in severity on the second or third day. Within a week or so, most symptoms disappear. The course of acute withdrawal varies depending on the specific drug. For instance, the withdrawal from meperidine (Demerol) begins more quickly after the last dose, peaks in severity within 10–12 hours, and may end within 4–5 days. In contrast, withdrawal from longer-acting opioids such as methadone may not begin until 1–3 days after the last dose and may last from 1 to 2 weeks.

The two most common methods of managing opioid withdrawal are 1) short-term substitution of a long-acting opioid for the opioid of choice and gradual withdrawal and 2) medication of symptoms.

Substitution and withdrawal. Once people have developed physical tolerance to and dependence on opioids, they will experience withdrawal on cessation or even reduction of drug use. One way to minimize the withdrawal is to substitute a long-acting opioid for the opioid of choice, administering gradually decreasing doses. Substituting a longer-acting opioid for a shorter-acting opioid decreases the number of times per day that the drug has to be administered.

Methadone, a long-acting synthetic opioid, is ideally suited for detoxification and withdrawal. It can be substituted for the drug of choice at about the same level, and the dosage can be maintained and then gradually reduced. In a hospital setting, where there can be close medical supervision, a 20% reduction each day of the total daily dosage is well tolerated by patients and causes little discomfort.[4] In outpatient settings, methadone withdrawal is generally accomplished over a 3-week period. Methadone is generally administered in liquid and tablet forms.

Symptomatic treatment of withdrawal. Opioid detoxification can also be medically managed by treating the symptoms of withdrawal. In other words, because opioid withdrawal includes insomnia, anxiety, gastrointestinal distress, and pain, physicians can administer drugs that will decrease these symptoms and signs.[6]

For example, the sedative-hypnotic chloral hydrate, the benzodiazepine flurazepam (Dalmane), or the antihistamine tripelennamine can be prescribed for insomnia. To decrease anxiety, physicians may prescribe the barbiturate phenobarbital, the benzodiazepine chlordiazepoxide (Librium), or other benzodiazepines. For treatment of gastrointestinal distress, physicians may prescribe the antispasmodic dicyclomine, the antiemetics (antinausea drugs) trimethobenzamide (Tigan) or metoclopramide (Reglan), or a belladonna and barbiturate combination for withdrawal-related irritable bowel syndrome. Physicians may administer propoxyphene (Darvon) for muscle aches and pain.

Over the past few years, there has been increased use of the antihypertensive drug clonidine to treat opioid withdrawal. Long-term use of opioids inhibits activity of nerves that contain norepinephrine (noradrenaline). This is especially true in the locus coeruleus, a part of the brain that contains more than half of all noradrenergic nerves in the central nervous system.[24] During opioid withdrawal, the noradrenergic nerves become hyperactive, causing many of the symptoms of opioid withdrawal. Clonidine decreases the firing of these nerves, thus reducing many, but not all, opioid withdrawal symptoms.[25] In particular, clonidine reduces muscle and bone pain,[26] diarrhea and abdominal cramps,[27] and anxiety and insomnia.[20] Opioid detoxification with clonidine can be successfully accomplished over 10–14 days.

To shorten the length of time needed for opioid detoxification, clonidine is often used in association with the opioid antagonist naltrexone. Naltrexone (which is described more fully later in this chapter) is a drug that reverses and blocks the effects of opioids.

When given to people who are currently taking opioids, naltrexone causes an immediate withdrawal syndrome. However, when clonidine is administered at the same time as naltrexone, the opioid withdrawal symptoms can be minimized. Clonidine and naltrexone are often used simultaneously because together they cause rapid detoxification. Indeed, detoxification from the longer-acting opioid methadone can be accomplished within 4 or 5 days.[28]

Detoxification in Perspective

It is critical to differentiate the medical management of withdrawal from the treatment of addiction itself. Withdrawal is primarily the physical result of chronic drug use. Thus, detoxification is merely the medical management of the physical aspects of chronic drug use.

The goal of detoxification is to get the patient drug free. The goal of addiction treatment is to keep the patient drug free. Thus, detoxification is merely the beginning, not the end, of addiction treatment.

As addicted people become detoxified, they often feel better than they have in years. However, physical well-being returns before psychological, emotional, and cognitive processes return to normal. In other words, patients may feel better physically but continue to have distorted emotions and thought processes. As a result, they may mistakenly believe that they are "cured" and require no further treatment. For this reason, during the detoxification period patients can be at high risk for leaving treatment and relapsing.

■ Medication-Assisted Recovery

In much the same way that detoxification does not constitute treatment of the addiction itself, medications are no substitute for recovery. Indeed, there are no pharmacologic "cures" for addiction. However, medications can be important adjuncts to the recovery process.

In general, medication-assisted recovery refers to the temporary use of prescribed medication that pharmacologically discourages or blocks the effects of impulsive use of psychoactive drugs. Although these medications are not substitutes for drug refusal skills, they can provide an extra measure of relapse prevention, especially during times of high risk for relapse, such as the Christmas holidays.

The drug disulfiram (Antabuse) causes an adverse effect when alcohol is consumed, and naltrexone (Trexan) reduces the pleasurable effects of opioids. These drugs are adjuncts to recovery; they should not be prescribed in the absence of a full program of recovery.

Disulfiram (Antabuse)

Imagine becoming violently ill shortly after having a beer. That is generally what disulfiram does. Disulfiram does not block alcohol intoxication but makes it extremely uncomfortable and unenjoyable.

When alcohol is consumed, it is converted in the liver to a chemical called acetaldehyde, which is then further broken down and eliminated. Disulfiram interferes with the metabolism of alcohol and causes acetaldehyde to accumulate rapidly in the bloodstream, rather than be further metabolized. Acetaldehyde is toxic and causes temporary but severe physical discomfort.

People who regularly take disulfiram and then consume alcohol technically experience acetaldehyde poisoning, which is distressing but not lethal. Symptoms include flushing, headache, nausea, vomiting, dizziness, and palpitations. Additional symptoms may include weakness, vertigo, decreased blood pressure, throbbing in the head and neck, chest pain, and labored breathing.[29] These unpleasant symptoms generally begin within an hour of drinking alcohol (while taking disulfiram) and can last for several hours.

The general purpose of disulfiram is to provide the alcoholic person with one additional, compelling reason not to drink. The disulfiram-alcohol interaction is one way to deter impulsive alcohol use. When disulfiram is considered to be an aversive therapy or a punishment, patients tend to resent or refuse to take the medication and may hide the pills and drink. In contrast, when disulfiram is considered to be an element of a healthy and full program of recovery, people view the drug as something that can help them resist the urge to drink, enhance their confidence in remaining sober, and help them to remain sober.[30]

Disulfiram may be of particular value to people who are 40 years of age or older, have a long drinking history, are relapse-prone but in treatment, are socially stable and motivated, attend Alcoholics Anonymous, are uninsightful, and are compulsive but capable of following rules.[31]

Disulfiram can help people "buy time" by providing an additional short-term influence over the decision to remain abstinent while the alcoholic patient establishes a full program of recovery. Adding disulfiram to a full program of recovery can strengthen recovery during times of severe stress, such as during the holiday season or divorce proceedings or after loss of a job. Disulfiram should always be considered as a pharmacologic complement to recovery, not a replacement for recovery itself.

Naltrexone (Trexan)

Imagine self-injecting a syringe of heroin, expecting to become euphoric in a few moments, and nothing happens. That is what naltrexone does.

Opioid agonists are drugs that occupy the opioid receptor site, inhibit pain transmission, and produce opioid-like effects such as analgesia without loss of consciousness and euphoria at high doses. *Opioid antagonists* have the opposite effects of opioids.

Opioid antagonists also fit into the opioid receptor sites. In fact, they block opioids from occupying the receptor sites and remove opioids that are currently occupying the receptor sites. Indeed, if opioid receptor sites are being occupied by opioid neurotransmitters, the opioid antagonists will actually reverse the opioid activity.

For people taking the opioid antagonist naltrexone, the administration of opioids will have no effect: no analgesia or euphoria. For this reason, naltrexone is often prescribed for opioid-addicted people. Like disulfiram, naltrexone is useful as an adjunct to recovery. Unlike disulfiram, naltrexone does not produce unpleasant effects when combined with opioids. Rather, the expected opioid effect simply does not occur. In other words, naltrexone blocks the reinforcing effects of opioids, decreasing the likelihood of repeated opioid use.[20]

Patients who are most likely to benefit from naltrexone therapy include married people who have established careers and family support for sobriety and who are well motivated for recovery.[32] In general, naltrexone is administered once daily or three times per week. Like disulfiram, the use of naltrexone outside a full program of recovery generally results in a poor outcome.

■ Dual Disorders: Medications Used for Psychiatric Disorders[*]

Patients with the dual disorders of addiction and a psychiatric disorder may be prescribed medications for their psychiatric problems. Some of these medications are psychoactive and represent a serious threat to sobriety, whereas others are not. Thus, the following section is designed to familiarize the reader with medications that are prescribed for anxiety, depression, bipolar disorder, and a few other psychiatric problems. In addition, mention will be made of medications that are psychoactive and should generally be avoided by people in recovery from addiction.

As a reminder, the term *psychoactive* as used in this book specifically describes the ability of a chemical to produce rapid changes in mood, emotion, and behavior.

In other words, a psychoactive drug—especially if taken in high doses—causes an experience that is generally described by the user as pleasurable or euphoric. Further, when people take the drug, they experience its effects shortly after the drug enters the brain (the speed with which it enters the brain may vary depending on the route of administration).

Generalized Anxiety and Panic Disorders

In general, anxiety describe clusters of physical and psychological manifestations of fear. Anxiety disorders describe groupings of symp-

---

[*]For a thorough review of medications used in treating psychiatric disorders, see *Review of General Psychiatry*, 3rd Edition. Edited by Goldman HH. Norwalk, CT, Appleton & Lange, 1992.

toms and signs of anxiety, panic, and phobias. For example, generalized anxiety disorder is described as excessive or unrealistic anxiety, worry, and apprehension about two or more life circumstances. These symptoms are accompanied by symptoms of autonomic hyperactivity, motor tension, and vigilance and scanning.[33]

The main characteristics of panic disorder are recurrent panic attacks, which are periods of intense fear or discomfort with pronounced alterations of physiological functions leading to fears of death or losing control. Panic disorder often includes tachycardia or palpitations, a smothering sensation, dizziness or fainting, trembling, sweating, nausea, choking, chest pains, depersonalization, and fears of losing control of behavior.[33]

Some of the medications that may be prescribed for anxiety disorders include the benzodiazepines, buspirone, beta-blockers, antihistamines, antidepressants, and clonidine.[34]

Benzodiazepines. Benzodiazepines are commonly used to treat anxiety disorders. For the average psychiatric patient, the benzodiazepines are ideally used for the short-term treatment of symptoms and signs of anxiety. For such a patient, the benzodiazepines are appropriately prescribed and can be safely used. However, these medications are psychoactive, mood-altering drugs. Thus, for patients with an anxiety disorder plus addiction, the benzodiazepines represent a serious threat to sobriety and abstinence from mood-altering drugs.

Benzodiazepines commonly used to treat anxiety disorders include alprazolam (Xanax), chlordiazepoxide (Libritabs, Librium), clorazepate (Tranxene), diazepam (Valium), halazepam (Paxipam), lorazepam (Ativan), and prazepam (Centrax).

Buspirone. Buspirone (BuSpar) is also commonly used to treat anxiety disorders. Buspirone is most frequently used to treat generalized anxiety disorders, chronic anxiety symptoms, anxiety with depressive symptoms, and anxiety in elderly patients. Buspirone differs from the benzodiazepines in that it decreases symptoms and signs of anxiety, but it is not a sedative-hypnotic. Buspirone is not psychoactive, not mood altering, and not euphorigenic. Buspirone is the recommended antianxiety medication for anxious patients in recovery.[34]

Beta-blockers. Beta-blockers are drugs that are best known for the treatment of hypertension, cardiac arrhythmias, and angina pectoris. They are occasionally prescribed for the treatment of the physical manifestations of anxiety such as tachycardia and tremor. They are often used to treat performance anxiety or to prevent physical manifestations of anxiety during anticipated stressful situations. The beta-blocker most commonly used for these purposes is propranolol (Inderal), although atenolol (Tenormin) is also used. Because tolerance builds rapidly to the drugs' effectiveness in decreasing symptoms of physical anxiety, they are generally used for short periods of time. Beta-blockers are not psychoactive and do not jeopardize recovery.

Antihistamines. Many of the older-generation antihistamines produce mild sedation as a side effect. For this reason, some physicians prescribe them for anxiety or insomnia. Tolerance to the anxiolytic and hypnotic effects of antihistamines develops rapidly. Thus, they are generally useful for short periods of time. Examples include diphenhydramine (Nytol, Benadryl), doxylamine (Unisom), and pyrilamine (Quiet World). Although these older antihistamines exert mild sedative effects, they are not euphorigenic. Nevertheless, their use may prove to be difficult for some people in recovery from addiction. It should be noted that some antihistamines taken in combination with other drugs can cause adverse affects.

Antidepressants. Most antidepressants substantially reduce the frequency and severity of panic attacks and often prevent them altogether. In addition, antidepressants have been used in the treatment of mixed depression and anxiety and in chronically anxious patients with sleep disturbances. Examples include the tricyclic antidepressants clomipramine (Anafranil), desipramine (Norpramin), doxepin (Adapin, Sinequan), and imipramine (Tofranil). Also, another group of antidepressants known as the monoamine oxidase inhibitors (e.g., phenelzine [Nardil]) have been used to treat panic disorders, especially those characterized by phobias. In therapeutic doses, the anti-

301

depressants are not psychoactive or euphorigenic, and they do not represent a risk to recovery.

Clonidine. The antihypertensive drug clonidine (Catapres) has been used to treat anxiety and panic. Because tolerance to clonidine's antianxiety and antipanic effects develops rapidly, it is generally reserved for short-term use. Clonidine is not psychoactive or euphorigenic and will not jeopardize recovery.

Major Depression and Bipolar Disorder

The term *mood* can be described as pervasive and sustained emotion that may affect all aspects of an individual's life and perception of the environment. Mood disorders are pathologically elevated or depressed mood disturbances that include full or partial manic or depressive syndromes.

The central feature of major depression is the presence of one or more major depressive episodes. These episodes involve a depression in mood with an accompanying loss of pleasure or indifference to most activities, most of the time, for at least a 2-week period. This deviation from normal mood may include significant changes in energy, sleep patterns, ability to concentrate, and weight. People may experience psychomotor retardation (lethargy) or agitation, persistent feelings of worthlessness or inappropriate guilt, and recurrent thoughts of death.[33]

Bipolar disorder, which used to be called manic depression, involves one or more episodes of mania, often in conjunction with one or more depressive episodes. Manic episodes are periods of unusually elevated, euphoric, expansive, or irritable mood that are severe enough to cause significant impairment in occupational or social functioning or apparent harm to oneself or others. Manic episodes may be marked by a decreased need for sleep, talkativeness, flight of ideas, distractibility, grandiosity, and immoderate involvement in activities that are pleasurable yet have negative consequences.[33]

Antidepressants. Psychoactive drugs such as cocaine and alcohol cause rapid changes in mood, emotion, and behavior. For example, people who feel sad and depressed occasionally use cocaine to feel better. In fact, cocaine causes a rapid emotional swing upward. For the next few minutes, these people do not feel sad or depressed. Indeed, they may feel euphoric. In this example, cocaine has an antidepressant effect because it elevates people's mood and emotion and stimulates behavior.

In contrast, the antidepressants work not by elevating people's mood but by inhibiting or stopping people's mood from becoming severely depressed. They inhibit the onset of severe depression or reduce the severity of depression.

These drugs have a long-term effect on mood. But unlike drugs such as cocaine or alcohol, they are not psychoactive because they do not cause a rapid change in mood, emotion, or behavior shortly after being consumed. Antidepressants often take a week or more to produce an effect and may take 1 or 2 months to produce a complete effect. They are not euphorigenic, although toxic doses can cause episodes of dysphoria. Some of the antidepressants such as fluoxetine (Prozac) have a mild stimulant effect in some patients, a phenomenon that needs to be evaluated. Overall, the antidepressants are not a threat to sobriety. They include the tricyclic antidepressants, the monoamine oxidase inhibitors, and a few assorted antidepressants.

The tricyclic antidepressants include amitriptyline (Elavil), amoxapine (Asendin), clomipramine (Anafranil), desipramine (Norpramin), doxepin (Sinequan), imipramine (Tofranil), nortriptyline (Pamelor, Aventyl), protriptyline (Vivactil), and trimipramine (Surmontil). They are used to relieve symptoms of major depressive episodes; bipolar disorder, depressed type; and other depressive problems. They are often used to treat mixed depression and agitation or anxiety.

The monoamine oxidase inhibitors include isocarboxazid (Marplan), phenelzine (Nardil), and tranylcypromine (Parnate). In general, they are used to treat "atypical depression," which is characterized by excessive sleeping, excessive eating, somatic complaints, and dysphoria. They are also used as a second-line drug when treatment with other antidepressants has failed.

Trazodone (Desyrel) is an antidepressant used to treat major depressive episodes with or without prominent anxiety. It is also used to treat certain types of chronic pain. Bupropion (Wellbutrin) and fluoxetine (Prozac) are used to treat major depressive disorder. Maprotiline (Ludiomil) is used to treat patients with major depressive disorder and bipolar disorder. Selegiline (Eldepryl) is better known as an adjunct to treating Parkinson's disease. It is used by some physicians to treat depression.

Mood regulators. In addition to the antidepressants, a few unrelated drugs are used to treat mood disorders, especially mania or the manic phases of bipolar disorder. The most popular of these drugs is lithium (e.g., Eskalith, Lithonate).

Much as antidepressants can inhibit episodes of depression, lithium can inhibit episodes of mania. Indeed, lithium is generally described as an antimanic drug because it can diminish active episodes of mania as well as help to minimize the intensity and frequency of subsequent manic episodes. Lithium is the standard treatment for manic episodes and for bipolar disorder in which mania is a predominant feature.

Lithium can be used alone or in combination with antidepressants for the treatment of depression. In particular, lithium helps to augment the effects of antidepressants for patients who are not responsive to antidepressants alone. In general, it takes 1–3 weeks for the full effect of lithium to occur.

The drug carbamazepine (Tegretol) is perhaps best known as an anticonvulsant. However, some physicians use carbamazepine alone or in combination with lithium or antidepressants to treat bipolar disorder. It often takes about 1 week for the full effect of carbamazepine to occur. Neither lithium nor carbamazepine is psychoactive or euphorigenic. Like the antidepressants, they do not threaten sobriety or recovery.

Benzodiazepines. Lithium is more than 95% effective in the management of acute mania, and it is the drug of choice for maintenance therapy.[35] However, it does have a slow onset of action. For this reason, some physicians prescribe the rapid-acting benzodiazepine lorazepam (Ativan) or other benzodiazepines for short-term management of an acute manic episode. Although appropriate for nonaddicted patients, the benzodiazepines are psychoactive medications and represent a threat to sobriety and recovery.

■ Methadone Maintenance[*]

Methadone (Dolophine, Methadose) is a synthetic opioid analgesic similar in potency to morphine. Indeed, it can be used for the management of severe pain. As described earlier, it is routinely used for detoxification and withdrawal from opioids. Methadone is also used as a legal substitute for illicit opioids. This process of substitution and sustained administration of methadone is called methadone maintenance therapy.

Methadone is longer lasting than most opioids. Thus, it can be administered less frequently and is highly effective when orally administered. Because methadone is a psychoactive, mood-altering opioid, tolerance, dependence, and addiction to methadone are expected. Indeed, the general principle of methadone maintenance is to substitute pharmaceutically prepared, physician-administered methadone for the chronic use of prescription opioids, heroin, or clandestinely prepared opioids.

Thus, methadone maintenance treatment differs from a drug-free treatment and recovery philosophy. However, methadone maintenance treatment is an accepted part of addiction medicine, and it does provide a treatment alternative for those people addicted to opioids who are unwilling to stop using them. The goal of methadone maintenance is the substantial reduction and, ideally, the cessation of opioid use.[36] For many patients, methadone maintenance is accompanied by a reduction in the use of other drugs. What follows is an overview of the benefits of methadone maintenance.

---

[*]For a thorough review of issues relating to methadone maintenance, see "Opioid Dependence and Methadone Maintenance Treatment." *Journal of Psychoactive Drugs* 23:99–232, 1991 (special issue).

Reduction in criminal behavior. Opioid addiction may cost many hundreds of dollars each day. To sustain this addiction, many opioid-addicted people sell opioids for a profit, keeping some for personal use. Some people steal and sell to afford a regular opioid supply. Because methadone is legal, patients who receive methadone are not required to engage in criminal activity to sustain an opioid addiction.

Vocational stabilization. For people addicted to opioids (especially those who sell opioids or steal to get opioids), each day is a struggle to obtain drugs. On days when opioids cannot be found, these people experience opioid withdrawal. When the criminal aspects of opioid addiction are interrupted and methadone is provided on a daily basis, people addicted to opioids are able to obtain legitimate employment and contribute to society.

Social stabilization. Participation in a methadone maintenance treatment program allows opioid-addicted people to pursue healthy social activities and resume family responsibilities. Indeed, this participation is associated with improvements in family relationships and a decrease in family problems.[37]

Entry and engagement in the health care system. For some people, methadone maintenance is one of the few contacts they have with the medical and psychiatric health care delivery system. Through this contact they can receive medical, psychiatric, psychological, legal, and vocational assistance. Indeed, methadone maintenance results in improvements in general health.[38]

Reduction of needle-borne disease. Methadone maintenance significantly reduces the use of illicit opioids and diminishes the use of needles for opioid administration. As a result, methadone maintenance is playing an important role in limiting the spread of acquired immunodeficiency syndrome (AIDS), needle-borne hepatitis, and other diseases among opioid addicts.

Reduction of hazards for pregnant opioid-addicted women. When a pregnant woman uses heroin, she subjects herself and her fetus to numerous hazards. In addition to the possibility of passing needle-borne disease to the fetus, heroin addiction most often involves a series of episodes of opioid use followed by episodes of withdrawal. Maternal opioid withdrawal can cause fetal death. Thus, methadone maintenance is usually recommended for opioid-addicted women who become pregnant. Methadone maintenance provides ongoing access to opioids rather than the physical trauma of repeated withdrawal episodes. Also, participation in a methadone maintenance treatment program provides access to maternal and prenatal care.[39]

Recovery from opioid addiction. For many people addicted to opioids, methadone maintenance represents an opportunity for psychosocial stabilization and normalization over a period of several months or longer. Increasingly, methadone maintenance programs offer Twelve-Step meetings such as Narcotics Anonymous specifically for methadone-maintained patients. By offering these and other support services, methadone maintenance treatment programs are better able to help opioid-addicted people cease taking methadone.

A Few Thoughts About Medications

Medications are inherently neither good nor bad. Some medications can eliminate or diminish distressing or dangerous psychiatric symptoms. Some medications can be invaluable for managing withdrawal and drug craving. At the same time, use of psychoactive medications by high-risk patients results in compulsive use. Also, psychoactive medications can cause changes in patients' feelings and thoughts that can compromise recovery.

It is critical to remember that addicted people have often searched for drug solutions to many of life's problems and have consistently failed to find them. Therefore, the use of medications by people with substance use disorders can be appropriate only in the context of a full program of recovery and in close cooperation with a physician who is knowledgeable about addiction medicine and psychiatric treatment.

■ Summary

The central treatment goal of recovery is learning to live a comfortable and responsible life without the use of psychoactive drugs. At the same time, treatment for addiction and psychiatric disorders often involves the use of medication, some of it psychoactive. There are points during addiction treatment—such as during acute withdrawal—when use of this medication may be appropriate for some patients. However, psychoactive medication is incompatible with the goal of a drug-free recovery.

Psychoactive medications such as the benzodiazepines are appropriately used during the treatment of acute withdrawal from sedative-hypnotics, including benzodiazepine withdrawal itself. Although psychoactive medications are appropriate to manage the acute sedative-hypnotic withdrawal, nonpsychoactive medications such as propranolol, buspirone, and clonidine can be used during the subacute or prolonged sedative-hypnotic withdrawal syndrome.

Because stimulant withdrawal includes a reduction of the level of several neurotransmitters, medications that normalize neurotransmitter levels will help to reduce withdrawal symptoms. These medications include antidepressants and products that contain amino acids. Management of opioid withdrawal can consist of either short-term substitution of another opioid and gradual withdrawal or medication of symptoms. Methadone, a long-acting synthetic opioid, can be substituted for the opioid of abuse and the dosage gradually reduced. Alternatively, physicians can prescribe medications that treat the symptoms of withdrawal, such as insomnia, anxiety, gastrointestinal distress, and pain. Thus, several medications may be used, including benzodiazepines for insomnia, phenobarbital or benzodiazepines for anxiety, assorted medications for gastrointestinal distress, and an opioid for muscle pain. In addition, clonidine and naltrexone can be used together to produce a relatively rapid opioid detoxification.

Some alcoholic people take disulfiram, which makes them violently ill when they drink alcohol. Disulfiram does not block alcohol intoxication, but rather makes people feel nauseated. Naltrexone is an opioid antagonist that blocks and reverses opioid activity. While a patient is taking naltrexone, opioids have virtually no effect and do not cause euphoria. The use of disulfiram or naltrexone is best described as an adjunct to a full program of treatment and recovery.

People with dual disorders often need pharmacologic treatment for their psychiatric problem. Some of the medications used for anxiety disorders include the benzodiazepines, buspirone, beta-blockers, antihistamines, antidepressants, and clonidine. The benzodiazepines are psychoactive and are a threat to sobriety. The other medications have no psychoactive effect or a very mild one, and they are not euphorigenic.

The primary medications used to treat major depression and bipolar disorder include antidepressants such as the tricyclic antidepressants and monoamine oxidase inhibitors and mood stabilizers such as lithium. These medications are not psychoactive, mood altering, or euphorigenic. However, some of them will cause dysphoria at toxic doses.

Methadone maintenance is an accepted form of treatment in addiction medicine, although it differs from a drug-free treatment philosophy. However, methadone maintenance followed by methadone detoxification often leads to abstinence from opioids. The benefits of methadone maintenance include a reduction in criminal behavior, vocational and social stabilization, engagement with the health care system, and reduction of needle-borne disease. Methadone maintenance is the treatment of choice for opioid-addicted women who become pregnant, because opioid withdrawal can cause fetal death.

■ References

1. Smith DE, Landry MJ: Psychoactive substance use disorders: drugs and Alcohol, in Review of General Psychiatry, 3rd Edition. Edited by Goldman HH. Norwalk, CT, Appleton & Lange, 1992, pp 172–188
2. The United States Pharmacopeial Convention: USP DI Drug Information for the Health Care Professional, 11th Edition. Rockville, MD, United States Pharmacopeial Convention, 1991
3. Landry MJ, Smith DE, McDuff DR, et al: Benzodiazepine dependence and withdrawal: identification and medical management. Journal of the American Board of Family Practice 5:1–9, 1992

4. Jaffe JH: Drug addiction and drug abuse, in Goodman and Gilman's The Pharmacological Basis of Therapeutics, 8th Edition. Edited by Goodman LS, Gilman A. New York, Pergamon, 1990, pp 522–573

5. Kranzler HR, Orrok B: The pharmacotherapy of alcoholism, in American Psychiatric Press Review of Psychiatry, Vol 8. Edited by Tasman A, Hales RE, Frances AJ. Washington, DC, American Psychiatric Press, 1989, pp 359–379

6. Haight Ashbury Free Clinics: Detoxification Protocol for the Drug Detoxification, Rehabilitation, and Aftercare Project. San Francisco, CA, Haight Ashbury Free Clinics, 1990

7. Sees KL, Clark HW: Use of clonidine in nicotine withdrawal. Journal of Psychoactive Drugs 20:263–268, 1988

8. Svensson TH, Bunney BS, Aghajanian GK: Inhibition of both noradrenergic and serotonergic neurons in brain by the alpha adrenergic agonist clonidine. Brain Research 92:291–306, 1975

9. Uhde TW, Stein MB, Vittone BJ, et al: Behavioral and physiologic effects of short-term and long-term administration of clonidine in panic disorder. Archives of General Psychiatry 46:170–177, 1989

10. Udelman JD, Udelman DL: Concurrent use of buspirone in anxious patients during withdrawal from alprazolam therapy. Journal of Clinical Psychiatry 51 (suppl):46–50, 1990

11. Dougherty RJ, Gates RR: The role of buspirone in the management of alcohol withdrawal: a preliminary investigation. Journal of Substance Abuse Treatment 7:189–192, 1990

12. Meyer RE: Anxiolytics and the alcoholic patient. Journal of Studies on Alcohol 47:269–273, 1986

13. Bruno F: Buspirone in the treatment of alcoholic patients. Psychopathology 22 (suppl):49–59, 1989

14. Volpicelli JR, Alterman AI, Mayashida M, et al: Naltrexone in the treatment of alcohol dependence. Archives of General Psychiatry 49:876–880, 1992

15. Schuckit MA: Guidelines for the treatment of alcoholic withdrawal. Psychiatry Letter 6:13–20, 1987

16. Blum K, Trachtenberg MC: Neurogenic deficits caused by alcoholism: restoration by SAAVE, a neuronutrient intervention adjunct. Journal of Psychoactive Drugs 20:297–313, 1988

17. Wright C, Talbott GD: The use of carbohydrate-electrolyte supplements in residential treatment of chemical dependence. Journal of Psychoactive Drugs 20:337–348, 1988

18. Milhorn HT: Chemical Dependence: Diagnosis, Treatment, and Prevention. New York, Springer-Verlag, 1990

19. Karan LD, Haller DL, Schnoll SH: Cocaine, in Clinical Textbook of Addictive Disorders. Edited by Frances RJ, Miller SI. New York, Guilford, 1991, pp 121–145

20. Herridge P, Gold MS: Pharmacological adjuncts in the treatment of opioid and cocaine addicts. Journal of Psychoactive Drugs 20:233–242, 1988

21. Tennent FS: Cocaine withdrawal step by step. Emergency Medicine 20:65–68, 1987

22. Daigle RD, Clark HW, Landry MJ: A primer on neurotransmitters and cocaine. Journal of Psychoactive Drugs 20:283–295, 1988

23. Horne DE: Clinical impressions of SAAVE and Tropamine. Journal of Psychoactive Drugs 20:333–336, 1988

24. Agren H: Clonidine treatment of the opiate withdrawal syndrome: a review of clinical trials of a theory. Acta Psychiatrica Scandinavica Supplement 327:91–113, 1986

25. Gossop M: Clonidine and the treatment of the opiate withdrawal syndrome. Drug and Alcohol Dependence 21:253–259, 1988

26. Milne B, Cervenko F, Jhamandas K, et al: Intrathecal clonidine: analgesia and effects on opioid withdrawal. Anesthesiology 62:34–38, 1985

27. Gold MS, Roehrich H: Treatment of opiate withdrawal with clonidine. ISI Atlas of Science: Pharmacology 1:29–32, 1987

28. Charney DS, Heninger GR, Kleber HD: The combined use of clonidine and naltrexone as a rapid, safe, and effective treatment of abrupt withdrawal from methadone. American Journal of Psychiatry 143:831–837, 1986

29. Alcoholism and Drug Addiction Research Foundation: Drugs and Drug Abuse: A Reference Text. Toronto, Canada, Addiction Research Foundation, 1987

30. Kwentus J, Sheffel W: The use of disulfiram and naltrexone, in Handbook of Hospital Based Substance Abuse Treatment. Edited by Lerner WD, Barr MA. New York, Pergamon, 1990, pp 154–168

31. Banys P: The clinical use of disulfiram (Antabuse): a review. Journal of Psychoactive Drugs 20:243–261, 1988

32. Jaffe JH, Epstein S, Ciraulo DA: Opioids, in Clinical Manual of Chemical Dependence. Edited by Ciraulo DA, Shader RI. Washington, DC, American Psychiatric Press, 1991, pp 95–133

33. American Psychiatric Association: Diagnostic and Statistical Manual of Mental Disorders, 3rd Edition, Revised. Washington, DC, American Psychiatric Association, 1987

34. Landry MJ, Smith DE, Steinberg JR: Anxiety, depression, and substance use disorders: diagnosis, treatment, and prescribing practices. Journal of Psychoactive Drugs 23:397–416, 1991

35. Davis GC, Goldman B: Somatic therapies, in Review of General Psychiatry, 3rd Edition. Edited by Goldman HH. Norwalk, CT, Appleton & Lange, 1992, pp 370–390

36. Goldstein A: Heroin addiction: neurobiology, pharmacology, and policy. Journal of Psychoactive Drugs 23:123–133, 1991

37. Sorensen JL, Gibson DR, Wermuth L, et al: Family difficulties and drug abuse treatment. Unpublished manuscript, 1988

38. Senay ED: Methadone maintenance treatment. International Journal of the Addictions 20:803–821, 1985

39. Zweben JA, Sorensen JL: Misunderstanding about methadone. Journal of Psychoactive Drugs 20:275–281, 1988

Chapter 13

A Special Look at Alcoholism

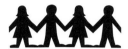

Modern medical research is beginning to clarify the nature of addiction to alcohol. Indeed, research reveals that alcoholism is a heterogeneous biopsychosocial disease. The origins of this disease may be polygenetic anomalies that cause neurotransmitter imbalances in the reward centers of the brain, periods of chronic stress, long periods of excessive drinking, or a combination of two or more causes. In either case, psychosocial influences are likely to be triggering factors. In cases of severe alcoholism—for example, when there is an association with a defective dopamine D$_2$ receptor gene—the disease is likely to be fatal unless the individual receives treatment. The most effective treatment for alcoholism, and indeed for addiction to any psychoactive drug, combines early intervention, education, counseling, self-help programs, neurofeedback, a healthy diet, and pharmacological adjuncts that improve nutrition, particularly brain nutrition.

Kenneth Blum, Ph.D.
Director, Laboratory of Pharmacogenetics
Division of Addictive Diseases
University of Texas Health Science Center
San Antonio, Texas

■ Alcoholism in Perspective

Although drugs such as crack cocaine are frequently in the news spotlight, alcohol is a far more deadly killer. Alcohol is responsible for the deaths of 150,000 Americans or more annually—over 400 people per day—compared to about 7,000 deaths annually from all illicit drugs combined.

There has been far more research on addiction to alcohol than on addiction to other psychoactive drugs—perhaps for a good reason: people use, abuse, and become addicted to alcohol far more often than they use, abuse, and become addicted to all other drugs combined, especially illicit drugs. Table 13–1 compares the use of alcohol, cigarettes, and any illicit drugs with respect to lifetime use (i.e., having ever used), use within the past year, and use within the past month.

The National Institute on Drug Abuse sponsors a National Household Survey on Drug Abuse to provide estimates of drug use trends

Table 13–1. Estimated number and percentage of alcohol, cigarette, and illicit drug users in U.S. households

| Drug | Time period | | |
	Lifetime	Past year	Past month
Any illicit drug	72,496,000 36%	27,971,000 14%	14,479,000 7.3%
Cigarettes	149,005,000 75.1%	67,831,000 34.2%	57,121,000 28.8%
Alcohol	168,498,000 85%	135,071,000 68%	105,845,000 53.4%

Note. Lifetime use indicates those people who have ever used a specific drug during their lifetime. Past year use describes people who have used a specific drug during the past year. Past month use is a relatively good measure of current drug use patterns of monthly or more use.
Source. Adapted from the National Institute on Drug Abuse: *National Household Survey on Drug Abuse: Main Findings 1988*. Rockville, MD, National Institute on Drug Abuse, 1990.

in the United States. This survey estimated that about 7.5% of the total household population ages 12 and older were daily drinkers, consuming alcohol on 20 or more days during the past month.[1] Males are more than twice as likely as females to be daily drinkers, and whites are about twice as likely as African Americans and Hispanics to be daily drinkers.

The survey also studied "heavy drinking," which was defined as drinking five or more drinks per occasion on five or more days in the past month. Of those ages 12 and older, 4.9% were heavy drinkers, with heavy drinking most common among those ages 18–25. Males were about four times more likely than females to be heavy drinkers. An estimated 10.5 million Americans are alcoholic, and an additional 7.2 Americans are alcohol abusers.[2] A similar study estimated that 13.5% of the U.S. population has experienced alcoholism or alcohol abuse.[3] Alcoholism is more common than addiction to other drugs in large part because more people drink alcohol than use other drugs.

■ Explanations for Alcoholic Behavior

Throughout history, and especially during the past 100 years, there have been numerous models for explaining alcoholic behavior. This fact is not surprising, because there have always been competing models to explain the world as well as human behavior. Some of these explanations include describing alcoholism in terms of moral corruption or as the result of psychological, sociological, behavioral, or biological problems.

Some of the earliest explanations of alcoholic behavior suggested that people who had alcoholic problems were morally corrupt, evil, or bad. Indeed, alcoholic people often break moral and ethical guidelines. However, moral and ethical problems are more likely the result, rather than the cause, of alcoholism. Similarly, some people might describe alcoholic people as lacking willpower.

As early as the 1920s and 1930s, some psychoanalysts and psychologists believed that addiction to alcohol and other drugs was caused by the self-medication of problematic feelings, thoughts, and behaviors. Indeed, there is evidence that some people do self-medicate their anxiety, depression, and other psychiatric symptoms. However, the self-medication model is a better explanation for some people's introduction to alcohol use, rather than fully explaining alcoholism per se.

The study of sociology places a high priority on the interaction among people. Thus, sociology emphasizes the cultural attitudes about the use of alcohol, the role of peer pressure, and modeling of the drinking behavior by others. Sociology also emphasizes the role of demographics (e.g., urban versus rural environment), socioeconomic variables, and other social issues. In general, a sociological perspective may be best for determining environmental stressors that may lead to drug use, cultural support for drug use, and the type of drug that is most accessible.

Behavioral models of alcoholism have placed an emphasis on the positive and negative reinforcement aspects of drug use. *Positive reinforcement* describes the increased likelihood of a repeated behavior if that behavior is associated with some type of reward or pleasant experience. Thus, the use of alcohol for some people is particularly rewarding because they interpret the experience as positive and pleasurable.

In contrast, *negative reinforcement* describes the increased likelihood of a repeated behavior if that behavior helps the subject to avoid a negative experience or unpleasant situation. Thus, the use of alcohol to avoid or reduce a negative experience such as withdrawal involves the negative reinforcement of alcohol. In addition, the behavioral approach helps to explain how alcohol use becomes associated with internal and external cues, thus partially explaining alcohol craving.

Few experts currently believe that the biological aspects of alcoholism can completely explain the addictive process. However, the contributions of neurochemistry and genetics are helping to describe the risk factors for acquiring alcoholism. For instance, current research may reveal that some alcoholic people are deficient in specific neurochemicals. In addition, the study of genetics is helping to describe individuals at higher risk for developing alcoholism when exposed to alcohol.

The Disease Model of Alcoholism

The disease model of alcoholism has been a significant aspect of medical thought for about 200 years. Benjamin Rush, a Philadelphia physician (died 1813) who signed the Declaration of Independence, concluded that alcohol was indeed a drug, habitual drunkenness was involuntary, and complete abstinence should be a major aspect of treatment.

Historically, the description of alcoholism as a disease stood in contrast to moral explanations in which character defects were believed to lead to sinful drinking behavior that the individual needed to subdue through willpower. More recently, the disease model of alcoholism (or addiction) has stood in contrast to models that explained alcoholism as primarily a behavioral problem, primarily a social problem, primarily a biological or neurochemical problem, or as a symptom of an underlying primary psychiatric disorder.

The disease model of alcoholism and addiction relies heavily on multidisciplinary research and incorporates information gained through psychological, sociological, behavioral, genetic, biological, and neurochemical studies. As knowledge about alcoholism and addiction expands, the disease model evolves. At present, it represents a cohesive model that helps to explain alcoholism and addiction to other drugs, and it is the basis for guiding addiction treatment efforts.

Currently, the disease model is the prevailing model that most thoroughly explains alcoholism and the addictive process. Organizations that embrace this model for describing and understanding alcoholism include the American College of Physicians, the American Medical Association, the American Psychiatric Association, the American Public Health Association, the American Hospital Association, the American Psychological Association, the American Society on Addiction Medicine, the National Association of Social Workers, the National Council on Alcoholism and Drug Dependence, and the World Health Organization.

Addiction to alcohol is remarkably similar to addiction to other drugs, once pharmacologic differences are considered.[4] In particular, addiction to alcohol, like addiction to cocaine or marijuana, can be described as a primary, progressive, chronic disease with genetic,

317

psychosocial, and environmental factors influencing its development and outcome. It is often fatal, and it is characterized by continuous or periodic impaired control over drinking, preoccupation with drinking, use of alcohol despite adverse consequences, and distortions in thinking such as denial.[5]

Although anyone can become addicted to alcohol, certain particularly vulnerable individuals are predisposed to developing alcoholism. Because these individuals are at higher risk, early and intensive efforts should be made to provide preventive and educational services for them. The disease model of alcoholism or addiction describes individuals who are expected to experience a more rapid onset of addiction and a more rapidly progressing addiction than other people. The disease model does not imply that "lower-risk" individuals can safely use alcohol or other drugs.

What Is a Disease?

It is useful to examine the medical concept of disease and its relation to alcoholism. Diseases are described in terms of identifiable, objective, and often measurable *signs* (observations that a physician can make), as well as subjective *symptoms* (aches, pains, and problems that a patient experiences and describes to a physician). Certain symptoms, signs, laboratory findings, and other test results are peculiar to specific diseases and are found in most people who have the same disease. Thus, a physician can observe characteristic signs, make a note of the patient's complaints and symptoms, establish a tentative diagnostic hypothesis, and possibly test that hypothesis with various tests.

Identifying characteristic clusters or groupings of symptoms and signs is important because they can predict the likely course of the disease. Thus, recognizing certain patterns of signs and symptoms can help to identify current and future stages of a disease.

Medical and psychiatric diseases and disorders can be described as involuntary pathologies—meaning that some aspect of health has become abnormal or unhealthy, but not as the direct result of choice or willfulness. That is, people do not choose to develop diseases. For example, cigarette smokers and asbestos workers may have chosen to smoke or work around asbestos, but they did not choose to develop lung cancer.

In relation to addiction to alcohol and other drugs, the issue of involuntary behavior is an emotional and often misunderstood topic. Although addiction involves behavior (e.g., drinking), it also involves a loss of control over that behavior. Thus, alcoholic people may choose to drink alcohol, and they certainly choose to experience their initial exposures to alcohol. However, alcoholic people do not choose to experience loss of control over their alcohol use; they do not choose to experience powerful compulsions to drink; and they do not choose to use alcohol despite adverse consequences and potent internal decisions not to drink.

Alcoholism: A Biopsychosocial Disease

Like acquired immunodeficiency syndrome (AIDS), alcoholism is a disease that affects every area of people's lives. The onset of alcoholism is influenced by various biological, psychological, and sociological factors. Once the alcoholism has emerged, it will in turn affect biological, psychological, and social areas of a person's life. Thus, all of these areas must be addressed in the treatment and recovery process. For this reason, alcoholism can be called a biopsychosocial disease.

The impairment of cognitive health in alcoholic people can be both short-term and long-term. Obviously, alcohol intoxication is a short-term impairment of cognition and thinking. People may experience amnesic episodes called alcoholic blackouts or milder versions of these episodes called brownouts. Many alcoholic people have problems with short-term memory and poor concentration. Many alcoholic patients also have specific deficits in problem solving, abstract thinking, concept shifting, psychomotor performance, and difficult memory tasks.[6-8] Long-term, high-dose alcohol users may have neurological problems that can take months and years to disappear fully. For the most severely alcoholic patients, serious organic cerebral impairment is a common complication, occurring in about 10% of patients.[9] During treatment, alcoholic people often make very poor decisions, including the decision to leave treatment against medical advice. Often, such a decision is simply the result of alcohol craving, frustrations, and distorted thinking as the brain heals itself.

Alcoholic people often have problems perceiving their environment accurately. They may experience psychological distortions such as misperceptions and misinterpretations of sensory information. Milder psychological effects include irritability and frustration. Mood changes are frequently part of alcoholism. Periods of intense anxiety can alternate with periods of depression on a regular basis.

The emotional health of alcoholic people is often characterized by extremes, especially negative emotions. Thus, they often are filled with anger, hate, and resentments. They frequently lack love, joy, warmth, and intimacy. Because of alcoholism-induced problems, some alcoholic people have not experienced hope in a long time, and hope will need to be nurtured during the treatment and recovery process.

The social health of alcoholic people often deteriorates quickly, and this deterioration may be noticed by family, friends, and co-workers. As the drive for alcohol becomes stronger, the quest for social interaction weakens. Old friends may be ignored and new drinking friends may emerge. As the alcoholism progresses, problems at work, with the family, and with friends often become worse. Legal and financial problems may emerge or escalate.

As the obsession with alcohol increases, alcoholic people tend to become progressively more self-centered. As they focus more intently on alcohol, they are unable to see much of the world around them, including their family. This blindness to the needs of others may be in contrast to a pre-alcoholic philosophy of caring and concern for others.

Alcoholic people often feel hopeless. Irrespective of specific religious beliefs (if any), they may feel that there is no higher or spiritual purpose to their lives. They may feel that there is no Power greater than themselves to help them solve their problems. It is for this reason that groups like Alcoholics Anonymous promote the concept of a Higher Power, as well as stress the importance of helping others.

The alcohol-induced deterioration of physical health is often a gradual process, measured over years. Thus, physical health is often the last aspect of health to deteriorate. For this reason, people may continue working despite serious alcoholism-related dysfunction in other areas of their life. In other words, they may appear physically healthy despite raging alcoholism.

Physical health is also the first aspect of health to return to normal after abstinence or detoxification. In fact, rapid physical recovery often leads to alcoholism relapse or leaving treatment against medical orders, because the alcoholic person feels better physically. Most serious alcohol-related medical problems are associated with late-stage alcoholism, with the exception of accidents.

Approximately one-third of the people with high-dose, chronic alcoholism develop Laënnec's cirrhosis of the liver. Cirrhosis is a disease in which the liver becomes covered with fiberlike tissue, causing the liver to break down and become filled with fat. This condition causes the liver to stop functioning properly. The liver can restore itself, unless too much damage has occurred. About half of the patients who develop cirrhosis die within 5 years.

Alcohol use can cause organic mental syndromes, which are problems caused by the brain experiencing trauma, such as exposure to alcohol. Some of these problems include acute intoxication, idiosyncratic intoxication, alcoholic blackout, alcohol withdrawal, and withdrawal delirium. Chronic alcohol-induced organic mental syndromes include alcohol amnestic disorder and dementia associated with alcoholism, including Wernicke-Korsakoff's syndrome.

Alcohol, especially wine, stimulates the stomach to secrete gastric acid, causing stomach inflammation and peptic ulcers. Alcoholic people also frequently have diarrhea and an impaired ability to absorb nutrients through the intestines.

Chronic alcohol use frequently causes high blood pressure, increasing the risks of strokes and heart attacks. Alcohol can also damage heart muscle directly, causing a heart muscle disease called cardiomyopathy. Alcohol also inhibits the manufacture of red and white blood cells, causing anemia and a weakened resistance to infection.

Shortly after alcohol enters the blood system, a significant rise in sex hormones occurs. However, at high doses of alcohol, the hormone levels fall. Sexual dysfunction may occur, including a lack of orgasm for both sexes, and males may lose the ability to sustain an erection. Alcoholism is a major cause of male impotence and general loss of sexual desire and ability.

Chronic alcoholism is associated with an increase of cancers in the gastrointestinal tract. Throat and mouth cancers are among the more prominent of these, especially when the alcoholic person also smokes cigarettes. In addition, alcoholism is associated with a higher incidence of liver, stomach, and colon cancer. Women may have a higher risk of breast cancer with low-dose, chronic alcohol use. Table 13–2 summarizes the effects of alcohol on health.

Table 13–2. Alcoholism and health

Health area	Health consequences
Cognitive	Intoxication
	Blackouts
	Memory impairment
	Concentration
	Neurological deficits
	Poor decisions
Psychological	Distortions in thinking
	Misperceptions
	Misinterpretations
	Mood changes
	Anxiety
	Depression
Emotional	Negative emotions
	Anger, hate, resentments
	Lack joy, warmth, intimacy
Social	Old friends ignored
	New drinking friends
	Work-based problems
	Family problems
	Legal problems
	Financial problems
Spiritual	Self-centered
	Blind to needs of others
	Hopelessness

■ The Genetics of Alcoholism

People have long realized that alcoholism—or certain kinds of alcoholism—runs in families. Alcoholic people are often able to identify one or more family members who are also alcoholic. An important question to ask is: Why does alcoholism run in some families? There are two broad possibilities: nature or nurture. In other words, are people taught to become alcoholic, perhaps learning it from others (nurture)? Or is there a hereditary influence that puts some people at higher risk for becoming alcoholic (nature)?

In real life, human behaviors are rarely governed entirely by nature or nurture. Rather, people may be influenced by hereditary factors that are in turn influenced by environmental factors, and vice versa. In other words, there is an interplay between nature and nurture. A shorthand way of relating this interplay to alcoholism is to say that alcoholism = genetics + environment.

To understand the role of genetics in the development of alcoholism, it is necessary to artificially separate genetic influences from environmental influences. Genetic studies are designed to minimize or control environmental influences in order to spotlight the role of genetics. A number of very different studies have been designed with this goal in mind. These studies include twin studies, family studies, animal studies, biological marker studies, and adoption studies.

Genetic Studies: Types and Goals

Research studies have confirmed that alcoholism tends to run in families in a pattern that is consistent with a genetically transmitted susceptibility. This genetically influenced vulnerability is in turn influenced by environmental variables.

One area of genetic research on alcoholism involves *twin studies*. In these studies researchers compare rates of alcoholism in identical and nonidentical twins. Identical twins develop from a single fertilized ovum (egg). The fertilized ovum divides into two identical cells, resulting in identical or monozygotic twins. These twins are genetically identical: they share exactly the same genes.

Alternatively, twins can originate from two separate ova fertilized by two separate spermatozoa. Such twins are nonidentical or dizygotic twins. They are as genetically distinct as nontwin brothers and sisters: they share about half of the same genes.

Thus, twin studies examine the rates of alcoholism in identical and nonidentical twin pairs. These studies ask two questions: What is the likelihood of an identical twin becoming alcoholic if the other twin is alcoholic? What is the likelihood of a nonidentical twin becoming alcoholic if the other twin is alcoholic? If alcoholism is genetically influenced, an identical twin who has an alcoholic twin should be more likely to become alcoholic than a nonidentical twin who has an alcoholic twin.[10]

Another research area involves *family studies,* which examine the family history of alcoholic people. These studies use individual alcoholic patients as a starting point and make note of alcoholic relatives in their families.

In regard to *animal research,* a genetic influence on alcoholism is suggested by the tendency of animals to self-administer alcohol. For example, if rats can be selectively bred for alcohol preference, then that preference suggests a genetic influence, albeit a manmade genetic influence.

Recently, there has been much research on possible *biological markers* for alcoholism. These scientists look for various physiological, behavioral, and biochemical differences between alcoholic people and nonalcoholic people, or between the sons and daughters of alcoholic people and control subjects.

In *adoption studies,* the prevalence of alcoholism is determined by comparing two groups of adoptees: offspring of alcoholic biological parents and offspring of nonalcoholic biological parents. Because both groups of adoptees are separated from their biological parents early in life and raised by nonalcoholic parents, adoption studies can separate the genetic influences from the environmental influences of the adoptive parents.

Twin studies.   Twin studies are based on the idea that if a trait such as alcoholism has genetic components, then people who are genetically identical (such as identical twins) should be more likely to share that trait than people who are genetically less close (nonidentical twins). The term *concordance* refers to the appearance of one or more traits in both members of a pair of twins.

A number of studies have analyzed information relating to the concordance rates between identical and nonidentical twins. Despite some differences among studies, twin studies generally support the existence of a higher concordance rate for alcoholism in identical twins compared with nonidentical twins.[11,12] On average, it appears that there is approximately a 60% concordance rate in identical twins and a 30% concordance rate in nonidentical twins.[13]

One of the first studies that looked at alcoholism in twins found a 74% concordance rate between identical twins. In other words, if one member of a pair of identical twins was alcoholic, the probability of the other twin being alcoholic was 74%.[14] This high concordance rate was in contrast to a 32% concordance rate for alcoholism between nonidentical twins.

In a study of virtually all of the male twins between the ages of 24 and 49 years in Finland, it was noted that there was a higher concordance rate for alcoholism between identical twins compared with nonidentical twins.[15] It was further noted that more social interaction between the twins was a factor in the high concordance rate, but this social interaction did not fully explain the strongly similar drinking habits. An analysis of the data reveals that genetics exhibited much influence on the frequency, quantity, and regularity of drinking at particular times.

Another recent and large project studied over 1,200 identical and 750 nonidentical Australian female twins.[16] One of the most important findings of this study was the evidence that marriage modified the impact of genetic factors. For instance, in twins under age 30, genetic differences accounted for 60% of the variance in drinking habits among unmarried twins, but for only 31% of the variance in married twins.

What do twin studies reveal regarding the genetics of alcoholism? In general, these studies describe the existence of a higher concordance rate for alcoholism in identical twins compared with nonidentical twins. They also point out that the genetic influence in twins is strong, but that the genetic influence is itself influenced by environmental factors.

Family studies. Although there are different types of family studies of alcoholism, the better studies conduct direct interviews with alcoholic people and their relatives, using standardized diagnostic criteria and a control group with which to compare these families. A handful of studies met these high criteria. Their results reveal that there is an average sevenfold increase in the risk of alcoholism among the first-degree relatives of alcoholic subjects compared with nonalcoholic control subjects.[17] (First-degree relatives are immediate blood relatives such as a father and a son.) Twenty-five percent of the fathers and 5% of the mothers of alcoholic subjects also have alcoholism. The relative risk of alcoholism is considerably greater in male relatives of alcoholic subjects.

One of the earliest and largest family studies examined about 1,000 alcoholic men and 166 alcoholic women. Alcoholism was identified in about 50% of the fathers, 6% of the mothers, 30% of the brothers, and 3% of the sisters. More recent studies noted somewhat lower rates of alcoholism in the fathers and brothers of alcoholic people, but in none of these studies were fewer than 25% of the fathers and brothers alcoholic, a rate at least five times greater than that for the male population in general.[18]

Although study results differ, the rates of alcoholism among male relatives range from 25% to 50%, and from 5% to 8% among female relatives. These results are consistent among studies that used a male or female alcoholic subject as a starting point.

Family studies also help to point out that there is a type of alcoholism that appears to run in families and a type that does not.[19] Alcoholism that runs in families is called *familial alcoholism*. Certain types of family studies focus on the differences between familial and nonfamilial alcoholism.

In general, people who have familial alcoholism have an earlier age at onset of alcoholic drinking, a short period of time between the first drink and alcoholism, greater severity of alcoholism, and poorer treatment outcomes.[20,21] They generally have more medical and legal problems, an increased lifetime prevalence of psychiatric problems, and a greater diversity of psychiatric disturbances among biological relatives.

Children with familial alcoholism are more prone to have a history of hyperactivity and behavioral problems. These children are more likely to engage in antisocial behavior. Further, these high-risk children with behavioral and antisocial problems are more likely to engage in behaviors that result in legal consequences, both as children and as adults.

An analysis of 32 familial alcoholism studies revealed that both male and female alcoholic patients more frequently come from homes in which their father, rather than their mother, is alcoholic.[22] Although female offspring of alcoholic mothers have higher-than-average alcoholism rates, male offspring of alcoholic mothers do not.

Animal studies. It might seem odd to study animals in order to understand human alcoholism, but animal studies provide researchers with valuable information about alcoholism, including its genetic aspects.[23] Most research animals such as rats and mice avoid drinking solutions that contain 10% or more alcohol when food and water are available. However, as early as 1959 researchers were able to breed genetic lines of mice that differed greatly in their preference for a 10% alcohol solution versus plain water.[24]

Rats bred selectively for alcohol preference satisfy an animal model of alcoholism.[25] They prefer alcohol solutions over plain water and solid food. They drink a human equivalent of more than a quart of distilled alcohol daily. They will attain very high blood alcohol concentrations and will work to obtain alcohol as a reward. They will self-administer alcohol directly into the stomach (through researcher-inserted tubing), indicating that they prefer alcohol for its pharmacologic effect, not for its taste, smell, or calories. They develop tolerance to and physical dependence on alcohol and retain this tolerance far longer than rats without alcohol preference. Also, after a period of alcohol deprivation, these rats drink alcohol to relieve withdrawal symptoms when it is available again.

Importantly, animal studies demonstrate biological differences between rats that prefer alcohol and rats that do not: there are variations in the level of the neurotransmitter serotonin in certain areas of the brain. Even alcohol-preferring rats that have not yet been exposed to alcohol consistently have lower levels of the neurotransmitters serotonin and dopamine in certain brain areas compared with rats that do not prefer alcohol.[26]

What can be learned from animal studies of alcoholism? First, alcohol-preferring animals display genetically influenced characteristics of human alcoholism. Second, these studies reveal genetic differences in brain chemistry that exist before exposure to alcohol. These differences also occur in humans.

Biological markers for alcoholism. To understand alcoholism better, researchers try to find ways in which alcoholic people differ from nonalcoholic people. They look for traits that alcoholic people have but that nonalcoholic people lack (or vice versa). In other words, researchers look for behavioral, physiological, and biochemical traits—often called biological markers—that are different in alcoholic and nonalcoholic people.

Research into biological markers is important because it helps to identify individuals who are particularly vulnerable to alcoholism. These high-risk individuals then can be exposed to intense prevention and education programs about alcoholism. Everyone should receive information about alcoholism and how to prevent it, but high-risk individuals should be exposed to this information earlier and more intensely.

The search for biological markers for alcoholism is important because a biological marker might actually be one of the causes of alcoholism. For instance, recent research that relates to the gene and chemical structure of a certain type of neurotransmitter receptor may have identified a difference between alcoholic people and nonalcoholic people.[27] Perhaps if scientists discovered how to alter the genes, they might be able to modify the risk for alcoholism. Of course, this is speculation.

Although a biological marker could predispose an individual to alcoholism and might be involved in its development, a marker could simply be present along with alcoholism, without having any effect on it.[28] In other words, a biological marker may frequently coexist with alcoholism, but not cause alcoholism or be caused by it. Biological markers for alcoholism are different from biological markers for alcohol consumption, which can document the effects of alcohol on the body.[29]

For a trait to be a useful biological marker for alcoholism, it should be common in people with alcoholism but infrequent in non-alcoholic people; it should persist even when the alcoholic person is not currently drinking; it should be more common among the first-degree (immediate blood) relatives of alcoholic people than among the general population; and it should be measurable and genetically transmitted.[30]

Some of these biological markers suggest an inborn tolerance to the effects of alcohol, implying that alcoholic people may lack the warning signals that nonalcoholic people use to help determine when to stop drinking. (This lack is in contrast to individuals who have intense responses to alcohol, such as those Asians who display a flushing response, tachycardia, and nausea—which may explain the low incidence of alcoholism among Asians.)

Compared with control groups without a family history of alcoholism, individuals with an alcoholic first-degree relative have diminished responses to alcohol, as measured by self-report and objective criteria.[31,32] In other words, those individuals with a first-degree alcoholic relative reported less euphoria than control subjects when both groups received the same amount of alcohol. In fact, those individuals felt less drunk, slurred their words less, and had better hand-eye coordination than control subjects.

Alcohol causes a decrease in coordination, a staggering walk, and poor balance. Sons of an alcoholic parent stagger and sway less than control subjects after consuming modest doses of alcohol.[33] These so-called "sway tests" suggest that people with alcoholism have a built-in tolerance or a lowered sensitivity to alcohol.

Scientists study brain electrical patterns as possible biological markers for alcoholism. An electroencephalogram (EEG) is a recording of electrical impulses produced by brain activity. Researchers have compared the EEG patterns of individuals at high risk for alcoholism (such as young sons of alcoholic parents) and the EEG patterns of control individuals not at risk. It was found that despite never having used alcohol or other drugs, sons of alcoholic people more frequently had certain EEG patterns (lower P3 waves) compared with sons of nonalcoholic people.[34,35] Abstinent alcoholic people also had this EEG pattern of lower P3 waves.[36] In addition, alcoholic people and sons of alcoholic people both displayed another EEG pattern (excessive beta-wave activity) not normally found in nonalcoholic people.[37]

Alcohol affects the hormonal system. Its effects on the hormonal system of alcoholic people and individuals with a family history of alcoholism differ from its effects on the hormonal system of individuals without a personal or family history of alcoholism. Blood levels of certain hormones that normally increase after alcohol ingestion (cortisol, prolactin, and adrenocorticotropic hormone [ACTH]) have been found to display different patterns of elevation in groups with and without a family history of alcoholism. Some hormones (cortisol and ACTH) have a diminished response to alcohol ingestion in individuals with a family history of alcoholism.[38,39] Another hormone (prolactin) rose to similar levels after standard doses of alcohol in male subjects with and without a positive family history for alcoholism, but the levels dropped more rapidly in men with a positive family history.[40,41]

There are additional markers for alcoholism, including differences in neurotransmitters such as serotonin and differences in certain enzymes (e.g., monoamine oxidase).[42]

Adoption studies. If a boy grows up in an alcoholic home and subsequently becomes alcoholic, does his alcoholism reflect a genetic influence, or did he somehow learn to become an alcoholic by watching his alcoholic parents? Adoption studies can compare genetically similar individuals who were raised in different environments. Adoption studies can also compare genetically different individuals who were raised in the same household.

Among the general population, there is about a 3%–5% risk of alcoholism among males and a 1% risk among females. As many as 25% of the sons with a family history of alcoholism may become alcoholic, whereas about 5% of the daughters with a family history of alcoholism are likely to become alcoholic. But how are these estimates obtained?

Adoption studies examine the incidence of adult alcoholism among the sons and daughters of alcoholic biological parents. These sons and daughters were generally adopted at a very young age (invariably before the age of 3 years) by nonalcoholic people. Thus, their predominant environmental and social influences came from their nonalcoholic adoptive parents. Several studies have consistently found that adopted-away sons of alcoholic people are three to four times more likely to become alcoholic than the adopted-away sons of nonalcoholic people.[43-45]

For example, a study of more than 5,000 Danish adoptees demonstrated that the sons of alcoholic people adopted by other families were more than three times as likely to become alcoholic compared with the adopted sons of nonalcoholic people.[46] In a similar study of more than 2,000 Swedish adoptees, male adoptees whose biological fathers were severely alcoholic had a 20% incidence of alcohol abuse, compared to a 6% incidence in the adopted sons of nonalcoholic people.[47]

Studies of daughters of alcoholic people have been less consistent, but studies have confirmed a genetic influence on alcoholism among women,[44] which is apparently transmitted through the mother. For example, one study documented that women who were born to alcoholic mothers but who were adopted during the first few months of life by nonrelatives were three times as likely to abuse alcohol as were women in the general population.[48]

■ Alcoholic Subtypes

Adoption studies provide compelling evidence that biological inheritance can be a fundamental factor in the development of alcoholism. Of equal importance, these studies have revealed the existence of two different types of inherited predisposition to alcoholism. One type of alcoholic family has alcoholism only among the male members. In contrast, other families have alcoholism in both men and women. Similarly, one type of alcoholism is strongly influenced by the sex of the individual and another type is strongly influenced by environmental factors. In other words, these adoption studies provided evidence for two different types of alcoholism. These alcoholism subtypes differ with respect to age at onset, drinking behavior, and personality traits.[49]

Table 13–3 indicates some of the differences between these two subtypes of alcoholism. Type 1 alcoholism is also called *milieu-limited* alcoholism, because it involves genetic factors plus strong environmental influences. (The term *milieu* means environment and social setting.) In contrast, type 2 or *male-limited* alcoholism is limited to males, is influenced strongly by genetics, is insignificantly influenced by environmental factors, and is associated with both parental alcoholism and parental antisocial behavior. Male-limited alcoholism is more likely to develop at an early age, whereas milieu-limited alcoholism is more likely to emerge after age 25.

The subtypes differ with respect to certain personality traits that, taken together, describe subtype personalities. These three traits are novelty seeking, harm avoidance, and reward dependence. The behavior of people with milieu-limited alcoholism is consistent with a "passive-dependent" personality. These people have a tendency to display inflexible and contemplative behavior and thus low novelty-seeking behavior. They have a tendency to avoid harm and risks.

People with milieu-limited alcoholism have significant concerns about the feelings and thoughts of others and experience guilt about their drinking behavior. They rank high in terms of reward dependence, meaning that they are often eager to help others and that they

Table 13–3. Subtypes of alcoholism

Variable	Type 1: milieu limited	Type 2: male limited
Sex	Males and females	Males only
Genetic influence	Necessary	Strong
Environmental influence	Strong	Weak
Age at onset	>25 years	<25 years
Guilt	Frequent	Rare
Harm avoidance	High	Low
Reward dependence	High	Low
Violence	Rare	Frequent
Arrests	Rare	Frequent
Novelty seeking	Low	High

can become emotionally dependent on others.

In comparison, male-limited alcoholic behavior is similar to the behavior of individuals with antisocial personality disorders. Male-limited alcoholic people have a tendency to display impulsive and excitable behavior. They display high novelty-seeking behavior; take physical, emotional, and financial risks; and do not place an emphasis on avoiding harm. They are often impetuous and uninhibited. They are not dependent on obtaining rewards from others and often have distant social relations. People with male-limited alcoholism tend to have frequent episodes of alcohol-influenced aggressiveness and alcohol-related legal problems.

Milieu-limited alcoholism is the more common type of genetically influenced alcoholism. It occurs in both men and women and accounts for most alcoholism among both sexes. The environment strongly influences both its occurrence and its severity. Milieu-limited alcoholism requires both a genetic predisposition and an environmental influence. An analysis of adoption studies revealed that if only one of these factors was present, the risk of alcoholism was about the same as that in the general population. However, if both factors were present, the risk was doubled and the severity was determined by the degree of environmental provocation.[18]

This form of alcoholism is usually not severe and is often not treated. It is associated with mild, untreated, adult-onset alcohol abuse in either biological parent, who generally have few alcohol-related legal problems. People with milieu-limited alcoholism are noted for their ability to occasionally abstain from alcohol for long periods. However, they have great difficulty in stopping drinking once they start. They often have anxious personality traits and develop a rapid dependence on and tolerance to the antianxiety effects

Table 13–4. Type 1: milieu-limited alcoholism

■ Men and women	■ Ability to abstain
■ Strong environmental influence	■ Loss of control once drinking
■ Adult onset	■ Anxious personality traits
■ Milder course	■ No criminality

of alcohol. Both women and men can have milieu-limited alcoholism, and either sex can genetically transmit the susceptibility to either a son or a daughter. This subtype of alcoholism is not related to an increase in criminal behavior.

Male-limited alcoholism is found only in men and accounts for about 25% of all male alcoholism in the general population. This subtype of alcoholism has a strong genetic influence and is largely unaffected by environmental influences. In fact, in families with male-limited susceptibility, alcoholism is nine times more frequent in the adopted sons regardless of environmental influences.

The male-limited alcoholism is usually associated with the development of alcohol-related problems early in life: during late childhood or early adolescence. These men often have frequent fights while drinking and get arrested for alcohol-related behavior. They are more likely to get tickets for drinking while driving and to cause alcohol-related automobile accidents. This form of alcoholism is difficult to treat.

Susceptibility to male-limited alcoholism is associated with severe alcoholism in the biological father, who also tends to have a history of serious criminal behavior. The susceptibility is not associated with alcoholism in the biological mother.

Women may inherit the same genetic factors that lead to male-limited alcoholism, but these factors do not lead to alcoholism in women. In fact, there is no evidence that this male-limited alcoholism can be transmitted to daughters. However, adopted-away daughters of biological fathers with male-limited alcoholism have a greater frequency of somatization disorder—that is, they have frequent complaints of medically unexplained pain or discomfort in various body

Table 13–5. Type 2: male-limited alcoholism

■ Strong genetic component	■ Severe course
■ Paternal alcoholism	■ Criminality
■ Early onset	■ Psychosocial problems

Note. Women who inherit the same genetic factors frequently develop somatization disorder, but not alcoholism.

areas. Interestingly, these women with somatization disorders share many of the personality characteristics of men with male-limited alcoholism. Both display high novelty-seeking behavior, are impulsive, and have quick tempers, but display low harm avoidance behavior and dependence-seeking behavior.

Understanding Genetic Influences

Nearly every study that explores some aspect of the genetic influence on alcoholism (and other drug addictions) identifies family history of alcoholism as the most significant risk factor for developing alcoholism. However, it is important to point out that some people who abuse alcohol and develop alcoholism do not have a family history of alcoholism. It is possible that environmental or psychological factors exert great influence on these people, or perhaps the family history of alcoholism exists but is unknown to them.

Similarly, not every person with a family history of alcoholism will become an alcoholic after drinking alcohol. There is a grave risk, but having a genetic predisposition for alcoholism is not a guarantee of automatically becoming alcoholic. What is inherited is not alcoholism. What is inherited is a predisposition for developing alcoholism.

Thus, people are not born alcoholic. Rather, some people are born with a genetically influenced increased probability of losing control over alcohol use, experiencing a compulsion to use alcohol, and continuing to use alcohol despite adverse consequences. However, people born without this genetic risk factor can be exposed to other risk factors that may also increase the probability of alcoholism. In other words, while important, hereditary is only one of several risk factors.

■ Summary

Alcohol use and addiction greatly exceed the use of and addiction to all illicit drugs combined. Throughout history, various models for explaining alcoholic behavior have been presented. These explanations include alcoholism as moral corruption, as a form of self-medication, as a consequence of sociological forces, as the result of positive and negative reinforcement, and as the result of biological abnormalities. Today, the disease model of alcoholism views alcoholism as a multidimensional problem influenced by biological, psychological, and sociological factors—and subsequently affecting those areas of life as well. In particular, alcoholism affects the individual's cognitive, psychological, emotional, social, spiritual, and physical health. Physical health is often the last area of health to deteriorate and the first area to return to normal.

Alcoholism research has revealed that genetic and environmental influences play a role in the expression and development of alcoholism. Various studies have explored the genetic influence on alcoholism: twin studies, family studies, animal studies, biological marker studies, and adoption studies. In general, these studies note that the single most important risk factor for developing alcoholism is having a family history of alcoholism. In particular, sons of alcoholic men are at a particularly high risk for becoming alcoholic. Also, genetic studies reveal that alcoholism itself is not inherited: people inherit a predisposition for becoming alcoholic.

Studies have also noted that there are two alcoholic subtypes. Milieu-limited alcoholism involves a genetic predisposition that is strongly influenced by environmental factors. Milieu-limited alcoholism occurs among both sexes, is often milder, has an adult onset, and often includes the ability to abstain occasionally but not to stop drinking once it has begun. People with milieu-limited alcoholism often have anxious and dependent personality traits, avoid risks and harm, and feel guilty about their drinking.

Male-limited alcoholism is found only in men, has a strong genetic influence but is largely unaffected by environmental factors, develops early in life, and is associated with criminal behavior and violence. These men often tend to take risks, engage in novelty-seeking behavior, and do not seek the approval of others. Women who inherit the genetic factors for male-limited alcoholism do not develop alcoholism, but rather develop somatization disorders with complaints of medically unexplained pain and discomfort. They often share personality traits with men who have male-limited alcoholism.

■ References

1. National Institute on Drug Abuse: National Household Survey on Drug Abuse: Main Findings 1988. Rockville, MD, National Institute on Drug Abuse, 1990

2. National Institute on Alcohol Abuse and Alcoholism: Seventh Special Report to the U.S. Congress on Alcohol and Health. Rockville, MD, National Institute on Alcohol Abuse and Alcoholism, 1990

3. Regier DA, Farmer ME, Rae DS, et al: Comorbidity of mental disorders with alcohol and other drug abuse: results from the Epidemiologic Catchment Area (ECA) study. Journal of the American Medical Association 264:2511–2518, 1990

4. Kosten TR, Rounsaville BJ, Babor TF, et al: Substance-use disorders in DSM-III-R: evidence for the dependence syndrome across different psychoactive substances. British Journal of Psychiatry 151:834–843, 1987

5. Morse RM, Flavin DK: The definition of alcoholism. Journal of the American Medical Association 268:1012–1014, 1992

6. Parsons OA, Leber WR: The relationship between cognitive dysfunction and brain damage in alcoholics: causal, interactive, or epiphenomenal? Alcoholism: Clinical and Experimental Research 5:326–343, 1981

7. Eckardt MJ, Martin PR: Clinical assessment of cognition in alcoholism. Alcoholism: Clinical and Experimental Research 10(2):123–127, 1986

8. Tabakoff B, Petersen RC: Brain damage and alcoholism. The Counselor 6(5):13–16, 1988

9. Horvath TB: Clinical spectrum and epidemiologic features of alcoholic dementia, in Alcohol, Drugs, and Brain Damage. Edited by Rankin JG. Toronto, Canada, Addiction Research Center, 1975, pp 1–16

10. Pickens RW, Svikis DS: Genetic influences in human substance abuse. Journal of Addictive Diseases 10:205–213, 1991

11. Partanen J, Bruun K, Markkanen T: Inheritance of Drinking Behavior: A Study on Intelligence, Personality, and the Use of Alcohol of Adult Twins. Helsinki, Finland, Finnish Foundation for Alcoholic Studies, 1966

12. Pickens RW, Svikis DS, McGue M, et al: Heterogeneity in the inheritance of alcoholism. Archives of General Psychiatry 48:19–28, 1991

13. Schuckit MA: Genetics and the risk of alcoholism. Journal of the American Medical Association 254:2614–2617, 1985

14. Kaij L: Alcoholism in Twins: Studies on the Etiology and Sequelae of Abuse of Alcohol. Stockholm, Sweden, Alonquist & Winkell Publishers, 1960

15. Kaprio J, Koskenvuo M, Langinvainio H, et al: Genetic influences on use and abuse of alcohol: a study of 5638 Finnish twin brothers. Alcoholism (NY) 11:349–356, 1987
16. Heath AC, Jardine R, Martin NG: Interactive effects of genotype and social environment on alcohol consumption in female twins. Journal of Studies on Alcohol 59:38–48, 1989
17. Merikangas KR: The genetic epidemiology of alcoholism. Psychological Medicine 20:11–22, 1990
18. Goodwin DW: Is Alcoholism Hereditary? New York, Ballantine, 1988
19. Goodwin DW: Studies of familial alcoholism: a growth industry, in Longitudinal Research in Alcoholism. Edited by Goodwin DW, Van Dusen KT, Mednick SA. Boston, MA, Kluwer-Nijhoff Publishing, 1984, pp 97–105
20. Penick EC, Powell BJ, Bingham SF, et al: A comparative study of familial alcoholism. Journal of Studies on Alcohol 48:136–146, 1987
21. Alford GS, Jouriles EN, Jackson SC: Differences and similarities in development of drinking between alcoholic offspring of alcoholics and alcoholic offspring of non-alcoholics. Addictive Behaviors 16:341–347, 1991
22. Pollock VE, Schneider LS, Gabrielli WF Jr, et al: Sex of parent and offspring in the transmission of alcoholism: a meta-analysis. Journal of Nervous and Mental Disease 175:668–673, 1987
23. Froehlich JC, Li T-K: Animal models for the study of alcoholism: utility of selected lines. Journal of Addictive Diseases 10:61–71, 1991
24. McClearn GE, Rodgers DA: Differences in alcohol preference among inbred strains of mice. Journal of Studies on Alcohol 20:691–695, 1959
25. Li T-K, Lockmuller JC: Why are some people more susceptible to alcoholism? Alcohol, Health and Research World 13:310–315, 1989
26. Murphy JM, McBride WJ, Lument L, et al: Regional brain levels of monoamines in alcohol-preferring and -nonpreferring lines of rats. Pharmacology, Biochemistry and Behavior 16:145–149, 1982
27. Noble EP, Blum D, Ritchie T, et al: Allelic association of the D2 dopamine receptor gene with receptor-binding characteristics in alcoholism. Archives of General Psychiatry 48:648–654, 1991
28. Tabakoff B, Hoffman PL: Genetics and biological markers of risk for alcoholism. Public Health Reports 103:690–698, 1988
29. Rosman AS, Lieber CS: Biochemical markers of alcohol consumption. Alcohol Health and Research World 14:210–218, 1990
30. Begleiter H, Porjesz B: Potential biological markers in individuals at high risk for developing alcoholism. Alcoholism (NY) 12:488–493, 1988

31. Schuckit MA: Subjective responses to alcohol in sons of alcoholics and controls. Archives of General Psychiatry 41:879–884, 1984
32. Lipscomb TR, Nathan PE: Blood alcohol level discrimination: the effects of family history of alcoholism, drinking pattern, and tolerance. Archives of General Psychiatry 37:571–577, 1980
33. Schuckit MA: Ethanol-induced changes in body sway in men at high alcoholism risk. Archives of General Psychiatry 42:375–379, 1985
34. Begleiter H, Porjesz B, Bihari B, et al: Event-related brain potentials in boys at risk for alcoholism. Science 225:1493–1496, 1984
35. Begleiter H, Porjesz B, Rawlings R, et al: Auditory recovery function and P3 in boys at high risk for alcoholism. Alcohol 4:315–321, 1987
36. Porjesz B, Begleiter H, Bihari B, et al: Event-related potentials to high incentive stimuli in abstinent alcoholics. Alcohol 4:283–287, 1987
37. Gabrielli WF, Mednick SA, Volavka J, et al: Electroencephalograms in children of alcoholic fathers. Psychophysiology 19:404–407, 1982
38. Schuckit MA: Differences in plasma cortisol after ethanol in relatives of alcoholics and controls. Journal of Clinical Psychiatry 45:374–379, 1984
39. Schuckit MA, Risch SC, Gold EO: Alcohol consumption, ACTH level, and family history of alcoholism. American Journal of Psychiatry 145:1391–1395, 1984
40. Schuckit MA, Parker DC, Rossman LR: Ethanol-related prolactin responses and risk for alcoholism. Biological Psychiatry 39:137–140, 1983
41. Schuckit MA, Gold E, Risch SC: Changes in blood prolactin levels in sons of alcoholics and controls. American Journal of Psychiatry 144:854–859, 1987
42. Pandey GN: Biochemical markers of predisposition to alcoholism. Alcohol Health and Research World 14:204–209, 1990
43. Cloninger CR, Bohman M, Sigvardsson S: Inheritance of alcohol abuse. Archives of General Psychiatry 38:861–868, 1981
44. Cadoret RJ, Gath A: Inheritance of alcoholism in adoptees. British Journal of Psychiatry 132:252–258, 1978
45. Goodwin DW, Schulsinger F, Moller N, et al: Drinking problems in adopted and nonadopted sons of alcoholics. Archives of General Psychiatry 31:164–169, 1974
46. Goodwin DW, Schulsinger F, Hermansen L, et al: Alcohol problems in adoptees raised apart from alcoholic biological parents. Archives of General Psychiatry 28:238–243, 1973
47. Bohman M: Some genetic aspects of alcoholism and criminality: a population of adoptees. Archives of General Psychiatry 35:269–276, 1978

48. Bohman M, Sigvardsson S, Cloninger CR: Maternal inheritance of alcohol abuse. Archives of General Psychiatry 38:965–969, 1981
49. Cloninger CR: Neurogenetic adaptive mechanisms in alcoholism. Science 236:410–416, 1987

Final Thoughts

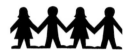

Human behavior is a reflection of the complex, multidimensional biopsychosocial phenomenon called life. It should come as no surprise that destructive and maladaptive behavior suggests the presence of multidimensional processes gone awry or excessive influence in certain biopsychosocial dimensions, such as environment or heredity.

The Human Genome Project has recently isolated a gene that predisposes people to colon cancer. There may be a day when the genes for addiction are isolated, helping to identify people at high risk for addiction to alcohol and other drugs. But people will continue to drink alcohol and use other drugs. Addicted people will still develop unhealthy defense mechanisms that make it difficult for them to identify their self-destructive behaviors.

There may be a day when a pharmaceutical company creates the pharmacologic cure for addiction. But people will still seek mood-altering experiences. Some people will still use psychoactive drugs to dissolve an invisible barrier between themselves and other people.

There may be a day when it seems that a quantum leap has occurred regarding the effectiveness of addiction treatment. But most people who need that treatment will still not want to go, and they may participate in treatment only after a crisis.

Whether they are family members, friends, or health care professionals, people involved in the lives of addicted individuals can gain the skills required to understand the addiction process, to coax addicted individuals into treatment, and to support their recovery. Although the crises that surround addiction can be maddening, interventions and the initiation of treatment can be the dawn of a new hope for addicted people and their families. Far beyond the mere cessation of destructive and maladaptive behavior, the recovery process is the ladder that helps people to reach their human potential. Learning about the drugs of abuse and the processes of treatment and recovery is an integral part of that process.

Appendix

Resources

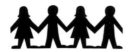

A wide variety of resources are available to addicted people and family members. These include agencies that provide referrals for treatment and resources for education, information, and literature. There are numerous self-help programs for addicted people and family members, many of which are based on the Twelve-Step model of Alcoholics Anonymous. Also, there are specialized support groups for addicted professional people, such as those for addicted physicians and nurses. Some organizations and programs are of particular interest to people with dual disorders. Finally, there are numerous self-help clearinghouses to help people locate or even organize a local self-help program.

■ Treatment Referrals

The yellow pages of the local phone book should list the treatment programs available within that region. The local affiliates of the National Council on Alcoholism and Drug Dependence will also provide information about local treatment resources.

National Association of Lesbian and Gay Alcoholism Professionals
(213) 381–8524

National Council on Alcoholism and Drug Dependence
Call directory assistance for local affiliates or (800) 622–2255

National Information Center on Deafness
800 Florida Avenue, N.E.
Washington, DC 20002
(202) 651–5051 (voice)
(202) 651–5052 (TTY)

National Institute on Drug Abuse
Treatment and Referral Hotline
(800) 662–HELP

Substance and Alcohol Intervention Services for the Deaf
50 West Main Street
Room 215
Rochester, NY 14614
(716) 475–4978
(716) 475–4970 (TTY)

Women in Crisis
360 West 125th Street
New York, NY 10011
(212) 316–5200

■ Twelve-Step Self-Help Programs for Addicted People

Irrespective of the treatment setting for addiction to alcohol and other drugs, self-help programs are central and essential components of treatment and recovery. In most urban areas, various self-help groups are available every day of the year. They are free, although donations of a dollar are routine to help pay for rent, coffee, and educational materials.

These self-help programs are modeled after the Twelve Steps of Alcoholics Anonymous and are casually referred to as the Twelve-Step programs. National addresses are provided below, but local affiliates are generally listed in the white pages of the phone book. Callers often reach an answering service or a machine that will list the location and times of meetings.

Alcoholics Anonymous
Box 459
Grand Central Station
New York, NY 10017
(212) 870–3400
(212) 686–5454 (TTD)

Cocaine Anonymous
3740 Overland Avenue, Suite H
Los Angeles, CA 90034
(310) 559–5833

Drugs Anonymous/Pills Anonymous
P.O. Box 473
Ansonia Station
New York, NY 10023
(212) 874–0700

Marijuana Addicts Anonymous
P.O. Box 1969
Bowling Green Station
New York, NY 10274
(212) 459–4423

Marijuana Anonymous
P.O. Box 2912
Van Nuys, CA 91404
(213) 964–2370

Narcotics Anonymous
P.O. Box 9999
Van Nuys, CA 91409
(818) 780–3951

■ Self-Help Programs for Family Members

There are a variety of self-help groups for family members of addicted people. Local affiliates can be found in the white pages of the phone book or by contacting national headquarters. Many of these are Twelve-Step programs, modeled after Alcoholics Anonymous; these are marked by an asterisk (*) below.

Adult Children of Alcoholics
World Service Organization
P.O. Box 3271
Torrance, CA 90510
(310) 534–1815

*Al-Anon and Alateen
Family Group Headquarters
P.O. Box 862
Midtown Station
New York, NY 10018-0862
(212) 302–7240
(800) 356–9996

Children of Alcoholics Foundation
P.O. Box 4185
Grand Central Station
New York, NY 10163
(213) 316–3916

*Cocanon Family Groups
P.O. Box 64742-66
Los Angeles, CA 90064
(310) 859–2206

*Codependents Anonymous

P.O. Box 33577
Phoenix, AZ 85067-3577
(602) 277–7991

*Families Anonymous

P.O. Box 528
Van Nuys, CA 91408
(818) 989–7841

*Nar-Anon Family Groups

P.O. Box 2562
Palos Verdes, CA 90274
(213) 547–5800

ToughLove

P.O. Box 1069
Doylestown, PA 18901
(215) 348–7090
(800) 333–1069

■ Resources for Addicted Professionals

Member organizations (such as the American Medical Association) often have committees or departments that focus on the needs of their members who are addicted. Some organizations may have a highly structured protocol and process for dealing with addicted members. Some organizations have volunteer members who provide assistance to family members and may help organize an intervention. Organizations may be most helpful through their state or local affiliates.

Airline Pilots Association

Aeromedical Office
12000 East 47th Avenue, Suite 117
Denver, CO 80239
(303) 371–0425

American Academy of Physician Assistants
Sub-Committee on Impaired Practitioners
950 North Washington Street
Alexandria, VA 22314
(703) 836–AAPA

American Bar Association
Commission on Impaired Lawyers
750 Lakeshore Drive
Chicago, IL 60611
(312) 988–5345

American Dental Association
Council on Dental Practice
211 East Chicago Avenue
Chicago, IL 60611
(312) 440–2622

American Judicature Society
25 East Washington Street, Suite 1600
Chicago, IL 60202
(312) 558–6900

American Medical Association
Department of Substance Abuse
Physician Assistance Program
535 Dearborn Street
Chicago, IL 60610
(312) 464–5066

American Nurses Association
Impaired Nursing Practice
600 Maryland Street, S.W., Suite 100 West
Washington, DC 20024
(202) 554–4444, ext. 300

American Osteopathic Association

Membership Department
142 East Ontario Street
Chicago, IL 60611
(800) 621–1773

American Psychiatric Association

Office of Education
Committee on the Impaired Physician
1400 K Street, N.W.
Washington, DC 20005
(202) 682–6130

American Psychological Association

Committee on Impaired Psychologists
1200 17th Street, N.W.
Washington, DC 20036
(202) 336–5500

American Veterinary Medical Association

930 North Meacham Road
Schaumburg, IL 60196
(800) 248–2862

Canadian Medical Association

Department of Health Care and Promotion
Physicians at Risk
1867 Alta Vista Drive
Ottawa, Canada K1G 068
(613) 731–9331
(800) 267–9703

Impaired Nurses Network

National Nurses Society on Addiction
2506 Gross Pointe Road
Evanston, IL 60201
(708) 966–5010

National Association of Social Workers
7981 Eastern Avenue
Silver Spring, MD 20910
(800) 638–8799

■ Resources for People With Dual Disorders

The following is a list of self-help groups, support groups, and educational organizations that may be of value to people with dual disorders. Some of these are Twelve-Step support groups and are marked with an asterisk (*). Some of these groups are more educational in nature and can provide information about specific psychiatric problems, such as phobias or depression. Some of these organizations are national and some are local.

Anxiety Disorders Association of America
6000 Executive Boulevard #513
Rockville, MD 20852
(301) 231–9350

Depression Awareness Recognition and Treatment
5600 Fishers Lane, Room 14C-03
Rockville, MD 20857
(301) 443–4140

*Depressives Anonymous
198 Broadway
New York, NY 10038
(212) 964–8934

*Emotional Health Anonymous
P.O. Box 429
Glendale, CA 91209–0429
(818) 240–3215

*Emotions Anonymous

P.O. Box 4245
Saint Paul, MN 55104
(612) 647–9712

GROW, Inc.

301 West White Street
Box 3667
Champaign, IL 61821
(217) 352–6989

Manic and Depressive Support Group, Inc.

P.O. Box 1747
Madison Square Station
New York, NY 10159
(212) 533–MDSG

National Alliance for the Mentally Ill

1901 North Fort Meyer Drive, Suite 500
Arlington, VA 22209
(703) 524–7600

National Council of Community Mental Health Centers

12300 Twinbrook Parkway, Suite 320
Rockville, MD 20852
(301) 984–6200

National Depressive and Manic Depressive Association

222 South Riverside Plaza, Suite 2812
Chicago, IL 60606
(312) 993–0066

National Institute on Mental Health

5600 Fishers Lane
Rockville, MD 20857
(301) 443–4513

National Mental Health Association
1021 Prince Street
Alexandria, VA 22314
(703) 684–7722

National Mental Health Consumer's Association
311 South Juniper Street, Room 902
Philadelphia, PA 19107
(215) 735–2465
(215) 735–6082 (self-help clearinghouse)

Obsessive-Compulsive Disorder Foundation
P.O. Box 70
Milford, CT 06460
(203) 878–5669

U.S. Veterans Administration
Mental Health and Behavioral Sciences Services
810 Vermont Avenue, N.W., Room 915
Washington, DC 20410
(202) 389–3416

■ Education, Information, and Literature

Numerous organizations provide education about drugs of abuse, addiction, codependence, treatment, recovery, relapse, and prevention. These organizations include government, nonprofit, and for-profit agencies. Their material may be geared for addicted people, families, health care professionals, or the interested public and may be free, inexpensive, or costly. The educational materials may include pamphlets, books, information sheets, lists of other resources, and videotapes. In addition, all of the Twelve-Step programs provide written material at local group meetings and through national headquarters.

Addiction Research Foundation

Marketing
33 Russell Street
Toronto, Ontario
Canada M5S 2S1
(416) 595–6059

Alcohol, Drug Abuse, and Mental Health Administration

5600 Fishers Lane
Rockville, MD 20857
(301) 443–3783

Alcohol Research Group

Research and Technical Library
1816 Scenic Avenue
Berkeley, CA 94709
(510) 642–5208

American Council for Drug Education

204 Monroe Street, Suite 110
Rockville, MD 20850
(301) 294–0600
(800) 659–3784
(301) 294–0603 (fax)

American Psychiatric Press, Inc.

1400 K Street, N.W.
Washington, DC 20005
(800) 368–5777

Association for Medical Education and Research in Substance Abuse

Brown University, Box G
Providence, RI 02912
(401) 863–1109

Center for Alcohol Studies

Smithers Hall
Rutgers University
Allison Road
Piscataway, NJ 08854
(908) 932–2190

Children of Alcoholics Foundation

P.O. Box 4185
Department RC
Grand Central Station
New York, NY 10163
(212) 316–3916

CNS Productions

Videos and Films
P.O. Box 311
116 C Street
Ashland, OR 97520
(800) 888–0617

Committee on Problems of Drug Dependence, Inc.

3420 North Broad Street
Philadelphia, PA 19140
(215) 221–3298

Do It Now Foundation

Written Literature
P.O. Box 27658
Tempe, AZ 85285
(602) 491–0393

Employee Assistance Professionals Association

4601 North Fairfax Drive
Arlington, VA 22203
(703) 522–6272
(703) 522–4585 (fax)

Hazelden Foundation

Educational Materials
P.O. Box 176
Center City, MN 55012
(800) 257–0070
(800) 328–9000 (Minnesota)

Hispanic Health Council

96-98 Cedar Street
Hartford, CT 06106
(203) 527–0856

Institute on Black Chemical Abuse

2614 Nicollet Avenue
Minneapolis, MN 55408
(612) 871–7878

The Johnson Institute

510 First Avenue North
Minneapolis, MN 55403-1607
(800) 247–0484

National Asian Pacific American Families Against Substance Abuse

6303 Friendship Court
Bethesda, MD 20817
(301) 530–0945

National Association for Children of Alcoholics

11426 Rockville Pike, Suite 100
Rockville, MD 20882
(301) 468–0985

National Clearinghouse for Alcohol and Drug Information

Center for Substance Abuse Prevention
P.O. Box 2345
Rockville, MD 20852
(800) 729–6686
(301) 468–2600
(301) 468–6433 (fax)
(301) 230–2867 (TDD)

National Council on Alcoholism and Drug Dependence

12 West 21st Street
New York, NY 10010
(212) 206–6770
(800) 622–2255

National Institute on Alcohol Abuse and Alcoholism

5600 Fishers Lane, Room 16-105
Rockville, MD 20857
(301) 443–3885

National Institute on Drug Abuse

5600 Fishers Lane, Room 10-05
Rockville, MD 20857
(301) 443–6480

Parents Resource Institute for Drug Education

The Hurt Building
50 Hurt Plaza, Suite 210
Atlanta, GA 30303
(404) 577–4500

Max A. Schneider, M.D., Education Division

3311 E. Kirkwood Avenue
Orange, CA 92669
(714) 639–0062

Substance Abuse Librarians and Information Specialists
Alcoholism and Drug Abuse Institute
3937 15th Avenue, N.E.
Seattle, WA 98105
(206) 543–0397

■ Self-Help Clearinghouses

Many of the U.S. states and Canadian provinces have regional self-help clearinghouses. These regional clearinghouses refer callers to local self-help groups for a multitude of problems. These include but are not limited to self-help groups on drug addiction, nicotine addiction, codependence, eating disorders, sexual compulsions, compulsive spending, incest, sexual abuse, physical abuse, mental disorders, mental retardation, physical disabilities, and acquired immunodeficiency syndrome (AIDS). These self-help groups may be for individuals with problems or for the family members of those individuals.

The clearinghouses can refer you to local groups or provide information about starting your own group. Call directory assistance in the state capital or a large city in your state to get phone numbers of regional clearinghouses. A few examples are listed below.

National Self-Help Clearinghouse
City University of New York
Graduate Center, Room 1206A
33 West 42nd Street
New York, NY 10036
(212) 642–2944

Self-Help Center
1600 Dodge Avenue, Suite S-122
Evanston, IL 60201
(708) 328–0470

Self-Help Clearinghouse

Saint Clares Riverside Medical Center
Denville, NJ 07834
(201) 625-9565
(201) 625–9053 (TDD)
CompuServ 70275,1003

Index

*Page numbers printed in **boldface** type refer to tables or figures.*